HODGKIN'S LYMPHOMA

Edited by **Nima Rezaei**

Hodgkin's Lymphoma
Edited by Nima Rezaei

Published by InTech
Janeza Trdine 9, 51000 Rijeka, Croatia

Publishing Process Manager Bojan Rafaj

Technical Editor Teodora Smiljanic

Cover Designer InTech Design Team

Additional hard copies can be obtained from orders@intechopen.com

Hodgkin's Lymphoma, Edited by Nima Rezaei
p. cm.
ISBN 978-953-51-0402-5

For EU product safety concerns:
IN TECH d.o.o., Prolaz Marije Krucifikse Kozulić 3, 51000 Rijeka, Croatia,
info@intechopen.com or visit our website at intechopen.com.

Meet the editor

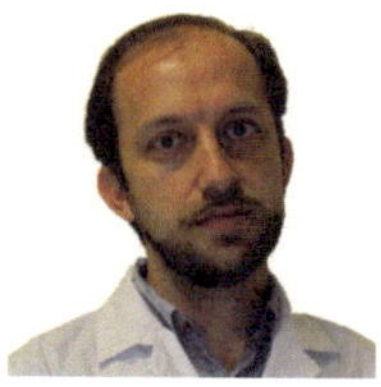

Nima Rezaei, born in 1976, received his Medical Degree from Tehran University of Medical Sciences in 2002. He received his M.Sc. and Ph.D. degrees in the field of Clinical Immunology and Genetic Medicine from the University of Sheffield in 2007 and 2009, respectively, as well as a short-term fellowship, awarded by the ESID, in the Paediatric Immunology and BMT Unit of the Newcastle General Hospital. He is already the Chief Executive Director of the Children's Medical Center Hospital, the Pediatrics Center of Excellence in Iran as well as the Deputy President of the Research Center for Immunodeficiencies. He has presented more than 200 lectures/posters in congresses and has published more than 250 articles in international scientific journals during last decade.

Contents

Preface

Hodgkin's lymphoma, previously known as Hodgkin's disease, is recognized as B cell derived cancer of lymphatic system. Although the disease had been described about 180 years ago, its exact causes and pathophysiology still remains unknown. However, there have been some progresses in identifying some genetic and environmental risk factors in development of lymphoma. Considering recent advances in treatment of patients with lymphoma during last two decades, the disease is considered as a curable disease, but it is still a controversial subject.

The current book consists of 11 chapters. Recent insights into the biology of Hodgkin's lymphoma, including historical aspects, epidemiology, pathophysiology, genetic defects, and prognostic indicators are explained in the chapters 1-3. Chapter 4 is a translational chapter from tumor microenvironment to immunotherapeutic approach, followed by the chapters 5-9, explaining treatment of early stage, advanced, and refractory Hodgkin's lymphoma as well as MALT lymphoma, respectively. The chapter 10 briefly explains some adverse effects of chemotherapy and radiotherapy in the affected patients, while the final chapter is focused on survivorship in Hodgkin's lymphoma. These chapters are intended to help physicians as well as medical students to learn and understand the pathophysiology of Hodgkin's lymphoma as well as practical approach to diagnosis and management in clinical practice.

The book is the result of valuable contribution of 20 scientists in this field and I would like to acknowledge the expertise of all contributors, for generously giving their time and considerable effort in preparing their respective chapters. I hope the book will be welcomed by the physicians, who wish to learn more about Hodgkin's lymphoma.

Nima Rezaei, MD, PhD
Research Center for Immunodeficiencies,
Children's Medical Center,
Tehran University of Medical Sciences, Tehran,
Iran

Part 1

Recent Insights into the Biology of Hodgkin's Lymphoma

1

Recent Insights into the Biology of Hodgkin's Lymphoma

Diponkar Banerjee

Department of Pathology and Laboratory Medicine, British Columbia Cancer Agency, Canada

1. Introduction

Hodgkin's lymphoma (HL) is currently recognized as B cell derived lymphoma with histological and biomarker-based distinction from other types of B cell derived lymphoma (Swerdlow, S.H. et al., 2008). HL had a worldwide incidence of 67,887cases in 2008, with an age standardized rate of 1.0 per 100,000 (both genders) (*http://globocan.iarc.fr/*). Some of the information in this chapter has already been part of an earlier review article (Banerjee, D., 2011) and is cited again for the sake of completeness, but this chapter also provides some historical or current data that was not included that review.

2. Historical aspects of Hodgkin's Lymphoma

The earliest description of Hodgkin's lymphoma (HL) in an autopsy patient is attributed to Malpighi who described an 18 year old female with prominent splenic nodules in his 1666 publication (Malpighi, M., 1666). Thomas Hodgkin, whose name is now associated with this disease, was very careful to mention this fact in the published version of his paper "On some morbid appearances of the absorbent glands and spleen" (Hodgkin, T., 1832) read to the Royal Medical and Chirurgical Society of London on January 10th and 24th, 1832. The paper was read not by Hodgkin but by the Society secretary Robert Lee. This was because Hodgkin was not a member of the Society at the time and therefore was prohibited from presenting the paper in person or even being present in the room during Lee's reading of his paper.

Although the compound microscope had been invented in 1590 by spectacle-makers Zacharias Janssen and his son Hans (Uluç, K. et al., 2009), its use in pathology was non existent in Malpighi's time. It is thus impossible to verify that Malpighi had indeed described what we now recognize as Hodgkin's lymphoma. Even Hodgkin, who actually knew about light microscopy, having used it in a study published with Lister (Hodgkin, T. & Lister, J.J., 1827), did not use a microscope to study this disease. This is due to the fact that tissue processing, staining, and histopathology were not established techniques at the time. Two of Hodgkin's original 7 cases were subsequently proven to be true examples of Hodgkin's lymphoma by Fox (Fox, H., 1926) and again by Poston, this time demonstrating that the neoplastic cells indeed expressed CD15 (Poston, R.N., 1999). Case IV is likely to be an example of a peripheral T cell lymphoma with rare CD15+ Reed Sternberg-like cells. It is possible the other 4 cases were also HL but no tissue was available for histology or immunohistochemistry at the time of Poston's study.

Hodgkin's description of his 7 cases remained in obscurity for years even after being rediscovered and attributed to him by Bright (Bright, R., 1838) and Wilks (Wilks, S., 1856). It was through Wilks' persistence that the disease was later recognized as Hodgkin's disease (Wilks, S., 1859). Wilks had to put the term "Hodgkin's disease" in the title of his paper to make the point (Wilks, S., 1865).

Most of the cases that Hodgkin described were patients who died soon after admission to hospital with terminal disease. He did have an opportunity to treat one of the 7 patients with cascarilla and soda to "improve his general health" and iodine "as an agent most likely to affect the glands" but noted dryly in his report that the treatment "appeared to be productive of no advantage, on which account it is probable the patient withdrew himself from my observation" (Hodgkin, T., 1832).

The first description of the histopathological features of HL was published by Theodor Langhans, (Langhans, T., 1872). Six years later, Greenfield published the histopathological features of HL in the English language (Greenfield, W., 1878). The detailed description of the characteristic multinucleated cells in this disease was described by Carl Sternberg (Sternberg, C., 1898) and Dorothy Reed (Reed, D., 1902) and are now called Reed-Sternberg cells. Gall and Mallory established HL as a neoplastic process (Gall, E. & Mallory, T., 1942). The first definitive evidence of the neoplastic nature of HL came in 1967 with the publication about the cytogenetics of HL (Seif, G.S. & Spriggs, A.I., 1967), further supported by a 1975 publication that showed clonal growth of Hodgkin cells (Boecker, W.R. et al., 1975).

The histopathological classification of HL has undergone several changes over the years. The first attempt to classify HL was by Jackson and Parker who in 1947 proposed three categories – paragranuloma, granuloma and sarcoma subtypes (Jackson, H. & Parker, F., 1947). Smetana and Cohen published the results of a retrospective review of mortality rates of HL cases culled from the records of the Armed Forces Institute of Pathology, classified according to the Jackson and Parker classification (Smetana, H.F. & Cohen, B.M., 1956). They did not describe how these patients had been treated.

Further refinement of HL classification came with the publications of Lukes and Butler (Lukes, R.J. et al., 1966; Lukes, R.J. & Butler, J.J., 1966), who divided HL into 6 groups: lymphocytic and/or histiocytic, (L & H), nodular, lymphocytic and/or histiocytic (L & H), diffuse, nodular sclerosis (NS), mixed, diffuse fibrosis and reticular. This was later simplified at the Rye Conference into 4 categories: Lymphocyte predominance (LP), Nodular sclerosis (NS), Mixed cellularity (MC), and Lymphocytic depletion (LD) (Lukes, R. et al., 1966). The first system to separate nodular lymphocyte predominance from classical HL was published in 1994 as part of the Revised European-American lymphoma (REAL) classification system, including the addition of a provisional entity of lymphocyte-rich classical HL (Harris, N.L. et al., 1994). The 2001 and 2008 WHO classification systems accepted the new category which is no longer a provisional one (Jaffe, E.S. et al., 2001; Swerdlow, S.H. et al., 2008). Recently, a comprehensive update of the histopathology and immunohistochemistry findings in HL has been published (Eberle, F.C. et al., 2009).

The therapy of HL has also undergone numerous changes, starting with Thomas Hodgkin's attempts with cascarilla and soda and iodine combination therapy on one patient (Hodgkin, T., 1832). Fowler's solution (potassium arsenite), a panacea concocted in 1786 by Thomas Fowler (Sears, D.A., 1988) for all sorts of chronic conditions, was used to treat HL (Waxman, S. & Anderson, K.C., 2001). It turns out that this was effective. In 1937 Hendrick and Burton from the University of Toronto published a case report of a young male patient with HL who had a remarkable response to colloidal arsenic (Hendrick, A.C. & Burton, E.F., 1937). More recently, Mathas et al. have shown that sodium arsenite rapidly down regulates constitutive IκB kinase (IKK) as well as NF-κB activity and induces apoptosis in Hodgkin Reed-Sternberg (HRS) cell lines containing functional IκB proteins and that arsenic trioxide induces tumour reduction in xenograft models of HL (Mathas, S. et al., 2003). The use of nitrogen mustard for the chemotherapy of HL was introduced by in 1946 (Goodman, L.S. et al., 1946), with reports from others on the results of nitrogen mustard on HL in the forties (Alpert, L.K. & Peterson, S.S., 1947; Dameshek, W. et al., 1949).

Immunotherapy was attempted in 1928 (Wallhauser, A. & Whitehead, J.M., 1928). Three HL patients were treated with saline extracts from affected lymph nodes by subcutaneous injections. Two of the 3 patients achieved complete remission, while the third relapsed after initial response, but responded to a second round of injections. This report encouraged Hanrahan to try the same approach in 1930 with 9 patients but with less spectacular results (Hanrahan, E.M., 1930). Hanrahan used a preservative, tricresol (a mixture of three isomeric phenols derived from toluene: ortho-, meta- or para-methylphenol), in the extract, so one could speculate that whatever the active substance was in the HL tissue extract might have been damaged by tricresol.

Radiotherapy for HL was reported in 1932 (Chevalier, P. & Bernard, J., 1932) and firmly established as an effective therapeutic modality by Vera Peters of the Ontario Cancer Institute (Peters, M.V., 1960, 1965, 1966; Peters, M.V. & Middlemiss, K.C., 1958).

Modern therapy of HL has been described in recent reviews (Boleti, E. & Mead, G.M., 2007; Edwards-Bennett, S.M. et al., 2010; Eichenauer, D.A. et al., 2009; Federico, M. et al., 2009; Mendler, J.H. et al., 2008; Oflazoglu, E. et al., 2008) and not further discussed here.

3. The cell of origin and the pathobiology of HRS cells

The neoplastic cells of classical HL (cHL) (Hodgkin/Reed-Sternberg cells or HRS cells) are usually derived from germinal centre B cells, and rarely are of T cell origin; those of nodular lymphocyte predominance (NLPHL) HL (LP cells) cases are always of germinal centre B cell origin (Brauninger, A. et al., 2006; Caporaso, N.E. et al., 2009; Kuppers, R., 2009; Küppers, R., 2009; Kuppers, R. et al., 2002; Mani, H. & Jaffe, E.S., 2009; Marafioti, T. et al., 2000; Seitz, V. et al., 2000).

Despite the fact that cHL HRS cells are derived from germinal centre or post-germinal centre B cells, they lack B cell markers including the B cell receptor (BCR) (Schwering, I. et al., 2003) as they lose their B cell programming (Hertel, C.B. et al., 2002) through several mechanisms including promoter DNA methylation (Doerr, J.R. et al., 2005; Ushmorov, A. et al., 2006), inhibition of transcription factor E2A by HLH proteins ABF-1 and Id2 resulting in reprogramming of neoplastic B cells (Mathas, S. et al., 2006), loss of PU.1 expression associated with defective immunoglobulin gene transcription (Jundt, F. et al., 2002), down-regulation of BOB.1/OBF.1 and Oct2 (Stein, H. et al., 2001) and upregulation of NOTCH1, a negative regulator of the B cell program (Jundt, F. et al., 2008). At the same time non-B cell lineage proteins are upregulated (Atayar, C. et al., 2005; Dorfman, D.M. et al., 2005).

The LP cells in NLPHL are derived from antigen-activated germinal centre B cells (Braeuninger, A. et al., 1997), express functional IgV genes with intraclonal diversification

(Mottok, A. et al., 2005; Schmitz, R. et al., 2009), BCL6 protein (Falini, B. et al., 1996), and GCET1 (centerin), a germinal centre B cell associated serpin (Montes-Moreno, S. et al., 2008). In contrast to H/RS cells, LP cells retain most of their B cell programming; however, LP cells also show selective loss of the B cell phenotype such as down regulation of CD19, CD37, PAG and LCK (Dogan, A. et al., 2000; Masir, N. et al., 2006; Tedoldi, S. et al., 2007). The mechanism is not related to promoter methylation of the encoding genes (Tedoldi, S. et al., 2007).

3.1 The role of the Epstein Barr virus in HL

The Epstein-Barr virus was first identified in 1964 by Epstein, Achong and Barr (Epstein, M. et al., 1964). Up to 40-60% of cHL cases may contain the EBV genome (Kapatai, G. & Murray, P., 2007), but since EBV infects 90% of the adult population worldwide (Cohen, J., 2000), and is a B lymphocytotropic virus, it may be a passenger, but not a driver in HL.

Comprehensive EBV-human protein interaction maps have been generated by Calderwood et al. (Calderwood, M.A. et al., 2007) who showed over 40 interactions between EBV proteins and over 170 interactions between EBV and human proteins.

4. Genetic defects in primary immunodeficiency disorders (PID) and HL

Mutations in the SH2D1A and ITK genes are associated with aberrant T and NK function that predisposes patients to serious EBV infections, and lymphoproliferative disease including HL in those that survive the initial fulminant infectious mononucleosis. Detailed reviews of these PIDs has been published recently (Rezaei, N., Hedayat, M., et al., 2011; Rezaei, N., Mahmoudi, E., et al., 2011) and some key points are summarized below.

4.1 SH2D1A

The small (128-amino acid) Src homology 2 domain protein 1A (SH2D1A, DSHP or SAP) is associated with X-linked lymphoproliferative disease (XLP). The patients respond to the Epstein-Barr virus (EBV) infection with a fulminant, frequently fatal infectious mononucleosis syndrome (Purtilo, D.T. et al., 1975; Rezaei, N., Mahmoudi, E., et al., 2011). Most cases of XLP are due to mutations in the SH2D1A gene, which codes for the adaptor molecule called Signaling Lymphocytic Activation Molecule (SLAM; CD150)-associated protein (SAP) (Rezaei, N., Mahmoudi, E., et al., 2011). Patients with XLP and Sap null mice have defective natural killer and CD8+ T cell cytotoxicity, impairment of T cell cytokine production, activation-induced cell death, germinal centre formation and T NK cell development (Rezaei, N., Mahmoudi, E., et al., 2011). Survivors may develop agammaglobulinemia and B cell malignant lymphomas including HL (Rezaei, N., Hedayat, M., et al., 2011; Seemayer, T.A. et al., 1995). SH2D1A has been detected in 5 of 6 EBV negative classical HL cell lines including T cell derived HL cell lines (Kis, L.L. et al., 2003) and SH2D1A mRNA found in HRS cells in HL tissue (Nichols, K.E. et al., 1998). The lack of EBV in HL cell lines expressing SH2D1A protein is unexplained (Kis, L.L. et al., 2003).

4.2 IL-2–inducible T-cell kinase (ITK)

IL-2–inducible T-cell kinase (ITK) is a cytoplasmic non-receptor tyrosine kinase expressed in thymocytes, mature T cells, NK cells, iNKT cells, and mast cells (Au-Yeung, B.B. & Fowell, D.J., 2007; Au-Yeung, B.B. et al., 2006; Gadue, P. & Stein, P.L., 2002; Gomez-Rodriguez, J. et al.,

2007; Grasis, J.A. et al., 2003; Iyer, A.S. & August, A., 2008; Qi, Q. et al., 2011). ITK mutations lead to fatal EBV induced lymphoproliferative disease characterized as hemophagocytic lymphohistiocytosis (HLH) and HL (Huck, K. et al., 2009; Stepensky, P. et al., 2011).

5. Prognostic indicators derived from transcriptome, genome and host response patterns

5.1 Gene copy number variation in HRS cells

Complex chromosomal and genomic alterations occur in HRS cells of HL. My laboratory reported novel gains and losses of 9 novel regions in Hodgkin Lymphoma cell lines L428 and KMH2, which shared gains in chromosome cytobands 2q23.1-q24.2, 7q32.2-q36.3, 9p21.3-p13.3, 12q13.13-q14.1, and losses in 13q12.13-q12.3, and 18q21.32-q23. The genes located in these regions include cell cycle associated genes, MAPK signaling pathway genes, those encoding tight junction proteins, Jak/Stat signaling pathway genes and tumour suppressor gene ING3 (Fadlelmola, F. et al., 2008).

Steidl et al. compared patients that had failed primary treatment with those that responded as usual (Steidl, C., Telenius, A., et al., 2010). Gains of 16p11.2-13.3 were associated with treatment failure and shorter disease-specific survival. One of the genes mapping to this region is the multidrug resistance gene ABCC1 encoding multidrug resistance protein MRP1 (Leslie, E. et al., 2001; Rosenberg, M. et al., 2001), and functional studies indicate that this does play a role in chemoresistance (Steidl, C., Telenius, A., et al., 2010).

5.2 Gene expression studies

Devilard et al. using whole cells including the microenvironment, found a signature that can distinguish between good outcome Hodgkin's disease and bad outcome cases (Devilard, E. et al., 2002). Good outcome was associated with overexpression of genes involved in apoptotic induction and cell signaling pathways, including cytokines, whereas bad outcome was associated with overexpression of genes associated with fibroblast activation, angiogenesis, extracellular matrix remodeling, cell proliferation, and the down regulation of tumor suppressor genes.

Sánchez-Aguilera et al. identified 145 genes predictive of outcome (Sanchez-Aguilera, A. et al., 2006). Four different signatures were obtained by supervised hierarchical clustering, 2 of which were associated with the host immune response of tumor microenvironment and the other 2 with the HRS cells based on known expression in HL cell lines and normal germinal centre B cells.

Chetaille et al. studied 63 cHL cases (not enriched for HRS by microdissection, thus including cells from the microenvironment) using full transcriptome coverage and found 47 genes associated with adverse outcome, and 403 genes associated with favorable outcome (Chetaille, B. et al., 2009). Favorable outcome was associated with expressed genes of the "B-cell" cluster, whereas genes associated with unfavorable outcome were in the "extracellular matrix" cluster.

Global gene expression analysis of microdissected LP cells (L&H cells) from 5 cases of NLPHL has been reported by Brune et al. (Brune, V. et al., 2008). The gene expression signatures were closer to T cell-rich B cell lymphoma and classical HL than to diffuse large B cell lymphoma, Burkitt lymphoma, and follicular lymphoma. There is increased expression of ABCC1 in LP cells, which as already discussed, encodes multidrug resistance protein MRP1 (Leslie, E. et al., 2001) and is also amplified and overexpressed in primary treatment refractory cHL (Steidl, C., Telenius, A., et al., 2010).

5.3 Host microenvironment/immune response

An increased number of CD68+ macrophages is associated with a shortened progression-free survival, an increased risk of relapse after HDCT/ASCT, and shortened disease-specific survival. In multivariate analysis, CD68+ cells as a prognostic factor is superior to the International Prognostic Score for disease-specific survival. The absence of an increased number of CD68+ cells in patients with limited-stage disease predicted long-term disease-specific survival of 100% in cHL patients treated with current treatment protocols (Steidl, C., Lee, T., et al., 2010). The immunohistochemistry (IHC) assay for CD68, which is widely available in clinical laboratories, can identify patients with HL who are likely to be refractory to first line therapy and was noted to be the first predictive in-vitro test for cHL (DeVita, V.T., Jr. & Costa, J., 2010).

5.4 Mechanisms of chemoresistance

The multidrug resistance gene ABCC1 in overexpressed in LP and HRS cells and HRS cells contain increased copy number of the ABCC1 gene (Brune, V. et al., 2008; Steidl, C., Telenius, A., et al., 2010). HL tumor samples contain a population of cells that increase efflux of Hoechst 33342 dye and are resistant to gemcitabine, a commonly used drug for the treatment of refractory HL. These cells have the phenotype of HRS cells and express multidrug resistance genes ABCG2 and MDR1 (ABCB1) (Shafer, J.A. et al., 2010).

Genes encoding cytokine receptors (IL5RA, IL13RA1), markers expressed on antigen-presenting cells (CD40, CD80), as well as genes with known association to chemoresistance, such as myristoylated alanine-rich protein kinase C substrate, and PRAME (preferentially expressed antigen in melanoma) are upregulated in chemoresistant cells (Staege, M.S. et al., 2008).

Chemoresistance in HL is also related to XIAP (X-linked inhibitor of apoptosis) an NF-kappaB-independent target of bortezomib. Bortezomib sensitizes HL cells against a variety of cytotoxic drugs independent of NF-kappaB (Kashkar, H. et al., 2007).

6. How the HRS cell, an abnormal B cell clone, survives the normal apoptotic process and immune destruction

Normally B cells that fail to achieve productive or high affinity Ig gene rearrangements or lack BCR are destroyed during the germinal centre reaction (Gordon, J. et al., 1993; Guzman-Rojas, L. et al., 2002; Hollowood, K. & Goodlad, J.R., 1998; Zhang, Q.P. et al., 2005). There are several excellent reviews on the topic of the germinal centre reaction and mechanisms of B cell apoptosis and survival during a normal antigen driven reaction (Elgueta, R. et al., 2010; Goodnow, C.C. et al., 2010; Nutt, S.L. & Tarlinton, D.M., 2011; Oracki, S.A. et al., 2010;

Vikstrom, I. & Tarlinton, D.M., 2011; Vinuesa, C.G. et al., 2010), so only a brief summary is provided in this chapter.

6.1 The germinal center reaction

The biologic or physiologic purpose of the germinal centre reaction is to generate long-term humoral immunity in the adaptive immune system against antigens expressed by pathogens, while, at the same time, eliminating autoreactive clones. The end result is the generation of long-lived antibody-secreting plasma cells and memory B cells which can rapidly trigger subsequent waves of plasma cell production when the same antigen/s are encountered again. The germinal centre reaction is a complex cascade of events, highly regulated, requiring crosstalk and collaboration between B cells, follicular helper T cells and antigen presenting cells including dendritic cells, macrophages and follicular dendritic cells (Cattoretti, G. et al., 2005; Elgueta, R. et al., 2010; Guzman-Rojas, L. et al., 2002; Jardin, F. et al., 2007; Kosco-Vilbois, M.H., 2003; Park, C.S. & Choi, Y.S., 2005; Phan, R.T. & Dalla-Favera, R., 2004; Schenka, A.A. et al., 2005; Siepmann, K. et al., 2001; Spender, L.C. et al., 2009; Tarlinton, D.M. & Smith, K.G., 2000; Zhang, Q.P. et al., 2005).

6.2 The primary lymphoid follicle

Primary lymphoid follicles appear in the second trimester of fetal life in humans and are composed of antigen-naive recirculating B cells that migrate through meshworks of follicular dendritic cells (FDC) with a transit time of 24 hours (Howard, J.C. et al., 1972). These antigen-naive B cells have already undergone recombination of gene fragments, with a theoretical repertoire of $>10^{10}$ antigen binding receptors (Berek, C. & Milstein, C., 1988). When these B cells encounter an antigen, they increase their expression of the chemokine receptor CCR7 which facilitates their migration to the interface between T and B cells zones (Cyster, J.G., 2005; Okada, T. & Cyster, J.G., 2006). Here they can contact antigen-primed T cells, triggering a burst of proliferation of the activated B cells in the outer follicle, ultimately forming a germinal centre (Coffey, F. et al., 2009). HRS cells of cHL also express CCR7 which may explain why HRS cells tend to be located in interfollicular zones (Höpken, U.E. et al., 2002). LP cells are $CCR7^-$ and therefore remain in germinal centers.

6.3 Somatic hypermutation - Generation of higher affinity antibodies

Activated B cells undergo a process of affinity maturation in the germinal center reaction. Rearranged immunoglobulin (Ig) variable region genes undergo random point mutations by a process called somatic hypermutation (SHM) in which single nucleotide substitutions are introduced at a rate of one mutation per 1000 base pairs per generation (Berek, C. & Milstein, C., 1988). Both LP cells of NLPHL and HRS cells of cHL show evidence of SHM of Ig variable region genes (Liso, A. et al., 2006) and are therefore considered to be derived from antigen-activated B cells.

6.4 Selection of high affinity B cells

Since SHM is a random process, a wide range of antigen-binding affinities may result. A mechanism for ensuring that high affinity antigen receptor positive cells are preferentially selected is required for optimal function. The default event seems to be death by apoptosis through the Fas/CD95 pathway unless the cells are rescued by signals from other cell types. Fas/CD95 triggers elimination of low-affinity and self-reactive B cell clones that arise during the germinal centre reaction through apoptosis (Defrance, T. et al., 2002). Prior to apoptosis, rapid activation of caspase-8 occurs in association with CD95 death-inducing signaling complex (DISC). c-FLIP(L), which protects B cells from Fas/CD95 triggered apoptosis is rapidly lost from the CD95 DISC unless the B cells are exposed to the survival signal provided by CD40L from follicular T helper cells (Hennino, A. et al., 2001). In cHL, over 80% of cases show constitutive expression of c-FLIP which protects the HRS cells from Fas/CD95 triggered apoptosis without the need for CD40L survival signals (Mathas, S. et al., 2004; Thomas, R. et al., 2002; Uherova, P. et al., 2004).

6.5 The role of the follicular helper T cell (T_{FH})

The localization of T cells coexpressing HNK-1 (CD57) in the germinal centers (GC) of lymph nodes and spleens was reported by my laboratory (Banerjee, D. & Thibert, R.F., 1983). Although expressing HNK-1 (CD57), which was initially thought to be human natural killer cell specific, these cells were not cytotoxically active. Under certain circumstances, we found that these cells could either suppress or enhance immunoglobulin production by pokeweed mitogen-activated tonsillar B cells (Banerjee, D. et al., 1988). Such cells are now recognized to be specialized CD4+ T cells called follicular helper T cells (T_{FH}) that home to the germinal center and play a pivotal role in regulating the fate of B cell in the germinal centre reaction. They express cell surface antigens CD4, CD57, and CXCR5, produce IL-21, IL-6, IL-27, BCL-6, ICOS, CD40L, and PD-1 (Crotty, S., 2011). While germinal centre CD57+ CD4+ T cells have been shown to be a major T helper cell subset for GC-B cells in Ig synthesis, and have the capacity to induce activation-induced cytosine deaminase (AID) and class switch recombination (Kim, J.R. et al., 2005), the most effective subset of capable of inducing IgG production is the $CXCR5^{hi}$ $ICOS^{hi}$ CD4+ T cell. The presence or absence of CD57 does not appear to affect this function (Rasheed, A.U. et al., 2006).

Cells with the phenotype of T_{FH} are usually found in contact with of NLPHL LP cells (Nam-Cha, S.H. et al., 2009) forming characteristic rosettes. The expression of PD-1 is more frequent than that of CD57 by the T cell rosettes around LP cells (Churchill, H.R. et al., 2010). PD-1+ T cells are also reported in cHL and HRS cells express both ligands for PD-1 (CD279), B7-H1 (PDL1; CD274) and B7-DC (PDL2; CD273) (Yamamoto, R. et al., 2008). The function of PD-1+ T cells in HL is unknown. In normal germinal center reactions, PD-1 signals enhance B cell survival (Good-Jacobson, K.L. et al., 2010), thus it is possible that PD-1+ T_{FH} cells in both NLPHL and cHL provide additional survival signals. Another protective effect of PD-1 could be mediated through its inhibition of cytotoxic T cells via overexpressed PD-1 ligands CD273 or CD274 by the target cells of cytotoxic T cells (Norde, W.J. et al., 2011).

6.6 IL-21

HRS cells aberrantly express IL-21 and the IL-21 receptor. IL-21 activates STAT3 in HRS cells, up-regulates STAT3 target genes, and protects HRS cells from CD95 death receptor–induced apoptosis. In addition, IL-21 through up-regulation of the CC chemokine macrophage-inflammatory protein-3α (MIP-3α) attracts $CCR6+CD4+CD25+FoxP3+CD127_{lc}$ regulatory T cells to migrate close to the proximity of HRS cells, protecting them from immune attack (Lamprecht, B. et al., 2008).

6.7 IL-6

IL-6 is a pleiotropic cytokine (also called B-cell stimulatory factor-2, IFN-b2, 26-kDa protein, Hybridoma/plasmacytoma growth factor and hepatocyte stimulating factor HSF) with biological activities in immune regulation, hematopoiesis, inflammation and neoplasia (Kishimoto, T., 2010). HL cells express multiple cytokines, including interleukin-6 (IL-6) (Tesch, H. et al., 1992). Increased serum levels are associated with advanced disease and worse prognostic scores (Vener, C. et al., 2000). HL cells produce IL-6 through constitutional activation of the PI3K signaling pathway which promotes expression of *HLXB9*, an EHG homeobox gene family member, which in turn activates IL6 (Nagel, S. et al., 2005). Thus HL cells, and presumably HRS cells in vivo, do not solely depend upon T_{FH} for IL-6 supply but make their own, possibly benefiting from an autocrine loop.

6.8 BCL-6

The *BCL6* proto-oncogene encodes a nuclear transcriptional repressor. It is important in germinal center (GC) formation and regulates lymphocyte function, differentiation, and survival. BCL-6 suppresses p53 in GC B-cells and protects B-cell lines from apoptosis induced by DNA damage. BCL-6 is thought to allow GC B-cells to sustain the low levels of physiological DNA breaks related to somatic mutation (SM) and immunoglobulin class switch recombination (Jardin, F. et al., 2007). BCL-6 is also an important regulator of the T_{FH} cell program, being essential for CXCR5 expression and follicular homing by T_{FH} cells (Yu, D. et al., 2009).

BCL-6 expression is usually seen in NLPHL and about 30% of lymphocyte rich classical HL (LRCHL) but not other forms of cHL (Nam-Cha, S.H. et al., 2009). However, in another study, none of the cases of LRCHL expressed BCL-6 (Brauninger, A. et al., 2003).

6.9 Bfl-1

Bfl-1 is a NF-κB target gene from the Bcl-2 family of apoptosis-regulating proteins. Bfl-1 is expressed in HRS cells in clinical biopsies and also expressed in HL cell lines. Bfl-1 can protect cultured H/RS cells from apoptosis induced by pharmacological inhibitors of NF-κB (Hinz, M. et al., 2001; Loughran, S.T. et al., 2011).

7. Next generation whole genome sequencing and new insights into the pathobiology of HL

Technological improvements now allow the analysis of entire genomes and transcriptomes at a sufficient resolution to detect point mutations at high speed and reduced cost (Cronin, M. & Ross, J.S., 2011). Two recent discoveries that are relevant to HL are highlighted in this review.

7.1 MHC class II transactivator CIITA, PD-1 and PD-1 ligands

In 15% of cHL, a gene fusion involving the major histocompatibility complex (MHC) class II transactivator CIITA (MHC2TA) and several partners has been reported (Steidl, C. et al., 2011). Not only is one of the fusions (with an uncharacterized gene BX648577) associated with downregulation of HLA Class II expression which could help HRS cells evade immunosurveillance, CIITA also fuses with genes encoding CD274 (PDL1) and CD273 (PDL2), leading to overexpression of both these PD-1 ligands by HRS cells. This could have two beneficial effects on HRS cell survival, the first through PD-1 survival signals from T_{FH} cells to the neoplastic B cells and the second through inhibition of cytotoxic T cells as already discussed above.

7.2 EZH2

Mutations in *EZH2,* a polycomb group oncogene which encodes a histone methyltransferase, have been described in follicular lymphomas and diffuse large B cell lymphomas of germinal centre type. These mutations involve a single tyrosine (Y641) in the SET domain of the EZH2 protein reducing its enzyme action (Morin, R.D. et al., 2010). While HL cases were not included in this study, this protein may have a role in HL. Whereas the expression of the polycomb group gene encoded proteins BMI-1 and EZH2 genes is associated with resting or proliferating germinal centre B cells, respectively and not coexpressed, Hodgkin/Reed-Sternberg (H/RS) cells co-express BMI-1 and EZH2 (Dukers, D.F. et al., 2004; Raaphorst, F.M. et al., 2000).

8. New targets for potential therapeutic approaches

CD20, a B cell expressed phosphoprotein, is usually expressed by LP cells in NLPHL but variably positive in a minority of cHL cases as recently reviewed by Saini and others (Saini, K.S. et al., 2011). Despite CD20 negativity in most cases of cHL, patients refractory to all conventional HL therapies have responded to rituximab (Younes, A. et al., 2003). An excellent review of the myriad of potential targets for novel therapies for treatment refractory HL has been published by Younes (Younes, A., 2009), and some of these, and the rationale for their use have been summarized in one of my recent review articles (Banerjee, D., 2011).

My laboratory recently reported that a 21 kDa protein (Zhou, M. et al., 2008), which we subsequently identified as CYB5B, an outer mitochondrial membrane protein, is overexpressed in the cytoplasm and plasma membrane of HRS cells but not at the plasma membrane of normal reactive lymphocytes or bone marrow precursor cells (Murphy, D. et al., 2010). Gains in the CYB5B locus in HL cell lines KMH2 and L428 were detected. HL cell lines show increased CYB5B mRNA but reactive lymphocytes and bone marrow precursor cells show no increase in CYB5B mRNA in comparison to housekeeping genes. Due to its location at the plasma membrane of only neoplastic cells in cHL, diffuse large B cell lymphoma (DLBCL) and anaplastic large cell lymphoma (ALCL), CYB5B might be an attractive target for antibody based therapy as toxicity should be minimal since we have determined that normal, reactive lymphocytes and CD34+ bone marrow precursor cells do not express the protein at the plasma membrane (Murphy, D. et al., 2010). We are in the process of creating chimeric antibodies to determine whether they are effective in killing HRS cells in pre-clinical models.

9. Discussion

From Hodgkin's first report in 1832 on what we now call Hodgkin's Lymphoma, to this day, the pathobiology of HL continues to intrigue and surprise us with the myriad ways in which the LP and HRS cells defy all physiologic rules of B cell survival by exploiting the very signals that would normally stop undesirable B cells from surviving. The vast network of crosstalk and redundancy of pathways the tumour cells have successfully utilized keeps growing in complexity. These observations challenge our preconceived notions of cell lineage fidelity as defined by expressed cell surface proteins and other biomarkers. Indeed reprogramming and plasticity of B cells is a reality, thus neoplastic B cells derived from the germinal centre can assume various "identities" and confuse regulatory cells and pathways (Mathas, S., 2007). Eventually, classification of B cell lymphomas including HL will require, not just lineage determination and morphology-based classification and grading, but also the detailed mapping of aberrant pathways in sufficient resolution for us to understand all the potential nodes that could be novel therapeutic targets.

10. Conclusion

HL is a unique set of B cell lymphomas that are characterized by the exploitation of redundant pathways, and crosstalk between regulatory cells that promote the growth and survival of defective B cells which, under normal conditions, would die during the germinal centre reaction. While this may seem an insurmountable level of complexity, the potential for effective novel targeted therapies to deal with refractory disease will be possible to attain when a comprehensive map of pathway pathology is feasible in the future.

11. Acknowledgment

This study was funded through operating grants from the Canadian Institutes of Health Research, other financial support from the Trudi Desmond Memorial Fund, the British Columbia Cancer Agency, the Department of Pathology and Laboratory Medicine, University of British Columbia Endowment Fund, the Lymphoma Foundation Canada, and the British Columbia Cancer Foundation.

12. References

Alpert, L. K. & Peterson, S. S. (1947), "The use of nitrogen mustard in the treatment of lymphomata", *Bull U S Army Med Dep,* Vol. 7 No. 2, 187-194

Atayar, C., Poppema, S., Blokzijl, T., Harms, G., Boot, M. & van den Berg, A. (2005), "Expression of the T-cell transcription factors, GATA-3 and T-bet, in the neoplastic cells of Hodgkin lymphomas", *Am J Pathol,* Vol. 166 No. 1, 127-134 0002-9440 (Print) 0002-9440 (Linking).

Au-Yeung, B. B. & Fowell, D. J. (2007), "A key role for Itk in both IFN gamma and IL-4 production by NKT cells", *J Immunol,* Vol. 179 No. 1, 111-119 0022-1767 (Print) 0022-1767 (Linking).

Au-Yeung, B. B., Katzman, S. D. & Fowell, D. J. (2006), "Cutting edge: Itk-dependent signals required for CD4+ T cells to exert, but not gain, Th2 effector function", *J Immunol,* Vol. 176 No. 7, 3895-3899 0022-1767 (Print) 0022-1767 (Linking).

Banerjee, D. (2011), "Recent Advances in the Pathobiology of Hodgkin's Lymphoma: Potential Impact on Diagnostic, Predictive, and Therapeutic Strategies", *Adv Hematol,* Vol. 2011, 439456 1687-9112 (Electronic).

Banerjee, D., Baril, J., Bell, D. A., McFarlane, D. & Karim, R. (1988), "Suppression of immunoglobulin production by germinal centre HNK-1+ CD3+ cells.", *Adv Exp Med Biol,* Vol. 237, 421-425 0065-2598.

Banerjee, D. & Thibert, R. F. (1983), "Natural killer-like cells found in B-cell compartments of human lymphoid tissues.", *Nature,* Vol. 304 No. 5923, 270-272 0028-0836.

Berek, C. & Milstein, C. (1988), "The dynamic nature of the antibody repertoire.", *Immunol Rev,* Vol. 105, 5-26 0105-2896.

Boecker, W. R., Hossfeld, D. K., Gallmeier, W. M. & Schmidt, C. G. (1975), "Clonal growth of Hodgkin cells", *Nature,* Vol. 258 No. 5532, 235-236 0028-0836 (Print) 0028-0836 (Linking).

Boleti, E. & Mead, G. M. (2007), "ABVD for Hodgkin's lymphoma: full-dose chemotherapy without dose reductions or growth factors", *Ann Oncol,* Vol. 18 No. 2, 376-380 0923-7534 (Print) 0923-7534 (Linking).

Braeuninger, A., Kuppers, R., Strickler, J. G., Wacker, H. H., Rajewsky, K. & Hansmann, M. L. (1997), "Hodgkin and Reed-Sternberg cells in lymphocyte predominant Hodgkin disease represent clonal populations of germinal center-derived tumor B cells", *Proc Natl Acad Sci U S A,* Vol. 94 No. 17, 9337-9342 0027-8424 (Print) 0027-8424 (Linking).

Brauninger, A., Schmitz, R., Bechtel, D., Renne, C., Hansmann, M. L. & Kuppers, R. (2006), "Molecular biology of Hodgkin's and Reed/Sternberg cells in Hodgkin's lymphoma", *Int J Cancer,* Vol. 118 No. 8, 1853-1861 0020-7136 (Print) 0020-7136 (Linking).

Brauninger, A., Wacker, H. H., Rajewsky, K., Kuppers, R. & Hansmann, M. L. (2003), "Typing the histogenetic origin of the tumor cells of lymphocyte-rich classical Hodgkin's lymphoma in relation to tumor cells of classical and lymphocyte-predominance Hodgkin's lymphoma", *Cancer Res,* Vol. 63 No. 7, 1644-1651 0008-5472 (Print) 0008-5472 (Linking).

Bright, R. (1838), "Observations on abdominal tumors and in tumescence: illustrated by cases of disease of the spleen. With remarks on the general pathology of that viscus.", *Guy's Hosp. Rep.,* Vol. 3, 401-461

Brune, V., Tiacci, E., Pfeil, I., Doring, C., Eckerle, S., van Noesel, C. J., Klapper, W., Falini, B., von Heydebreck, A., Metzler, D., Brauninger, A., Hansmann, M. L. & Kuppers, R. (2008), "Origin and pathogenesis of nodular lymphocyte-predominant Hodgkin lymphoma as revealed by global gene expression analysis", *J Exp Med,* Vol. 205 No. 10, 2251-2268 1540-9538 (Electronic) 0022-1007 (Linking).

Calderwood, M. A., Venkatesan, K., Xing, L., Chase, M. R., Vazquez, A., Holthaus, A. M., Ewence, A. E., Li, N., Hirozane-Kishikawa, T., Hill, D. E., Vidal, M., Kieff, E. & Johannsen, E. (2007), "Epstein-Barr virus and virus human protein interaction maps", *Proc Natl Acad Sci U S A,* Vol. 104 No. 18, 7606-7611 0027-8424 (Print) 0027-8424 (Linking).

Caporaso, N. E., Goldin, L. R., Anderson, W. F. & Landgren, O. (2009), "Current insight on trends, causes, and mechanisms of Hodgkin's lymphoma", *Cancer J,* Vol. 15 No. 2, 117-123 1528-9117 (Print) 1528-9117 (Linking).

Cattoretti, G., Angelin-Duclos, C., Shaknovich, R., Zhou, H., Wang, D. & Alobeid, B. (2005), "PRDM1/Blimp-1 is expressed in human B-lymphocytes committed to the plasma cell lineage", *J Pathol,* Vol. 206 No. 1, 76-86 0022-3417 (Print) 0022-3417 (Linking).

Chetaille, B., Bertucci, F., Finetti, P., Esterni, B., Stamatoullas, A., Picquenot, J., Copin, M., Morschhauser, F., Casasnovas, O., Petrella, T., Molina, T., Vekhoff, A., Feugier, P., Bouabdallah, R., Birnbaum, D., Olive, D. & Xerri, L. (2009), "Molecular profiling of classical Hodgkin lymphoma tissues uncovers variations in the tumor microenvironment and correlations with EBV infection and outcome.", *Blood*, Vol. 113 No. 12, 2765-3775 1528-0020.

Chevalier, P. & Bernard, J. (Eds) (1932), *La maladie de Hodgkin (lymphogranulomatose maligne)*, Masson, Paris.

Churchill, H. R., Roncador, G., Warnke, R. A. & Natkunam, Y. (2010), "Programmed death 1 expression in variant immunoarchitectural patterns of nodular lymphocyte predominant Hodgkin lymphoma: comparison with CD57 and lymphomas in the differential diagnosis", *Hum Pathol*, Vol. 41 No. 12, 1726-1734 1532-8392 (Electronic) 0046-8177 (Linking).

Coffey, F., Alabyev, B. & Manser, T. (2009), "Initial clonal expansion of germinal center B cells takes place at the perimeter of follicles.", *Immunity*, Vol. 30 No. 4, 599-609 1097-4180.

Cohen, J. (2000), "Epstein-Barr virus infection.", *N Engl J Med*, Vol. 343 No. 7, 481-492 0028-4793.

Cronin, M. & Ross, J. S. (2011), "Comprehensive next-generation cancer genome sequencing in the era of targeted therapy and personalized oncology.", *Biomark Med*, Vol. 5 No. 3, 293-305 1752-0371.

Crotty, S. (2011), "Follicular helper CD4 T cells (TFH).", *Annu Rev Immunol*, Vol. 29, 621-663 1545-3278.

Cyster, J. G. (2005), "Chemokines, sphingosine-1-phosphate, and cell migration in secondary lymphoid organs.", *Annu Rev Immunol*, Vol. 23, 127-159 0732-0582.

Dameshek, W., Weisfuse, L. & Stein, T. (1949), "Nitrogen mustard therapy in Hodgkin's disease; analysis of 50 consecutive cases", *Blood*, Vol. 4 No. 4, 338-379 0006-4971 (Print) 0006-4971 (Linking).

Defrance, T., Casamayor-Pallejà, M. & Krammer, P. H. (2002), "The life and death of a B cell.", *Adv Cancer Res*, Vol. 86, 195-225 0065-230X.

Devilard, E., Bertucci, F., Trempat, P., Bouabdallah, R., Loriod, B., Giaconia, A., Brousset, P., Granjeaud, S., Nguyen, C., Birnbaum, D., Birg, F., Houlgatte, R. & Xerri, L. (2002), "Gene expression profiling defines molecular subtypes of classical Hodgkin's disease", *Oncogene*, Vol. 21 No. 19, 3095-3102 0950-9232 (Print) 0950-9232 (Linking).

DeVita, V. T., Jr. & Costa, J. (2010), "Toward a personalized treatment of Hodgkin's disease", *N Engl J Med*, Vol. 362 No. 10, 942-943 1533-4406 (Electronic) 0028-4793 (Linking).

Doerr, J. R., Malone, C. S., Fike, F. M., Gordon, M. S., Soghomonian, S. V., Thomas, R. K., Tao, Q., Murray, P. G., Diehl, V., Teitell, M. A. & Wall, R. (2005), "Patterned CpG methylation of silenced B cell gene promoters in classical Hodgkin lymphoma-derived and primary effusion lymphoma cell lines", *J Mol Biol*, Vol. 350 No. 4, 631-640 0022-2836 (Print) 0022-2836 (Linking).

Dogan, A., Bagdi, E., Munson, P. & Isaacson, P. G. (2000), "CD10 and BCL-6 expression in paraffin sections of normal lymphoid tissue and B-cell lymphomas.", *Am J Surg Pathol*, Vol. 24 No. 6, 846-852 0147-5185.

Dorfman, D. M., Hwang, E. S., Shahsafaei, A. & Glimcher, L. H. (2005), "T-bet, a T cell-associated transcription factor, is expressed in Hodgkin's lymphoma", *Hum Pathol*, Vol. 36 No. 1, 10-15 0046-8177 (Print) 0046-8177 (Linking).

Dukers, D. F., van Galen, J. C., Giroth, C., Jansen, P., Sewalt, R. G., Otte, A. P., Kluin-Nelemans, H. C., Meijer, C. J. & Raaphorst, F. M. (2004), "Unique polycomb gene expression pattern in Hodgkin's lymphoma and Hodgkin's lymphoma-derived cell lines", *Am J Pathol*, Vol. 164 No. 3, 873-881 0002-9440 (Print) 0002-9440 (Linking).

Eberle, F. C., Mani, H. & Jaffe, E. S. (2009), "Histopathology of Hodgkin's lymphoma", *Cancer J*, Vol. 15 No. 2, 129-137 1528-9117 (Print) 1528-9117 (Linking).

Edwards-Bennett, S. M., Jacks, L. M., Moskowitz, C. H., Wu, E. J., Zhang, Z., Noy, A., Portlock, C. S., Straus, D. J., Zelenetz, A. D. & Yahalom, J. (2010), "Stanford V program for locally extensive and advanced Hodgkin lymphoma: the Memorial Sloan-Kettering Cancer Center experience", *Ann Oncol*, Vol. 21 No. 3, 574-581 1569-8041 (Electronic) 0923-7534 (Linking).

Eichenauer, D. A., Bredenfeld, H., Haverkamp, H., Muller, H., Franklin, J., Fuchs, M., Borchmann, P., Muller-Hermelink, H. K., Eich, H. T., Muller, R. P., Diehl, V. & Engert, A. (2009), "Hodgkin's lymphoma in adolescents treated with adult protocols: a report from the German Hodgkin study group", *J Clin Oncol*, Vol. 27 No. 36, 6079-6085 1527-7755 (Electronic) 0732-183X (Linking).

Elgueta, R., de Vries, V. C. & Noelle, R. J. (2010), "The immortality of humoral immunity.", *Immunol Rev*, Vol. 236, 139-150 1600-065X.

Epstein, M., Barr, Y. & Achong, B. (1964), "A Second Virus-Carrying Tissue Culture Strain (Eb2) of Lymphoblasts from Burkitt's Lymphoma", *Pathol Biol (Paris)*, Vol. 12, 1233-1234 0369-8114.

Fadlelmola, F., Zhou, M., de Leeuw, R., Dosanjh, N., Harmer, K., Huntsman, D., Lam, W. & Banerjee, D. (2008), "Sub-megabase resolution tiling (SMRT) array-based comparative genomic hybridization profiling reveals novel gains and losses of chromosomal regions in Hodgkin Lymphoma and Anaplastic Large Cell Lymphoma cell lines.", *Mol Cancer*, Vol. 7, 2 1476-4598.

Falini, B., Bigerna, B., Pasqualucci, L., Fizzotti, M., Martelli, M. F., Pileri, S., Pinto, A., Carbone, A., Venturi, S., Pacini, R., Cattoretti, G., Pescarmona, E., Lo Coco, F., Pelicci, P. G., Anagnastopoulos, I., Dalla-Favera, R. & Flenghi, L. (1996), "Distinctive expression pattern of the BCL-6 protein in nodular lymphocyte predominance Hodgkin's disease", *Blood*, Vol. 87 No. 2, 465-471 0006-4971 (Print) 0006-4971 (Linking).

Federico, M., Luminari, S., Iannitto, E., Polimeno, G., Marcheselli, L., Montanini, A., La Sala, A., Merli, F., Stelitano, C., Pozzi, S., Scalone, R., Di Renzo, N., Musto, P., Baldini, L., Cervetti, G., Angrilli, F., Mazza, P., Brugiatelli, M. & Gobbi, P. G. (2009), "ABVD compared with BEACOPP compared with CEC for the initial treatment of patients with advanced Hodgkin's lymphoma: results from the HD2000 Gruppo Italiano per lo Studio dei Linfomi Trial", *J Clin Oncol*, Vol. 27 No. 5, 805-811 1527-7755 (Electronic) 0732-183X (Linking).

Fox, H. (1926), "Remarks on the presentation of microscopical preparations made from some of the original tissue described by Thomas Hodgkin, 1832.", *Ann. Med. Hist.*, Vol. 8, 370-374

Gadue, P. & Stein, P. L. (2002), "NK T cell precursors exhibit differential cytokine regulation and require Itk for efficient maturation", *J Immunol,* Vol. 169 No. 5, 2397-2406 0022-1767 (Print) 0022-1767 (Linking).

Gall, E. & Mallory, T. (1942), "Malignant Lymphoma: A Clinico-Pathologic Survey of 618 Cases.", *Am J Pathol,* Vol. 18 No. 3, 381-429 1525-2191.

Gomez-Rodriguez, J., Readinger, J. A., Viorritto, I. C., Mueller, K. L., Houghtling, R. A. & Schwartzberg, P. L. (2007), "Tec kinases, actin, and cell adhesion", *Immunol Rev,* Vol. 218, 45-64 0105-2896 (Print) 0105-2896 (Linking).

Good-Jacobson, K. L., Szumilas, C. G., Chen, L., Sharpe, A. H., Tomayko, M. M. & Shlomchik, M. J. (2010), "PD-1 regulates germinal center B cell survival and the formation and affinity of long-lived plasma cells.", *Nat Immunol,* Vol. 11 No. 6, 535-542 1529-2916.

Goodman, L. S., Wintrobe, M. M. & et al. (1946), "Nitrogen mustard therapy; use of methyl-bis (beta-chloroethyl) amine hydrochloride and tris (beta-chloroethyl) amine hydrochloride for Hodgkin's disease, lymphosarcoma, leukemia and certain allied and miscellaneous disorders", *J Am Med Assoc,* Vol. 132, 126-132 0002-9955 (Print) 0002-9955 (Linking).

Goodnow, C. C., Vinuesa, C. G., Randall, K. L., Mackay, F. & Brink, R. (2010), "Control systems and decision making for antibody production.", *Nat Immunol,* Vol. 11 No. 8, 681-688 1529-2916.

Gordon, J., Knox, K. & Gregory, C. D. (1993), "Regulation of survival in normal and neoplastic B lymphocytes", *Leukemia,* Vol. 7 Suppl 2, S5-9 0887-6924 (Print) 0887-6924 (Linking).

Grasis, J. A., Browne, C. D. & Tsoukas, C. D. (2003), "Inducible T cell tyrosine kinase regulates actin-dependent cytoskeletal events induced by the T cell antigen receptor", *J Immunol,* Vol. 170 No. 8, 3971-3976 0022-1767 (Print) 0022-1767 (Linking).

Greenfield, W. (1878), "Specimens illustrative of the pathology of lymphadenoma and leucothemia.", *Trans Pathol Soc London,* Vol. 29, 272–304

Guzman-Rojas, L., Sims-Mourtada, J. C., Rangel, R. & Martinez-Valdez, H. (2002), "Life and death within germinal centres: a double-edged sword", *Immunology,* Vol. 107 No. 2, 167-175 0019-2805 (Print) 0019-2805 (Linking).

Hanrahan, E. M. (1930), "Results of treatment by autogenous gland filtrate in Hodgkin's disease.", *Ann Surg,* Vol. 92 No. 1, 23-34 0003-4932.

Harris, N. L., Jaffe, E. S., Stein, H., Banks, P. M., Chan, J. K., Cleary, M. L., Delsol, G., De Wolf-Peeters, C., Falini, B., Gatter, K. C. & et al. (1994), "A revised European-American classification of lymphoid neoplasms: a proposal from the International Lymphoma Study Group", *Blood,* Vol. 84 No. 5, 1361-1392 0006-4971 (Print) 0006-4971 (Linking).

Hendrick, A. C. & Burton, E. F. (1937), "A Case of Hodgkin's Disease Treated with Colloidal Elemental Arsenic", *Can Med Assoc J,* Vol. 36 No. 5, 519-520 0008-4409 (Print) 0008-4409 (Linking).

Hennino, A., Bérard, M., Krammer, P. H. & Defrance, T. (2001), "FLICE-inhibitory protein is a key regulator of germinal center B cell apoptosis.", *J Exp Med,* Vol. 193 No. 4, 447-458 0022-1007.

Hertel, C. B., Zhou, X. G., Hamilton-Dutoit, S. J. & Junker, S. (2002), "Loss of B cell identity correlates with loss of B cell-specific transcription factors in Hodgkin/Reed-Sternberg cells of classical Hodgkin lymphoma", *Oncogene,* Vol. 21 No. 32, 4908-4920 0950-9232 (Print) 0950-9232 (Linking).

Hinz, M., Loser, P., Mathas, S., Krappmann, D., Dorken, B. & Scheidereit, C. (2001), "Constitutive NF-kappaB maintains high expression of a characteristic gene network, including CD40, CD86, and a set of antiapoptotic genes in Hodgkin/Reed-Sternberg cells", *Blood,* Vol. 97 No. 9, 2798-2807 0006-4971 (Print) 0006-4971 (Linking).

Hodgkin, T. (1832), "On some morbid appearances of the absorbent glands and spleen.", *Med. Chirurg. Trans.,* Vol. 17, 68–114

Hodgkin, T. & Lister, J. J. (1827), "Notice of some microscopic observations of the blood and animal tissues", *Phil. Mag.,* Vol. ns2, 130-138

Hollowood, K. & Goodlad, J. R. (1998), "Germinal centre cell kinetics", *J Pathol,* Vol. 185 No. 3, 229-233 0022-3417 (Print) 0022-3417 (Linking).

Höpken, U. E., Foss, H. D., Meyer, D., Hinz, M., Leder, K., Stein, H. & Lipp, M. (2002), "Up-regulation of the chemokine receptor CCR7 in classical but not in lymphocyte-predominant Hodgkin disease correlates with distinct dissemination of neoplastic cells in lymphoid organs.", *Blood,* Vol. 99 No. 4, 1109-1116 0006-4971.

Howard, J. C., Hunt, S. V. & Gowans, J. L. (1972), "Identification of marrow-derived and thymus-derived small lymphocytes in the lymphoid tissue and thoracic duct lymph of normal rats.", *J Exp Med,* Vol. 135 No. 2, 200-219 0022-1007.

Huck, K., Feyen, O., Niehues, T., Ruschendorf, F., Hubner, N., Laws, H. J., Telieps, T., Knapp, S., Wacker, H. H., Meindl, A., Jumaa, H. & Borkhardt, A. (2009), "Girls homozygous for an IL-2-inducible T cell kinase mutation that leads to protein deficiency develop fatal EBV-associated lymphoproliferation", *J Clin Invest,* Vol. 119 No. 5, 1350-1358 1558-8238 (Electronic) 0021-9738 (Linking).

Iyer, A. S. & August, A. (2008), "The Tec family kinase, IL-2-inducible T cell kinase, differentially controls mast cell responses", *J Immunol,* Vol. 180 No. 12, 7869-7877 0022-1767 (Print) 0022-1767 (Linking).

Jackson, H. & Parker, F. (Eds) (1947), *Hodgkin's disease and allied disorders.,* Oxford University Press, New York.

Jaffe, E. S., Harris, N. L., Stein, H. & Vardiman, J. (Eds) (2001), *World Health Organization Classification of Tumours: Pathology and Genetics of Tumours of Haematopoietic and Lymphoid Tissues,* IARC Press, 9283224116, Lyon.

Jardin, F., Ruminy, P., Bastard, C. & Tilly, H. (2007), "The BCL6 proto-oncogene: a leading role during germinal center development and lymphomagenesis", *Pathol Biol (Paris),* Vol. 55 No. 1, 73-83 0369-8114 (Print) 0369-8114 (Linking).

Jundt, F., Acikgoz, O., Kwon, S. H., Schwarzer, R., Anagnostopoulos, I., Wiesner, B., Mathas, S., Hummel, M., Stein, H., Reichardt, H. M. & Dorken, B. (2008), "Aberrant expression of Notch1 interferes with the B-lymphoid phenotype of neoplastic B cells in classical Hodgkin lymphoma", *Leukemia,* Vol. 22 No. 8, 1587-1594 1476-5551 (Electronic) 0887-6924 (Linking).

Jundt, F., Kley, K., Anagnostopoulos, I., Schulze Probsting, K., Greiner, A., Mathas, S., Scheidereit, C., Wirth, T., Stein, H. & Dorken, B. (2002), "Loss of PU.1 expression is associated with defective immunoglobulin transcription in Hodgkin and Reed-

Sternberg cells of classical Hodgkin disease", *Blood,* Vol. 99 No. 8, 3060-3062 0006-4971 (Print) 0006-4971 (Linking).

Kapatai, G. & Murray, P. (2007), "Contribution of the Epstein Barr virus to the molecular pathogenesis of Hodgkin lymphoma.", *J Clin Pathol,* Vol. 60 No. 12, 1342-1349 1472-4146.

Kashkar, H., Deggerich, A., Seeger, J. M., Yazdanpanah, B., Wiegmann, K., Haubert, D., Pongratz, C. & Kronke, M. (2007), "NF-kappaB-independent down-regulation of XIAP by bortezomib sensitizes HL B cells against cytotoxic drugs", *Blood,* Vol. 109 No. 9, 3982-3988 0006-4971 (Print) 0006-4971 (Linking).

Kim, J. R., Lim, H. W., Kang, S. G., Hillsamer, P. & Kim, C. H. (2005), "Human CD57+ germinal center-T cells are the major helpers for GC-B cells and induce class switch recombination.", *BMC Immunol,* Vol. 6, 3 1471-2172.

Kis, L. L., Nagy, N., Klein, G. & Klein, E. (2003), "Expression of SH2D1A in five classical Hodgkin's disease-derived cell lines", *Int J Cancer,* Vol. 104 No. 5, 658-661 0020-7136 (Print) 0020-7136 (Linking).

Kishimoto, T. (2010), "IL-6: from its discovery to clinical applications.", *Int Immunol,* Vol. 22 No. 5, 347-352 1460-2377.

Kosco-Vilbois, M. H. (2003), "Are follicular dendritic cells really good for nothing?", *Nat Rev Immunol,* Vol. 3 No. 9, 764-769 1474-1733 (Print) 1474-1733 (Linking).

Kuppers, R. (2009), "The biology of Hodgkin's lymphoma", *Nat Rev Cancer,* Vol. 9 No. 1, 15-27 1474-1768 (Electronic) 1474-175X (Linking).

Küppers, R. (2009), "Molecular biology of Hodgkin lymphoma.", *Hematology Am Soc Hematol Educ Program,* 491-496 1520-4383.

Kuppers, R., Schwering, I., Brauninger, A., Rajewsky, K. & Hansmann, M. L. (2002), "Biology of Hodgkin's lymphoma", *Ann Oncol,* Vol. 13 Suppl 1, 11-18 0923-7534 (Print) 0923-7534 (Linking).

Lamprecht, B., Kreher, S., Anagnostopoulos, I., Johrens, K., Monteleone, G., Jundt, F., Stein, H., Janz, M., Dorken, B. & Mathas, S. (2008), "Aberrant expression of the Th2 cytokine IL-21 in Hodgkin lymphoma cells regulates STAT3 signaling and attracts Treg cells via regulation of MIP-3alpha", *Blood,* Vol. 112 No. 8, 3339-3347 1528-0020 (Electronic) 0006-4971 (Linking).

Langhans, T. (1872), "Das maligne Lymphosarkum Pseudoleukamie", *Virchows Pathol Anat,* Vol. 54, 509–536

Leslie, E., Deeley, R. & Cole, S. (2001), "Toxicological relevance of the multidrug resistance protein 1, MRP1 (ABCC1) and related transporters.", *Toxicology,* Vol. 167 No. 1, 3-23 0300-483X.

Liso, A., Capello, D., Marafioti, T., Tiacci, E., Cerri, M., Distler, V., Paulli, M., Carbone, A., Delsol, G., Campo, E., Pileri, S., Pasqualucci, L., Gaidano, G. & Falini, B. (2006), "Aberrant somatic hypermutation in tumor cells of nodular-lymphocyte-predominant and classic Hodgkin lymphoma", *Blood,* Vol. 108 No. 3, 1013-1020 0006-4971 (Print) 0006-4971 (Linking).

Loughran, S. T., Campion, E. M., D'Souza, B. N., Smith, S. M., Vrzalikova, K., Wen, K., Murray, P. G. & Walls, D. (2011), "Bfl-1 is a crucial pro-survival nuclear factor-kappaB target gene in Hodgkin/Reed-Sternberg cells", *Int J Cancer* 1097-0215 (Electronic) 0020-7136 (Linking).

Lukes, R., Craver, L., Hal, l. T., Rappaport, H. & Ruben, P. (1966), "Report of the Nomenclature Committee", *Cancer Res,* Vol. 26, 1311

Lukes, R. J., Butler, J. & Hicks, E. B. (1966), "[The prognosis of Hodgkin's disease according to the histologic type and the clinical stage. Role of the reactions of the host]", *Nouv Rev Fr Hematol,* Vol. 6 No. 1, 15-22 0029-4810 (Print) 0029-4810 (Linking).

Lukes, R. J. & Butler, J. J. (1966), "The pathology and nomenclature of Hodgkin's disease", *Cancer Res,* Vol. 26 No. 6, 1063-1083 0008-5472 (Print) 0008-5472 (Linking).

Malpighi, M. (1666), "De Viscerum Structura Exercitatio Anatomica.", in. J. Montij, Bononiae, pp. 125-156.

Mani, H. & Jaffe, E. S. (2009), "Hodgkin lymphoma: an update on its biology with new insights into classification", *Clin Lymphoma Myeloma,* Vol. 9 No. 3, 206-216 1938-0712 (Electronic) 1557-9190 (Linking).

Marafioti, T., Hummel, M., Foss, H. D., Laumen, H., Korbjuhn, P., Anagnostopoulos, I., Lammert, H., Demel, G., Theil, J., Wirth, T. & Stein, H. (2000), "Hodgkin and reed-sternberg cells represent an expansion of a single clone originating from a germinal center B-cell with functional immunoglobulin gene rearrangements but defective immunoglobulin transcription", *Blood,* Vol. 95 No. 4, 1443-1450 0006-4971 (Print) 0006-4971 (Linking).

Masir, N., Marafioti, T., Jones, M., Natkunam, Y., Rudiger, T., Hansmann, M. L. & Mason, D. Y. (2006), "Loss of CD19 expression in B-cell neoplasms", *Histopathology,* Vol. 48 No. 3, 239-246 0309-0167 (Print) 0309-0167 (Linking).

Mathas, S. (2007), "The pathogenesis of classical Hodgkin's lymphoma: a model for B-cell plasticity.", *Hematol Oncol Clin North Am,* Vol. 21 No. 5, 787-804 0889-8588.

Mathas, S., Janz, M., Hummel, F., Hummel, M., Wollert-Wulf, B., Lusatis, S., Anagnostopoulos, I., Lietz, A., Sigvardsson, M., Jundt, F., Johrens, K., Bommert, K., Stein, H. & Dorken, B. (2006), "Intrinsic inhibition of transcription factor E2A by HLH proteins ABF-1 and Id2 mediates reprogramming of neoplastic B cells in Hodgkin lymphoma", *Nat Immunol,* Vol. 7 No. 2, 207-215 1529-2908 (Print) 1529-2908 (Linking).

Mathas, S., Lietz, A., Anagnostopoulos, I., Hummel, F., Wiesner, B., Janz, M., Jundt, F., Hirsch, B., Jöhrens-Leder, K., Vornlocher, H. P., Bommert, K., Stein, H. & Dörken, B. (2004), "c-FLIP mediates resistance of Hodgkin/Reed-Sternberg cells to death receptor-induced apoptosis.", *J Exp Med,* Vol. 199 No. 8, 1041-1052 0022-1007.

Mathas, S., Lietz, A., Janz, M., Hinz, M., Jundt, F., Scheidereit, C., Bommert, K. & Dorken, B. (2003), "Inhibition of NF-kappaB essentially contributes to arsenic-induced apoptosis", *Blood,* Vol. 102 No. 3, 1028-1034 0006-4971 (Print) 0006-4971 (Linking).

Mendler, J. H., Kelly, J., Voci, S., Marquis, D., Rich, L., Rossi, R. M., Bernstein, S. H., Jordan, C. T., Liesveld, J., Fisher, R. I. & Friedberg, J. W. (2008), "Bortezomib and gemcitabine in relapsed or refractory Hodgkin's lymphoma", *Ann Oncol,* Vol. 19 No. 10, 1759-1764 1569-8041 (Electronic) 0923-7534 (Linking).

Montes-Moreno, S., Roncador, G., Maestre, L., Martinez, N., Sanchez-Verde, L., Camacho, F. I., Cannata, J., Martinez-Torrecuadrada, J. L., Shen, Y., Chan, W. C. & Piris, M. A. (2008), "Gcet1 (centerin), a highly restricted marker for a subset of germinal center-derived lymphomas", *Blood,* Vol. 111 No. 1, 351-358 0006-4971 (Print) 0006-4971 (Linking).

Morin, R. D., Johnson, N. A., Severson, T. M., Mungall, A. J., An, J., Goya, R., Paul, J. E., Boyle, M., Woolcock, B. W., Kuchenbauer, F., Yap, D., Humphries, R. K., Griffith, O. L., Shah, S., Zhu, H., Kimbara, M., Shashkin, P., Charlot, J. F., Tcherpakov, M., Corbett, R., Tam, A., Varhol, R., Smailus, D., Moksa, M., Zhao, Y., Delaney, A., Qian, H., Birol, I., Schein, J., Moore, R., Holt, R., Horsman, D. E., Connors, J. M., Jones, S., Aparicio, S., Hirst, M., Gascoyne, R. D. & Marra, M. A. (2010), "Somatic mutations altering EZH2 (Tyr641) in follicular and diffuse large B-cell lymphomas of germinal-center origin.", *Nat Genet,* Vol. 42 No. 2, 181-185 1546-1718.

Mottok, A., Hansmann, M. L. & Bräuninger, A. (2005), "Activation induced cytidine deaminase expression in lymphocyte predominant Hodgkin lymphoma.", *J Clin Pathol,* Vol. 58 No. 9, 1002-1004 0021-9746.

Murphy, D., Parker, J., Zhou, M., Fadlelmola, F., Steidl, C., Karsan, A., Gascoyne, R., Chen, H. & Banerjee, D. (2010), "Constitutively overexpressed 21 kDa protein in Hodgkin lymphoma and aggressive non-Hodgkin lymphomas identified as cytochrome B5b (CYB5B).", *Mol Cancer,* Vol. 9, 14 1476-4598.

Nagel, S., Scherr, M., Quentmeier, H., Kaufmann, M., Zaborski, M., Drexler, H. G. & MacLeod, R. A. (2005), "HLXB9 activates IL6 in Hodgkin lymphoma cell lines and is regulated by PI3K signalling involving E2F3.", *Leukemia,* Vol. 19 No. 5, 841-846 0887-6924.

Nam-Cha, S. H., Montes-Moreno, S., Salcedo, M. T., Sanjuan, J., Garcia, J. F. & Piris, M. A. (2009), "Lymphocyte-rich classical Hodgkin's lymphoma: distinctive tumor and microenvironment markers", *Mod Pathol,* Vol. 22 No. 8, 1006-1015 1530-0285 (Electronic) 0893-3952 (Linking).

Nichols, K. E., Harkin, D. P., Levitz, S., Krainer, M., Kolquist, K. A., Genovese, C., Bernard, A., Ferguson, M., Zuo, L., Snyder, E., Buckler, A. J., Wise, C., Ashley, J., Lovett, M., Valentine, M. B., Look, A. T., Gerald, W., Housman, D. E. & Haber, D. A. (1998), "Inactivating mutations in an SH2 domain-encoding gene in X-linked lymphoproliferative syndrome", *Proc Natl Acad Sci U S A,* Vol. 95 No. 23, 13765-13770 0027-8424 (Print) 0027-8424 (Linking).

Norde, W. J., Maas, F., Hobo, W., Korman, A., Quigley, M., Kester, M. G., Hebeda, K., Falkenburg, J. H., Schaap, N., de Witte, T. M., van der Voort, R. & Dolstra, H. (2011), "PD-1/PD-L1 Interactions Contribute to Functional T-Cell Impairment in Patients Who Relapse with Cancer After Allogeneic Stem Cell Transplantation", *Cancer Res,* Vol. 71 No. 15, 5111-5122 1538-7445 (Electronic) 0008-5472 (Linking).

Nutt, S. L. & Tarlinton, D. M. (2011), "Germinal center B and follicular helper T cells: siblings, cousins or just good friends?", *Nat Immunol,* Vol. 12 No. 6, 472-477 1529-2916.

Oflazoglu, E., Kissler, K. M., Sievers, E. L., Grewal, I. S. & Gerber, H. P. (2008), "Combination of the anti-CD30-auristatin-E antibody-drug conjugate (SGN-35) with chemotherapy improves antitumour activity in Hodgkin lymphoma", *Br J Haematol,* Vol. 142 No. 1, 69-73 1365-2141 (Electronic) 0007-1048 (Linking).

Okada, T. & Cyster, J. G. (2006), "B cell migration and interactions in the early phase of antibody responses.", *Curr Opin Immunol,* Vol. 18 No. 3, 278-285 0952-7915.

Oracki, S. A., Walker, J. A., Hibbs, M. L., Corcoran, L. M. & Tarlinton, D. M. (2010), "Plasma cell development and survival.", *Immunol Rev,* Vol. 237 No. 1, 140-159 1600-065X.

Park, C. S. & Choi, Y. S. (2005), "How do follicular dendritic cells interact intimately with B cells in the germinal centre?", *Immunology,* Vol. 114 No. 1, 2-10 0019-2805 (Print) 0019-2805 (Linking).

Peters, M. V. (1960), "The place of irradiation in the control of Hodgkin's disease", *Proc Natl Cancer Conf,* Vol. 4, 571-584 0077-3670 (Print) 0077-3670 (Linking).

Peters, M. V. (1965), "Current Concepts in Cancer. 2. Hodgkin's Disease. Radiation Therapy", *JAMA,* Vol. 191, 28-29 0098-7484 (Print) 0098-7484 (Linking).

Peters, M. V. (1966), "Prophylactic treatment of adjacent areas in Hodgkin's disease", *Cancer Res,* Vol. 26 No. 6, 1232-1243 0008-5472 (Print) 0008-5472 (Linking).

Peters, M. V. & Middlemiss, K. C. (1958), "A study of Hodgkin's disease treated by irradiation", *Am J Roentgenol Radium Ther Nucl Med,* Vol. 79 No. 1, 114-121 0002-9580 (Print) 0002-9580 (Linking).

Phan, R. T. & Dalla-Favera, R. (2004), "The BCL6 proto-oncogene suppresses p53 expression in germinal-centre B cells", *Nature,* Vol. 432 No. 7017, 635-639 1476-4687 (Electronic) 0028-0836 (Linking).

Poston, R. N. (1999), "A new look at the original cases of Hodgkin's disease", *Cancer Treat Rev,* Vol. 25 No. 3, 151-155 0305-7372 (Print) 0305-7372 (Linking).

Purtilo, D. T., Cassel, C. K., Yang, J. P. & Harper, R. (1975), "X-linked recessive progressive combined variable immunodeficiency (Duncan's disease)", *Lancet,* Vol. 1 No. 7913, 935-940 0140-6736 (Print) 0140-6736 (Linking).

Qi, Q., Xia, M., Bai, Y., Yu, S., Cantorna, M. & August, A. (2011), "Interleukin-2-inducible T cell kinase (Itk) network edge dependence for the maturation of iNKT cell", *J Biol Chem,* Vol. 286 No. 1, 138-146 1083-351X (Electronic) 0021-9258 (Linking).

Raaphorst, F. M., van Kemenade, F. J., Blokzijl, T., Fieret, E., Hamer, K. M., Satijn, D. P., Otte, A. P. & Meijer, C. J. (2000), "Coexpression of BMI-1 and EZH2 polycomb group genes in Reed-Sternberg cells of Hodgkin's disease", *Am J Pathol,* Vol. 157 No. 3, 709-715 0002-9440 (Print) 0002-9440 (Linking).

Rasheed, A. U., Rahn, H. P., Sallusto, F., Lipp, M. & Müller, G. (2006), "Follicular B helper T cell activity is confined to CXCR5(hi)ICOS(hi) CD4 T cells and is independent of CD57 expression.", *Eur J Immunol,* Vol. 36 No. 7, 1892-1903 0014-2980.

Reed, D. (1902), "On the pathological changes in Hodgkin's disease with especial reference to its relation to tuberculosis.", *Johns Hopkins Hosp Rep,* Vol. 10, 133-136

Rezaei, N., Hedayat, M., Aghamohammadi, A. & Nichols, K. E. (2011), "Primary immunodeficiency diseases associated with increased susceptibility to viral infections and malignancies", *J Allergy Clin Immunol,* Vol. 127 No. 6, 1329-1341 e1322; quiz 1342-1323 1097-6825 (Electronic) 0091-6749 (Linking).

Rezaei, N., Mahmoudi, E., Aghamohammadi, A., Das, R. & Nichols, K. E. (2011), "X-linked lymphoproliferative syndrome: a genetic condition typified by the triad of infection, immunodeficiency and lymphoma", *Br J Haematol,* Vol. 152 No. 1, 13-30 1365-2141 (Electronic) 0007-1048 (Linking).

Rosenberg, M., Mao, Q., Holzenburg, A., Ford, R., Deeley, R. & Cole, S. (2001), "The structure of the multidrug resistance protein 1 (MRP1/ABCC1). crystallization and single-particle analysis.", *J Biol Chem,* Vol. 276 No. 19, 16076-16082 0021-9258.

Saini, K. S., Azim, H. A., Cocorocchio, E., Vanazzi, A., Saini, M. L., Raviele, P. R., Pruneri, G. & Peccatori, F. A. (2011), "Rituximab in Hodgkin lymphoma: is the target always a hit?", *Cancer Treat Rev,* Vol. 37 No. 5, 385-390 1532-1967.

Sanchez-Aguilera, A., Montalban, C., de la Cueva, P., Sanchez-Verde, L., Morente, M. M., Garcia-Cosio, M., Garcia-Larana, J., Bellas, C., Provencio, M., Romagosa, V., de Sevilla, A. F., Menarguez, J., Sabin, P., Mestre, M. J., Mendez, M., Fresno, M. F., Nicolas, C., Piris, M. A. & Garcia, J. F. (2006), "Tumor microenvironment and mitotic checkpoint are key factors in the outcome of classic Hodgkin lymphoma", *Blood,* Vol. 108 No. 2, 662-668 0006-4971 (Print) 0006-4971 (Linking).

Schenka, A. A., Muller, S., Fournie, J. J., Capila, F., Vassallo, J., Delsol, G., Valitutti, S. & Brousset, P. (2005), "CD4+ T cells downregulate Bcl-2 in germinal centers", *J Clin Immunol,* Vol. 25 No. 3, 224-229 0271-9142 (Print) 0271-9142 (Linking).

Schmitz, R., Stanelle, J., Hansmann, M. L. & Kuppers, R. (2009), "Pathogenesis of classical and lymphocyte-predominant Hodgkin lymphoma", *Annu Rev Pathol,* Vol. 4, 151-174 1553-4014 (Electronic).

Schwering, I., Brauninger, A., Klein, U., Jungnickel, B., Tinguely, M., Diehl, V., Hansmann, M. L., Dalla-Favera, R., Rajewsky, K. & Kuppers, R. (2003), "Loss of the B-lineage-specific gene expression program in Hodgkin and Reed-Sternberg cells of Hodgkin lymphoma", *Blood,* Vol. 101 No. 4, 1505-1512 0006-4971 (Print) 0006-4971 (Linking).

Sears, D. A. (1988), "History of the treatment of chronic myelocytic leukemia", *Am J Med Sci,* Vol. 296 No. 2, 85-86 0002-9629 (Print) 0002-9629 (Linking).

Seemayer, T. A., Gross, T. G., Egeler, R. M., Pirruccello, S. J., Davis, J. R., Kelly, C. M., Okano, M., Lanyi, A. & Sumegi, J. (1995), "X-linked lymphoproliferative disease: twenty-five years after the discovery", *Pediatr Res,* Vol. 38 No. 4, 471-478 0031-3998 (Print) 0031-3998 (Linking).

Seif, G. S. & Spriggs, A. I. (1967), "Chromosome changes in Hodgkin's disease", *J Natl Cancer Inst,* Vol. 39 No. 3, 557-570 0027-8874 (Print) 0027-8874 (Linking).

Seitz, V., Hummel, M., Marafioti, T., Anagnostopoulos, I., Assaf, C. & Stein, H. (2000), "Detection of clonal T-cell receptor gamma-chain gene rearrangements in Reed-Sternberg cells of classic Hodgkin disease.", *Blood,* Vol. 95 No. 10, 3020-3024 0006-4971.

Shafer, J. A., Cruz, C. R., Leen, A. M., Ku, S., Lu, A., Rousseau, A., Heslop, H. E., Rooney, C. M., Bollard, C. M. & Foster, A. E. (2010), "Antigen-specific cytotoxic T lymphocytes can target chemoresistant side-population tumor cells in Hodgkin lymphoma", *Leuk Lymphoma,* Vol. 51 No. 5, 870-880 1029-2403 (Electronic) 1026-8022 (Linking).

Siepmann, K., Skok, J., van Essen, D., Harnett, M. & Gray, D. (2001), "Rewiring of CD40 is necessary for delivery of rescue signals to B cells in germinal centres and subsequent entry into the memory pool", *Immunology,* Vol. 102 No. 3, 263-272 0019-2805 (Print) 0019-2805 (Linking).

Smetana, H. F. & Cohen, B. M. (1956), "Mortality in relation to histologic type in Hodgkin's disease", *Blood,* Vol. 11 No. 3, 211-224 0006-4971 (Print) 0006-4971 (Linking).

Spender, L. C., O'Brien, D. I., Simpson, D., Dutt, D., Gregory, C. D., Allday, M. J., Clark, L. J. & Inman, G. J. (2009), "TGF-beta induces apoptosis in human B cells by transcriptional regulation of BIK and BCL-XL", *Cell Death Differ,* Vol. 16 No. 4, 593-602 1476-5403 (Electronic) 1350-9047 (Linking).

Staege, M. S., Banning-Eichenseer, U., Weissflog, G., Volkmer, I., Burdach, S., Richter, G., Mauz-Korholz, C., Foll, J. & Korholz, D. (2008), "Gene expression profiles of Hodgkin's lymphoma cell lines with different sensitivity to cytotoxic drugs", *Exp Hematol,* Vol. 36 No. 7, 886-896 0301-472X (Print) 0301-472X (Linking).

Steidl, C., Lee, T., Shah, S. P., Farinha, P., Han, G., Nayar, T., Delaney, A., Jones, S. J., Iqbal, J., Weisenburger, D. D., Bast, M. A., Rosenwald, A., Muller-Hermelink, H. K., Rimsza, L. M., Campo, E., Delabie, J., Braziel, R. M., Cook, J. R., Tubbs, R. R., Jaffe, E. S., Lenz, G., Connors, J. M., Staudt, L. M., Chan, W. C. & Gascoyne, R. D. (2010), "Tumor-associated macrophages and survival in classic Hodgkin's lymphoma", *N Engl J Med,* Vol. 362 No. 10, 875-885 1533-4406 (Electronic) 0028-4793 (Linking).

Steidl, C., Shah, S. P., Woolcock, B. W., Rui, L., Kawahara, M., Farinha, P., Johnson, N. A., Zhao, Y., Telenius, A., Neriah, S. B., McPherson, A., Meissner, B., Okoye, U. C., Diepstra, A., van den Berg, A., Sun, M., Leung, G., Jones, S. J., Connors, J. M., Huntsman, D. G., Savage, K. J., Rimsza, L. M., Horsman, D. E., Staudt, L. M., Steidl, U., Marra, M. A. & Gascoyne, R. D. (2011), "MHC class II transactivator CIITA is a recurrent gene fusion partner in lymphoid cancers.", *Nature,* Vol. 471 No. 7338, 377-381 1476-4687.

Steidl, C., Telenius, A., Shah, S. P., Farinha, P., Barclay, L., Boyle, M., Connors, J. M., Horsman, D. E. & Gascoyne, R. D. (2010), "Genome-wide copy number analysis of Hodgkin Reed-Sternberg cells identifies recurrent imbalances with correlations to treatment outcome", *Blood* 1528-0020 (Electronic) 0006-4971 (Linking).

Stein, H., Marafioti, T., Foss, H. D., Laumen, H., Hummel, M., Anagnostopoulos, I., Wirth, T., Demel, G. & Falini, B. (2001), "Down-regulation of BOB.1/OBF.1 and Oct2 in classical Hodgkin disease but not in lymphocyte predominant Hodgkin disease correlates with immunoglobulin transcription.", *Blood,* Vol. 97 No. 2, 496-501 0006-4971.

Stepensky, P., Weintraub, M., Yanir, A., Revel-Vilk, S., Krux, F., Huck, K., Linka, R. M., Shaag, A., Elpeleg, O., Borkhardt, A. & Resnick, I. B. (2011), "IL-2-inducible T-cell kinase deficiency: clinical presentation and therapeutic approach", *Haematologica,* Vol. 96 No. 3, 472-476 1592-8721 (Electronic) 0390-6078 (Linking).

Sternberg, C. (1898), "Ueber eine Eigenartige unter dem Bilde der Pseudoleukaemie verlaufende Tuberculosis des lymphatischen Apparates.", *Ztschr Heilk,* Vol. 19, 21-30

Swerdlow, S. H., Campo, E., Harris, N. L., Jaffe, E. S., Pileri, S. A., Stein, H., Thiele, J. & Vardiman, J. W. (Eds) (2008), *WHO Classification of Tumours of Haematopoietic and Lymphoid Tissues.*, IARC Press, 9283224310, Lyon, France.

Tarlinton, D. M. & Smith, K. G. (2000), "Dissecting affinity maturation: a model explaining selection of antibody-forming cells and memory B cells in the germinal centre", *Immunol Today,* Vol. 21 No. 9, 436-441 0167-5699 (Print) 0167-5699 (Linking).

Tedoldi, S., Mottok, A., Ying, J., Paterson, J. C., Cui, Y., Facchetti, F., van Krieken, J. H., Ponzoni, M., Ozkal, S., Masir, N., Natkunam, Y., Pileri, S., Hansmann, M. L., Mason, D., Tao, Q. & Marafioti, T. (2007), "Selective loss of B-cell phenotype in lymphocyte predominant Hodgkin lymphoma", *J Pathol,* Vol. 213 No. 4, 429-440 0022-3417 (Print) 0022-3417 (Linking).

Tesch, H., Feller, A. C., Jücker, M., Klein, S., Merz, H. & Diehl, V. (1992), "Activation of cytokines in Hodgkin's disease.", *Ann Oncol,* Vol. 3 Suppl 4, 13-16 0923-7534.

Thomas, R., Kallenborn, A., Wickenhauser, C., Schultze, J., Draube, A., Vockerodt, M., Re, D., Diehl, V. & Wolf, J. (2002), "Constitutive expression of c-FLIP in Hodgkin and Reed-Sternberg cells.", *Am J Pathol,* Vol. 160 No. 4, 1521-1528 0002-9440.

Uherova, P., Olson, S., Thompson, M. A., Juskevicius, R. & Hamilton, K. S. (2004), "Expression of c-FLIP in classic and nodular lymphocyte-predominant Hodgkin lymphoma.", *Appl Immunohistochem Mol Morphol,* Vol. 12 No. 2, 105-110 1541-2016.

Uluç, K., Kujoth, G. C. & Başkaya, M. K. (2009), "Operating microscopes: past, present, and future.", *Neurosurg Focus,* Vol. 27 No. 3, E4 1092-0684.

Ushmorov, A., Leithauser, F., Sakk, O., Weinhausel, A., Popov, S. W., Moller, P. & Wirth, T. (2006), "Epigenetic processes play a major role in B-cell-specific gene silencing in classical Hodgkin lymphoma", *Blood,* Vol. 107 No. 6, 2493-2500 0006-4971 (Print) 0006-4971 (Linking).

Vener, C., Guffanti, A., Pomati, M., Colombi, M., Alietti, A., La Targia, M. L., Bamonti-Catena, F. & Baldini, L. (2000), "Soluble cytokine levels correlate with the activity and clinical stage of Hodgkin's disease at diagnosis.", *Leuk Lymphoma,* Vol. 37 No. 3-4, 333-339 1042-8194.

Vikstrom, I. & Tarlinton, D. M. (2011), "B cell memory and the role of apoptosis in its formation.", *Mol Immunol,* Vol. 48 No. 11, 1301-1306 1872-9142.

Vinuesa, C. G., Linterman, M. A., Goodnow, C. C. & Randall, K. L. (2010), "T cells and follicular dendritic cells in germinal center B-cell formation and selection.", *Immunol Rev,* Vol. 237 No. 1, 72-89 1600-065X.

Wallhauser, A. & Whitehead, J. M. (1928), "IMMUNOLOGICAL METHOD IN HODGKIN'S DISEASE: A PRELIMINARY REPORT", *Amcrican Journd ol' Surgery.,* Vol. v No. September, 229-233

Waxman, S. & Anderson, K. C. (2001), "History of the development of arsenic derivatives in cancer therapy", *Oncologist,* Vol. 6 Suppl 2, 3-10 1083-7159 (Print) 1083-7159 (Linking).

Wilks, S. (1856), "Cases of lardaceous disease and some allied affections. With remarks. ", *Guy's Hosp. Rep.*, Vol. 2, 103-132

Wilks, S. (1859), "Diseases, etc., of the ductless glands. I. The spleen.", *Trans. Pathol. Soc.London* Vol. 10, 259-263

Wilks, S. (1865), "Cases of enlargement of the lymphatic glands and spleen, (or, Hodgkin's disease), with remarks. ", *Guy's Hosp. Rep.*, Vol. 11, 56-67

Yamamoto, R., Nishikori, M., Kitawaki, T., Sakai, T., Hishizawa, M., Tashima, M., Kondo, T., Ohmori, K., Kurata, M., Hayashi, T. & Uchiyama, T. (2008), "PD-1-PD-1 ligand interaction contributes to immunosuppressive microenvironment of Hodgkin lymphoma", *Blood,* Vol. 111 No. 6, 3220-3224 0006-4971 (Print) 0006-4971 (Linking).

Younes, A. (2009), "Novel treatment strategies for patients with relapsed classical Hodgkin lymphoma.", *Hematology Am Soc Hematol Educ Program,* 507-519 1520-4383.

Younes, A., Romaguera, J., Hagemeister, F., McLaughlin, P., Rodriguez, M. A., Fiumara, P., Goy, A., Jeha, S., Manning, J. T., Jr., Jones, D., Abruzzo, L. V. & Medeiros, L. J. (2003), "A pilot study of rituximab in patients with recurrent, classic Hodgkin disease", *Cancer,* Vol. 98 No. 2, 310-314 0008-543X (Print) 0008-543X (Linking).

Yu, D., Rao, S., Tsai, L. M., Lee, S. K., He, Y., Sutcliffe, E. L., Srivastava, M., Linterman, M., Zheng, L., Simpson, N., Ellyard, J. I., Parish, I. A., Ma, C. S., Li, Q. J., Parish, C. R., Mackay, C. R. & Vinuesa, C. G. (2009), "The transcriptional repressor Bcl-6 directs T follicular helper cell lineage commitment.", *Immunity,* Vol. 31 No. 3, 457-468 1097-4180.

Zhang, Q. P., Xie, L. K., Zhang, L. J. & Tan, J. Q. (2005), "Apoptosis in human germinal centre B cells by means of CC chemokine receptor 3 expression induced by interleukin-2 and interleukin-4", *Chin Med J (Engl),* Vol. 118 No. 8, 665-670 0366-6999 (Print) 0366-6999 (Linking).

Zhou, M., Fadlelmola, F. M., Cohn, J. B., Skinnider, B., Gascoyne, R. D. & Banerjee, D. (2008). "Constitutive overexpression of a novel 21 kDa protein by Hodgkin lymphoma and aggressive non-Hodgkin lymphomas.", *Mol Cancer,* Vol. 7, 12 1476-4598.

Part 2

Advances in Classical Hodgkin's Lymphoma Biology: New Prognostic Factors and Outcome Prediction Using Gene Expression Signatures

2

Advances in Classical Hodgkin Lymphoma Biology: New Prognostic Factors and Outcome Prediction Using Gene Expression Signatures

Beatriz Sánchez-Espiridión, Juan F. García and Margarita Sánchez-Beato
Spanish National Cancer Research Centre (CNIO) & M.D. Anderson Cancer Center Madrid, Spain

1. Introduction

Transcriptional analysis of cancer is a powerful and increasingly useful tool in biomedical research. Many studies are revealing transcriptional patterns using gene expression profiling (GEP) analyses, increasing our knowledge of cancer pathogenesis, identifying signatures related to prognosis and revealing the variation in responses to therapy.

Gene-expression signatures have been identified for the most common types of non-Hodgkin lymphomas. These studies have demonstrated the ability of these technologies to identify pathogenic mechanisms, new molecular targets and biological processes involved in lymphomagenesis (Margalit, Somech et al. 2005). Thus, in the last decade molecular subtypes of diffuse large B-cell, namely germinal center B-cell and activated B-cell-like types, have been identified, each of which has their particular prognostic and therapeutic implications. Likewise, GEP studies have identified relevant molecular characteristics in follicular lymphomas (Alizadeh, Eisen et al. 2000; Alizadeh, Ross et al. 2001), primary mediastinal large B-cell lymphomas (Rosenwald, Wright et al. 2003), Burkitt lymphomas (Dave, Fu et al. 2006; Hummel, Bentink et al. 2006) or mantle cell lymphomas (Rosenwald, Wright et al. 2003). Specific therapeutic targets are likely to emerge from these insights into the molecular pathogenesis of the different lymphomas.

Regarding Hodgkin lymphoma (HL), GEP has provided vital clues and new insights into its pathogenesis (Devilard, Bertucci et al. 2002). More recently, GEP has also identified specific gene patterns related to tumor aggressivity and/or sensitivity to therapy (Sanchez-Aguilera, Montalban et al. 2006; Chetaille, Bertucci et al. 2009; Steidl, Lee et al. 2010).

DNA microarray assays require well-preserved RNA, which is usually extracted from frozen tissue, so this technology is not adequate for clinical applications. However, new strategies for translating this information into clinical practice are currently being investigated, through the identification of smaller gene signatures and validation of them for clinical practice using simple, robust, and conventional assays such as quantitative real time PCR (qRT-PCR) (Sanchez-Espiridion, Sanchez-Aguilera et al. 2009; Sanchez-Espiridion, Montalban et al. 2010).

In this chapter we review recent advances in the understanding of HL biology, new data and improvements in the clinical management of patients in the future, from the application of high-throughput molecular analyses, including gene and microRNA (miRNA) expression, immunohistochemistry and others.

2. Hodgkin lymphoma biology

HL is currently classified as two distinct disease entities, nodular lymphocyte-predominant HL (NLPHL) and classical HL (cHL), which differ in their clinical presentation, age distribution and prognosis. From a biological point of view, NLPHL has been defined as a different disease entity, characterized by a distinct gene-expression signature similar to indolent B-cell non-Hodgkin lymphoma (NHL)(Brune, Tiacci et al. 2008).

cHL represents a distinctive model of histological complexity, with a minor population of the characteristic Hodgkin and Reed-Sternberg (HRS) tumor cells diluted in a reactive inflammatory background composed of non-neoplastic B- and T-cells, macrophages, eosinophils, neutrophils and plasma cells. This microenvironment is very probably essential for HRS cell survival, as indicated by the difficulty of growing HRS cells in culture or in immunodeficient mice (for a review see (Herreros, Sanchez-Aguilera et al. 2008)).

Also, HRS cells are latently infected by Epstein-Barr virus (EBV) in 40-60% of patients, contributing to cHL pathogenesis (Khan 2006; Kapatai and Murray 2007).

The complex relationship between the HRS cells and their microenvironment is only partially understood, although important, if fragmentary, advances are being made. Essentially, this microenvironment represents an ineffective TH2-type immune response, in which a large number of chemokines and cytokines are involved (Skinnider and Mak 2002). HRS cells attract many cells into the lymphoma tissue, resulting in an inflammatory microenvironment that probably promotes the survival of HRS cells and helps them to escape attack from cytotoxic T or NK cells. A better understanding of these essential cellular interactions may inspire novel approaches for a targeted therapy of this malignancy.

2.1 HRS cells

The tumoral HRS cells are unique in the extent to which they have lost the characteristic B-cell–associated gene expression pattern. Deregulation of transcription factor networks plays a key role in this reprogramming process. These HRS cells show strong constitutive activity of the NF-kappaB transcription factors. Multiple mechanisms probably contribute to this deregulated activation, including signaling through particular receptors and genetic lesions, thus identifying NF-kappaB inhibition as an interesting therapeutic approach to this lymphoid malignancy (Kuppers 2009).

2.2 Hodgkin lymphoma microenvironment

There are various lines of evidence suggesting an active role of this "microenvironment" in tumor biology through bidirectional signaling between the HRS and inflammatory cells that promotes proliferation and survival of neoplastic cells (Kuppers 2009). A complex network of cytokines and cell-contact-mediated interactions between tumor and inflammatory cells are thought to be involved and may rescue HRS cells from the proapoptotic state arising from their characteristic BCR deficiency by providing alternative survival signals (Figure 1).

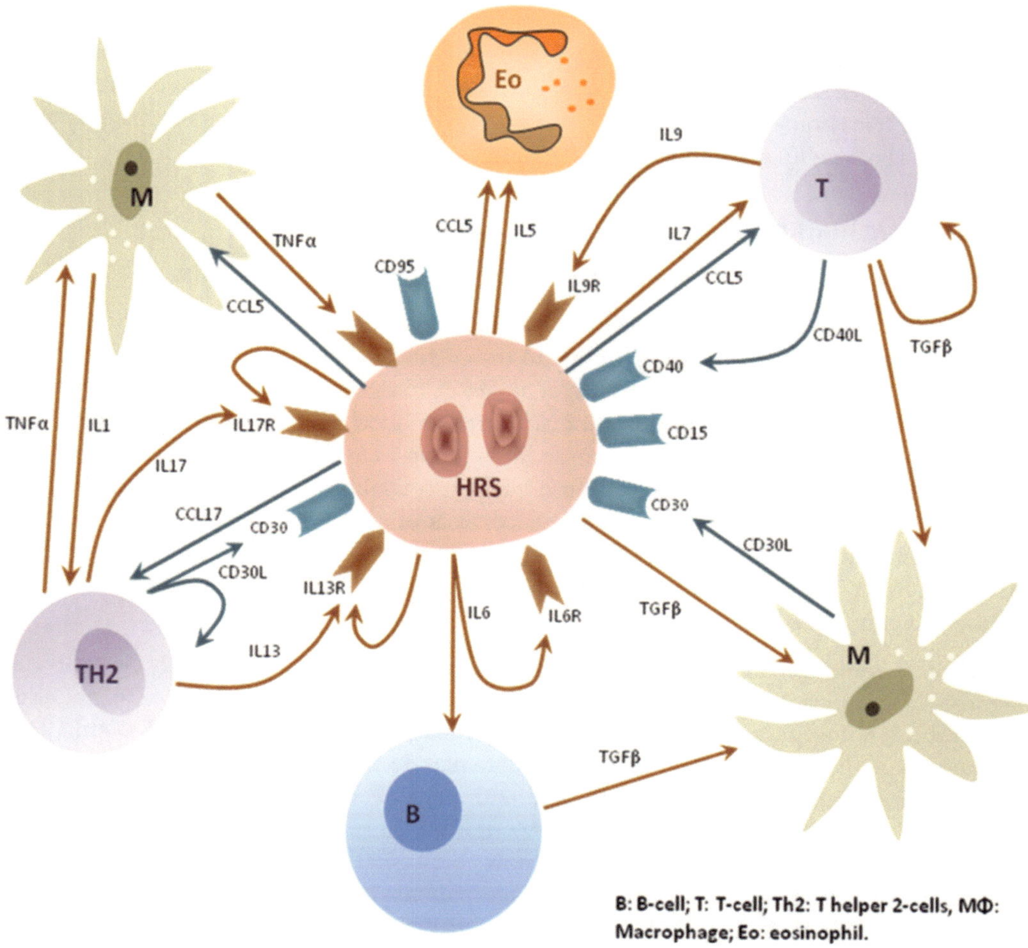

Fig. 1. Chemical crosstalk between HRS cells and the microenvironment. B: B-cell; T: T-cell; Th2: T-helper 2-cells, MΦ: Macrophage; Eo: Eosinophil.

This variable microenvironment gives rise to a prominent and abnormal immune reaction, for which reason the biology of HL can be considered unique among lymphomas. Many studies of HL have, therefore, focused on the cellular composition of this microenvironment, not only to gain more insight into the pathobiology of the disease, but also to explore whether these immune-related cells in some way contribute to outcome prediction.

The tumor microenvironment is an important factor in the development and progression of cancer. Recent evidence suggests that cellular composition can significantly modify clinical outcome in hematological malignancies and particularly in follicular lymphoma and cHL (Dave, Wright et al. 2004; Alvaro, Lejeune et al. 2005). The exact functional role of the microenvironment in the pathophysiology of cHL remains a matter of debate, especially with regard to the role of Th2 and T-reg cells, which have a paradoxically favorable prognostic value (Alvaro-Naranjo, Lejeune et al. 2005; Alvaro, Lejeune et al. 2005; Kelley, Pohlman et al. 2007). A growing number of immunohistochemical (IHC) studies have attempted to evaluate the composition and prognostic significance of the various cellular components, with particular interest in tumor-infiltrating lymphocytes. More recently, GEP studies based on DNA microarrays have demonstrated their ability to define more accurately the interaction pathways of HRS cells with nonmalignant reactive and stromal cells in cHL lymphoma tissues (see below). Therefore, a complete understanding of cHL, requires that both cellular components be considered.

3. Prognostic markers: Limitations and new challenges

3.1 The conventional international prognostic score: Current limitations

cHL is assumed to be a curable tumor, but a substantial proportion of patients with advanced disease do not respond favorably to the current standard chemotherapy regimens based on adriamycin (Canellos, Anderson et al. 1992). Historically, outcome in cHL patients has been predicted using standard clinical variables such as bulk disease, patient age, number of nodal sites and erythrocyte sedimentation rate. The most widely used and reproducible prognostic score is based on clinical and analytical parameters that make up the International Prognostic Score (IPS). This consists of seven clinical variables, including serum albumin less than 4 g/dl, hemoglobin less than 10.5 g/dl, male gender, age 45 or above, stage IV disease, white blood cell count at least 15,000/mm^3, and absolute lymphocyte count less than 600/mm^3.

This clinical measure, although widely accepted, still does not accurately identify, at diagnosis, a significant fraction of patients with very poor prognosis (Gobbi, Zinzani et al. 2001) and it´s not applicable to patients with early-stage HL (Hasenclever and Diehl 1998). Additionally, other study noted that the IPS score had no significant prognostic influence in modern series of patients and that only age and stage IV disease remained significant in multivariate analyses (Sanchez-Espiridion, Montalban et al. 2010). A re-evaluation of the IPS, together with the identification of new biological prognostic factors in larger populations of patients, is necessary to improve patients stratification into clearly defined risk groups for which risk-adapted therapeutic strategies are suitable.

3.2 Risk stratification and new approaches to clinical guidance: Biological prognostic factors and markers in cHL

HL is generally a curable tumor; so, research currently focuses on identifying patients with a low probability of cure who might benefit from more novel and/or intensive treatment strategies, and those with a better prognosis who are suitable for less toxic therapies. To establish a more rational risk-adapted treatment strategy the identification of truly high-risk populations requires supplementation with molecular markers. In this context, biological factors may serve as prognostic markers and provide novel targets for cHL therapy. Moreover, the addition of biological markers to the already recognized clinical prognostic factors (including those of the IPS) may improve patient risk stratification.

This chapter summarizes new insights into cHL biology in a clinical context and the role that new technologies have played in identifying biological markers with future prognostic and therapeutic applications.

Many markers have recently been identified as prognostic factors in HL, including surface receptors, intracellular proteins, cytokines, and genetic abnormalities (amplifications, deletions, epigenetic silencing), or alterations in miRNA in HRS cells and surrounding inflammatory cells. Technical advances such as microarray-based gene and miRNA expression profiling, RT-PCR platforms, comparative genomic hybridization (CGH), SNP arrays, microdissection and IHC studies have led to new discoveries (see below). Their integration with the classical parameters will further improve the understanding of the disease and the management of patients.

Gene expression profiling studies in cHL

It has been difficult to identify biological markers for several reasons, including the scarcity of large and confirmatory prospective trials, the lack of reproducibility and feasibility of assays and the negligible improvement upon already used clinical risk factors (IPS or others). The characteristic histological heterogeneity and scarcity of tumoral cells have also hindered molecular studies in HL. However, several studies have analyzed GEP in whole tissue sections and identified specific transcriptional patterns in the tumoral cells and the non-tumoral microenvironment. Additionally, other studies in HL have demonstrated differential gene expression patterns between HRS cells and normal mature B-cells, providing vital clues for understanding the pathogenesis of the disease (Kuppers, Klein et al. 2003).

DNA microarrays are currently the best developed and most widely used high-throughput molecular technique for identifying biological markers that rely on array-based gene expression analyses using whole-tissue sections. IHC staining has been used as a validation tool, but the technique has inherent limitations, such as the poor reproducibility of the results generated.

Gene expression studies in cHL initially focused on elucidating HRS cell-specific genes and the biological mechanisms underlying cHL pathogenesis (Kuppers, Klein et al. 2003). Subsequently, the relationship between cell microenvironment and HRS cells with clinical outcome was investigated (Devilard, Bertucci et al. 2002; Sanchez-Aguilera, Montalban et al. 2006; Chetaille, Bertucci et al. 2009) (Table 1). These studies reported prognostic signatures related to tumor HRS and microenvironment cells, identifying genes that, although not completely overlapping, did suggest the involvement of the same cellular subpopulations (macrophages, B-cells, T-cells) as those affecting clinical outcome (for a recent review (Bertucci, Chetaille et al. 2011)).

The first study to suggest the existence of correlations between gene expression profiles, mainly microenvironment-related genes, and prognosis was that of Devilard et al. (Devilard, Bertucci et al. 2002). They measured the mRNA expression levels of around 1,000 genes in 34 benign and malignant lymphoid samples including 21 cHL tissue samples and identified three molecular groups of HL. Samples from patients with bad outcomes clustered together, whereas the two other groups contained most of the good outcome cases. These good outcome cases overexpressed genes involved in apoptosis induction and cell signaling (including cytokines), while the bad outcome samples were characterized by upregulation of genes involved in fibroblast activation, angiogenesis, extracellular matrix remodeling, cell proliferation and downregulation of tumor suppressor genes. However, the number of genes and samples analyzed was small, thus preventing any robust conclusions being drawn.

Reference	cHL tumor samples	Microarray platform Nº of genes	Control samples	Gene signature associated with	Validation set	Multivariate analysis
Devilard, Bertucci et al. 2002	21 samples limited and advanced stages	~1000 genes	Cell lines Tissues (adenitis, lymphomas)	Sustained CR	No	No
Sanchez-Aguilera, Montalban et al. 2006	29 samples advanced stages	~9.348 genes	Cell lines	Sustained CR	250 samples IHC TMA	No
Chetaille, Bertucci et al. 2009	63 samples limited and advanced stages	~16.000 genes	Cell lines Tissues (adenitis, lymphomas)	Sustained CR	146 samples IHC TMA	EFS OS
Steidl, Lee et al. 2010	130 samples limited and advanced stages	~25.000 genes	No	Absence of P	166 samples IHC TMA	PFS OS

cHL: classical Hodgkin lymphoma; RS: Reed Sternberg, IHC: immunohistochemistry; TMA: Tissue microarray; EFS; event-free survival; CR: complete remission; P: progression; OS: Overall survival; PFS progression-free survival, DSS: disease-specific survival

Table 1. Gene expression profiling studies in cHL.

A second important study was published by our group (Sanchez-Aguilera, Montalban et al. 2006), which used gene expression analysis to identify specific gene signatures associated with favorable or unfavorable clinical outcomes. We identified a 145-gene signature related to poor treatment response. These genes were grouped into four clusters representing genes expressed either by the tumor cells (regulation of mitosis and cell growth/apoptosis) or the tumor microenvironment. Thus, some genes reflect cell populations that participate in previously reported immune responses (ten Berge, Oudejans et al. 2001; Alvaro, Lejeune et al. 2005), including those expressed by T-cells (CD8B1, CD3D, CD26, SH2D1A), macrophages (ALDH1A1, LYZ, STAT1) and plasmacytoid dendritic cells (ITM2A). Other genes are involved in extracellular matrix adhesion and remodeling of the extracellular matrix (TIMP4, SPON1, LAMB1). Genes involved in fibroblast function and chemotaxis, and molecules expressed either by antigen-presenting cells (CR1, HLA-DR3) or specific populations of B-cells (IRTA2, VDR) were also identified in this research. This study was the first to present evidence of the important role of tumor-associated macrophages within a prognostic context in HL. The other half of the genes identified were mainly expressed by the HRS cells and are involved in apoptosis regulation (CYCS, CASP14, HSPA1L), signal transduction (PDCD10, PRKACB), metabolism and cell growth (COX7A2, MYCN, DCK) and in the regulation of the mitotic checkpoint (MAD2L1, BUB1, STK6, CDC2, CHEK1, TOP2A). Additionally, the link with survival was validated for eight genes (ALDH1A1, STAT1, SH2D1A1, TOP2A, RRM2, PCNA, MAD2L1, CDC2) by IHC in an independent set of 235 samples. Finally, alterations in the regulation of the mitotic checkpoint in HRS cells were also validated.

In another study, Chetaille et al. (Chetaille, Bertucci et al. 2009) analyzed gene expression data from a set of 63 cHL tissue samples with both early and advanced stages, including control tissues (lymphadenitis) and cHL cell lines and cHL samples from patients. Available clinical data allowed the comparison of profiles from 41 cases with favorable outcome and 21 with unfavorable outcome, identifying a set of 450 genes associated with survival. The authors found that expression of genes associated with B-cells and apoptosis was associated with good prognosis, whereas genes involved in stroma remodeling were correlated with poor prognosis. An independent set of 146 samples was analyzed by IHC, enabling the prognostic significance of some of the identified markers including FOXP3, CD20 and TOP2A to be validated. These proved to have a remarkably strong prognostic value for BCL11A in the series. Additionally, a gene signature associated with the EBV status of samples was identified. This seems to be characteristic of the Th1 antiviral immune response, thus providing new clues about the differences between EBV+ and EBV- cases. The influence of EBV infections on HL and the knowledge obtained from GEP is discussed in more detail below.

Finally, a study performed by Steidl et al. (Steidl, Lee et al. 2010) reported the results of a retrospective study using IHC and GEP. Initial analyses of RNA isolated from 130 frozen specimens identified a GEP significantly associated with primary treatment failure that included increased gene signatures related to tumor-infiltrating macrophages, angiogenic cells, adipocytes, HRS cells, with overexpression of matrix metallopeptidases (like MMP1) and underexpression of gene signatures related to germinal center B-cells. A validation study using IHC showed that low percentages of CD68+ macrophages (< 5 percent) correlated with higher progression-free survival (PFS), with a 100 percent disease-specific survival (DSS) rate observed for patients with limited-stage disease (stages IA and IIA) and absence of tumor-infiltrating macrophages.

These data are consistent with a previous observation made by Chetaille et al. (Chetaille, Bertucci et al. 2009), which showed reduced presence of background small B-cells (≤ 10 percent) and overexpression of MMP1 associated with shorter survival. Interestingly, in multivariate analyses, CD68+ macrophages remained an independent adverse prognostic factor for DSS, outperforming the IPS.

RT-PCR models

It is now feasible to apply multigenic predictive molecular tests in a routine setting by using alternative techniques, like quantitative RT-PCR. An assay for patients with advanced cHL has recently been described that incorporates a limited number of genes and pathways from both tumor and microenvironment cell components, designed for routine formalin-fixed paraffin-embedded (FFPE) samples (Sanchez-Espiridion, Montalban et al. 2010). Thirty genes were chosen on the basis of the findings of two previous studies (Sanchez-Aguilera, Montalban et al. 2006; Sanchez-Espiridion, Sanchez-Aguilera et al. 2009) and their deployment in 282 FFPE samples enabled a prognostic model to be developed. The model included 11 genes from four functional pathways (apoptosis, cell cycle regulation, macrophage activation and interferon regulatory factor-IRF4). This 4-cluster/11-gene signature was included in a final algorithm (defined as molecular risk score, MRS) that was able to identify subgroups of patients with different probabilities of treatment failure.

One of the well established clinical variables (stage IV) was also included in the score, thus combining the main molecular characteristics of the treatment response-related tumors and tumor burden estimates into a single scoring system. The multivariate Cox model indicated that most patients with stage IV cHL and with a high MRS (≥ 0.3) will have a very poor outcome, with a 5-year FFS probability of 24.3 percent and overall survival (OS) probability of 76.3 percent (Sanchez-Espiridion, Montalban et al. 2010). This assay represented another interesting, although preliminary, attempt to translate gene profiling results into routine practice, providing a tool for further exploring and refining the already available biological and clinical prognostic markers.

Reference	Technique	HRS cells signatures	Microenvironmental signatures
Sanchez-Aguilera, Montalban et al. 2006	GEP	Cell cycle, apoptosis, signals transduction	Immune response, extracellular matrix, adhesion and cell-cell signaling
Chetaille, Bertucci et al. 2009	GEP	BCR signaling, apoptosis, cell metabolism	Stroma remodeling genes
Sanchez-Espiridion, Sanchez-Aguilera et al. 2009	RT-PCR array	Cell cycle (G2-M and G1 pathway), histones, chaperones and MAP kinase pathway	T-cell pathway, monocyte, macrophage
Sanchez-Espiridion, Montalban et al. 2010	RT-PCR array	Cell cycle, apoptosis	Macrophage activation, IRF4
Steidl, Lee et al. 2010	GEP	HRS cell-related genes	Macrophages, monocytes , metalloproteinases, angiogenic cells

GEP: gene expression profiling; RT-PCR: reverse-transcription polymerase chain reaction

Table 2. Gene expression signatures outcome related in cHL.

Comparative genomic hybridization (CGH) and SNP array studies

Several studies have assessed the association between SNPs and the risks of developing HL. One of these compared 200 HL cases and 220 controls to examine the relationship between genetic polymorphisms in cytokine genes and the susceptibility to developing HL (Monroy, Cortes et al. 2011). It describes a set of four genes (COX2, IL18, ILR4, IL10) out of 38 that are correlated with an increased risk of developing cHL. Once more, this highlights the importance of aberrant cytokine signaling in HL pathogenesis. The authors also showed that genetic variants in DNA repair genes are significantly associated with the risk of developing cHL

Array CGH (aCGH) studies showed genomic imbalances in cHL cases affecting several genes belonging to the main cell-survival pathways known to be activated in HL (JAK/STAT, NF-KB, API-Jun-B). However, the correlation between these genes and clinical outcomes was not calculated. A recent study by Steidl et al. (Steidl, Telenius et al. 2010) reported copy number gains on chromosome 16p as being less frequent in patients with primary refractory disease and strongly associated with prognosis after ABVD chemotherapy. These results could be related to the presence of the multidrug resistant gene ABCC1 located in this chromosomal region (16p13.11). In addition, frequent losses on 4q27 (IL2/IL21 genes) and 17p12, and gains on 19q13.3 (BCL3/RELB) have also been described as being associated with ABVD resistance (Slovak, Bedell et al. 2011).

Immunohistochemical markers and gene expression studies

Some of the markers identified by GEP have been identified as being of potential use, leading to their clinical application by IHC techniques, especially those associated with the complex reactive inflammatory infiltrate.

BCL2. The relationship between BCL2 expression and patient outcome in HL is a controversial issue with studies reporting BCL2 expression to be independently associated with reduced FFS in addition to other clinical prognostic variables (age over 45 years, stage IV disease, low albumin and elevated lactate dehydrogenase) (Rassidakis, Medeiros et al. 2002), whereas others have not demonstrated the same relationship (Montalban, Garcia et al. 2004).

p21 and p53. Similarly to BCL2, other markers like p21 and p53 have been associated with treatment outcomes (Sup, Alemany et al. 2005).

MMP11 is a marker of matrix metallopeptidases expressed by tumor-associated macrophages, found to be associated with treatment failure by GEP and IHC (Steidl, Lee et al. 2010) with good discriminatory power with respect to patient outcome. More than 1% MMP11 staining by IHC predicted reduced PFS survival in both univariate and multivariate analyses.

CD20 encodes a B-lymphocyte cell-surface antigen and has been evaluated by IHC in several studies (Chetaille, Bertucci et al. 2009; Steidl, Lee et al. 2010), which revealed a positive association of an increased number of tumor-infiltrating CD20+ cells with both prolonged PFS and DFS. Similar findings, in which high numbers of CD20+ cells present in the inflammatory background were correlated with improved event-free survival (EFS) and OS were reported by Chetaille (Chetaille, Bertucci et al. 2009). No correlation with the number of CD20+ HRS cells and patient outcome was found in Steidl's study (Steidl, Lee et al. 2010) or another one of 598 patients (Rassidakis, Medeiros et al. 2002). However, a small study performed by Portlock et al. (Portlock, Donnelly et al. 2004) in a set of 248 samples showed that both time to treatment and OS were significantly lower in patients treated with ABVD with CD20+ cells.

Tzankov et al. found that the presence of more than 10 percent of CD20+ HRS cells was associated with worse patient outcomes in patients treated from 1974 to 1980 whereas there was no effect on FFS in patients treated from 1981 to 1999 (Tzankov, Krugmann et al. 2003). Thus, the prognostic relevance of CD20 in HL might depend on other factors, such as the therapeutic modality and the criteria used to define CD20 positivity. As is the case with many other identified markers, these results need further validation in prospective studies to determine their reproducibility.

CD68 is a macrophage marker encoding a transmembrane glycoprotein that is strongly expressed by human monocytes and tissue macrophages. It is a member of the lysosomal/endosomal-associated membrane glycoprotein (LAMP) family. In the aforementioned study (Sinha, Adhikari et al. 2001) the initial finding of a tumor infiltrating macrophage gene signature associated with treatment failure prompted an additional IHC validation of CD68 expression relation with clinical outcome. In univariate analysis, the presence of a large number of infiltrating CD68+ cells was correlated with reduced PFS and DFS. Remarkably, this marker is better than the IPS in predicting DFS in multivariate analysis ($p=0.003$ *vs.* $p=0.030$) and as such is currently a matter under further investigation in many studies that are attempting to validate its predictive value (Kamper, Bendix et al. 2011).

Similar findings correlating the presence of tumor-infiltrating macrophages with adverse patient outcomes have also been described in follicular lymphoma (Dave, Wright et al. 2004; Farinha, Masoudi et al. 2005), suggesting that interactions between the malignant lymphoma cells and the microenvironment are critical to the pathogenesis and progression of these diseases.

Despite these results, the use of CD68 alone as a marker is currently a matter of interest, with several studies having produced contradictory results (Azambuja, Natkunam et al. 2011). Nevertheless, there is no doubt about their prognostic value in cHL.

CD163 is a monocyte/macrophage-specific protein in the scavenger receptor cysteine-rich superfamily that appears to be involved in anti-inflammatory functions believed to be predominantly associated with M2 (macrophages). This marker has been found to be correlated with outcome in several studies in a similar manner to CD68 (Steidl, Lee et al. 2010; Kamper, Bendix et al. 2011). However, it is considered to be more specific and thus more accurate for macrophage identification than CD68.

T-cells. The presence of T-cells in the inflammatory infiltrate also seems to influence patient outcomes and several studies have examined the ratio of regulatory T-cells ($CD4^{+}$, $CD25^{-}$ and FOXP3 expression) and cytotoxic T-cells ($TIA\text{-}1^{+}$ or granzyme B expression) in relationship to OS and DFS rates (Alvaro, Lejeune et al. 2005). The ratio of regulatory $FOXP3^{+}$ T-cells to cytotoxic T/NK (natural killer cells) with granzyme B expression independently predicts patient survival.

Other markers. A variety of other prognostic markers have been described in HL. Increased serum levels of soluble CD30 (Zanotti, Trolese et al. 2002), IL-10, BAFF, TNFα, TARC and VEGF have all been associated with adverse patient outcomes (Casasnovas, Mounier et al. 2007). In several studies, combining the CD30 level with the IPS gave improved predictive values (Ma, Ding et al. 2009; Renna, Mocciaro et al. 2009).

3.3 Influence of EBV

Finally, it is essential to mention studies concerning the role of EBV infection in cHL. Before the use of GEP by DNA arrays, only a few differences had been found between the EBV + and EBV- microenvironments, and these had not been comprehensively characterized.

GEP studies looking for EBV-induced alterations showed that Epstein-Barr nuclear antigen 1 (EBNA1) upregulated the expression of a chemokine (CCL20) in EBV+ cHL cells, ultimately leading to increased chemotaxis of T-regulatory cells (Baumforth, Birgersdotter et al. 2008). Additionally, Chetaille *et al.* (Chetaille, Bertucci et al. 2009) demonstrated that EBV+ and EBV- cHL cases can be clearly separated from each other by a robust gene signature involving innate immunity and antiviral responses in EBV+ cases. Thus, EBV+ cases overexpressed antiviral genes such as NS1BP, PLSCR1 and OAS, together with TLR8 receptor and MDA5 helicase, which are both, involved in the recognition of viruses and mediate innate immunity against viral infection. The molecular profile of EBV+ tumors (overexpression of IFNG, CXCL9, CXL10, and CXCL11/ITAC) also provided evidence of intratumoral Th1 activity in EBV+ cHL cases, which might be orchestrated by IFNG. Nonetheless, EBV+ patients did not have a better outcome, suggesting that the intratumoral immune reaction described is inadequate for eliminating tumor cells.

ITK (IL-2–inducible T-cell kinase) deficiency, a novel primary immunodeficiency disease characterized by severe EBV associated immune dysregulation commonly progresses to cHL with a variable treatment response (Rezaei, Hedayat et al. 2011). Additionally, three cases EBV-positive HL associated to this deficiency were subsequently found to harbor a homozygous nonsense mutation in the ITK gene (Stepensky, Weintraub et al. 2011). Additionally, the study of Steidl et al. (Steidl, Lee et al. 2010) showed that CD68 and CD163 markers were both associated with latent EBV infection of the malignant cells, thus highlighting the potential prognostic implications of EBV infection. Despite these results, the impact of EBV infection on clinical outcome remains unclear; more studies are needed to elucidate its exact role in cHL patients.

4. miRNAs: A new approach to elucidating the biology of Hodgkin's lymphoma

Several studies have demonstrated the role of miRNA deregulation in cancer pathogenesis and treatment response in several tumor models. Others confirm that miRNAs are good biomarkers for cancer diagnosis and prognosis, including hematological malignancies. miRNAs are small, noncoding RNAs that regulate the expression of multiple mRNAs by binding to the 3′ untranslated region (UTR) of their target genes. miRNAs are the best characterized members of a family of noncoding RNAs (ncRNAs) that are now the object of intense investigation. They function by targeting mRNA and inducing its degradation or inhibiting its translation. A number of studies suggest that miRNAs may regulate around 30% of the genome. As a consequence they are implicated in almost every cellular process, and, in fact miRNA expression has been shown to be tissue-specific, playing key roles in the control of the various biological processes such as differentiation, proliferation and others, all of which are involved in cancer pathogenesis. The deregulated expression of miRNA in tumoral samples compared with their normal counterparts, and their frequent genomic location in fragile chromosomal sites, also points to their role in the development of cancer. In fact, specific miRNA signatures have been identified for some tumor types, and they are thought to have tumor suppressor or oncogenic properties (for which reason they are termed "oncomirs"), as well as metastasis regulatory functions. miRNAs are encoded by intronic or intergenic regions. They are first transcribed to pri-miRNA, then processed to pre-miRNA by the Drosha complex, and subsequently exported to the cytoplasm, where the RNase Dicer cleavages them to generate a double strand molecule of 21-25 nucleotides. One of the two chains is then joined to the RNA-induced silencing complex (RISC), which interacts with Argonaute proteins and binds to 3'UTR on target mRNAs, inducing their degradation and/or blocking translation (Esquela-Kerscher and Slack 2006).

Altered miRNA expression has a role in hematopoietic malignancies. One of the first pieces of evidence of the role of miRNAs in cancer came from a study of B-cell chronic lymphocytic leukemia where miR-15 and miR-16 were downregulated due to hemi- or homozygous chromosomal deletion at 13q14 (Calin, Dumitru et al. 2002). As mentioned before, several miRNA loci reside on chromosomal fragile sites, which are frequently altered in cancer. These include the miR-15a/16 cluster, which is also deleted in pituitary adenomas, miR-143 and miR-145, which are located in the 5q33 that is deleted in lung cancer (Calin and Croce 2006), and the miR-17-92 cluster, which is frequently amplified in B-cell lymphomas (Ota, Tagawa et al. 2004; He, Thomson et al. 2005) and lung cancers (Hayashita, Osada et al. 2005). Expression of specific miRNAs is implicated in B-cell and hematological differentiation, and regulates germinal center formation (Kluiver, Kroesen et al. 2006; Thai, Calado et al. 2007; Zhou, Wang et al. 2007). It is possible that miRNA losses and gains have a significant role in MCL by regulating CCND1 mRNA expression (Chen, Bemis et al. 2008). Another study in MCL showed that the most essential pathways and genes in MCL pathogenesis are potentially targeted simultaneously by multiple miRNAs, suggesting that transcriptional regulation by miRNAs in MCL is the result of the concurrent deregulation of multiple miRNAs with related targets (Di Lisio, Gomez-Lopez et al. 2010).

Furthermore, they may constitute markers of differentiation stage, malignant transformation, sensitivity or resistance to specific drugs. Their capacity as prognostic markers has also been demonstrated in lymphomas. Montes-Moreno et al. have developed a model based on miRNA expression, valid for FFPE samples, that uses RT-PCR to predict OS and PFS in chemoimmunotherapy-treated DLBCL patients, improving the prediction just based on clinical variables (Montes-Moreno, Martinez et al. 2011).

Some attempts have been made to elucidate specific miRNA signatures for the characteristic HRS cells and their microenvironment. Preliminary work showed that miRNA losses and gains may explain some of the biological and clinical features of different lymphoma types, and recent analyses of miRNA expression in cHL-derived cell-lines and tumors have also demonstrated deregulated expression of some miRNAs in this malignancy. Overexpression of BIC/miR-155 has been found in cHL cell lines and samples by qRT-PCR analysis (Kluiver, Poppema et al. 2005) but not in other NHL types, except some PMBL and DLBCL samples. miRNA profiling of cHL-derived cell lines performed with qRT-PCR and microarrays has revealed specifically expressed miRNAs that include miR-17-92 cluster members, miR-16, miR-21, miR-24 and miR-155 (Gibcus, Tan et al. 2009) and a significant downregulation of miR-150 in cHL. The authors also demonstrated the targeting of IKBKE by miR-155, among others, in cHL cell lines; thus, miR-155 expression in HL might represent an attempt to reduce NFkappaB activity in this lymphoma. In primary tumors, comparison of miRNA profiles of microdissected HRS cells from cHL patients, four common cell lines (HDLM2, L540, KMH2 and L1236) and CD77+ germinal center B-cells (used as normal counterparts) yielded a distinct cHL signature of 12 overexpressed and three underexpressed miRNAs (Van Vlierberghe, De Weer et al. 2009) including some of the previously described miRNAs, including miR-21 and miR-155. Additionally, a 25-specific miRNA signature differentiating cHL and reactive lymphoid nodes was presented by

Navarro et al. (Navarro, Gaya et al. 2008). When studying cell lines, some of the miRNAs in the samples and cell lines were found to be different, suggesting that this could be due to the microenvironment or to the immortalization process of the cell lines. They also identified some miRNAs (miR-96, miR-128a, miR-128b) whose expression was related to the presence of EBV, although no prognostic implication of the identified specific EBV-related miRNAs was demonstrated.

These results imply that a small subset of miRNAs may define tumor entities better than microarray expression data from thousands of messenger RNAs, and suggest that miRNAs may play an important role in the biology of cHL, and may be useful in the development of therapies targeting miRNAs in tumor cells.

Although cHL-specific miRNA signatures have been proposed, their potential prognostic role remains unclear. There are few observations that link miRNA deregulation and clinical characteristics of the patients. Overexpression of miR-328 has been found in advanced cHL stages (III-IV stages) (Navarro, Gaya et al. 2008), and lower miR-138 levels. However, the potential prognostic role of miRNA signatures in cHL has not yet been sufficiently well investigated in larger series of patients.

Taken together, these findings suggest that miRNAs may play significant roles in HL pathogenesis, and could help to explain its biology, being additionally useful for patient risk stratification and development of new therapeutic approaches. Thus, the relevance of miRNA expression in cHL and its putative value for outcome prediction is worthy of further investigation.

Recently, our group has identified specific profiles from tumor cells and their non-tumoral microenvironment by miRNA expression studies. Initial analyses suggest that clinical outcome can be predicted by models that integrate miRNA signatures. These preliminary findings suggest a possible role for miR-21 and miR-30d as potential targets to overcome treatment resistance in cHL (Sánchez-Espiridión B, Figueroa V et al. 2011).

5. Perspectives

An increasing body of knowledge in cHL pathogenesis, and the complex relationship between the tumoral HRS cells and the microenvironment has been built up from gene and miRNA profiling studies. The correlations that these studies identify, spotlighting tumor-infiltrating macrophages in classic HL, reinforce the critical roles of microenvironmental and immunomodulatory interactions between RS and non-tumor cells, stromal, cytokine, and membrane molecules in disease pathobiology and treatment responsiveness. As we have seen in this chapter, these studies have led to remarkable discoveries such as the relevance of B-cells and macrophages in patient outcome, and to the identification of several new prognostic markers. All these results, including the optimization of new technologies such as RT-PCR in FFPE tissues and miRNA profiling, are clinically promising. However, further validation in large and independent series of patients is needed for them to be included as part of clinical routine. There is no doubt that their integration with results generated by other modern high-throughput molecular analyses (such as proteomics) will further improve our understanding of the disease and the patient management.

6. Acknowledgments

We would like to acknowledge all members of the former CNIO's Lymphoma Group. We also would thank AM Martin for their thoughtful discussion and help with the figure. This work was supported by grant PI10/00621 from FIS, Spain.

7. References

Alizadeh, A. A., M. B. Eisen, et al. (2000). "Distinct types of diffuse large B-cell lymphoma identified by gene expression profiling." *Nature* 403(6769): 503-11.

Alizadeh, A. A., D. T. Ross, et al. (2001). "Towards a novel classification of human malignancies based on gene expression patterns." *J Pathol* 195(1): 41-52.

Alvaro-Naranjo, T., M. Lejeune, et al. (2005). "Tumor-infiltrating cells as a prognostic factor in Hodgkin's lymphoma: a quantitative tissue microarray study in a large retrospective cohort of 267 patients." *Leuk Lymphoma* 46(11): 1581-91.

Alvaro, T., M. Lejeune, et al. (2005). "Outcome in Hodgkin's lymphoma can be predicted from the presence of accompanying cytotoxic and regulatory T cells." *Clin Cancer Res* 11(4): 1467-73.

Azambuja, D., Y. Natkunam, et al. (2011). "Lack of association of tumor-associated macrophages with clinical outcome in patients with classical Hodgkin's lymphoma." *Ann Oncol.*

Baumforth, K. R., A. Birgersdotter, et al. (2008). "Expression of the Epstein-Barr virus-encoded Epstein-Barr virus nuclear antigen 1 in Hodgkin's lymphoma cells mediates Up-regulation of CCL20 and the migration of regulatory T cells." Am J Pathol 173(1): 195-204.

Bertucci, F., B. Chetaille, et al. (2011). "Gene Expression Profiling for In Silico Microdissection of Hodgkin's Lymphoma Microenvironment and Identification of Prognostic Features." *Adv Hematol* 2011: 485310.

Brune, V., E. Tiacci, et al. (2008). "Origin and pathogenesis of nodular lymphocyte-predominant Hodgkin lymphoma as revealed by global gene expression analysis." *J Exp Med* 205(10): 2251-68.

Calin, G. A. and C. M. Croce (2006). "Genomics of chronic lymphocytic leukemia microRNAs as new players with clinical significance." *Semin Oncol* 33(2): 167-73.

Calin, G. A., C. D. Dumitru, et al. (2002). "Frequent deletions and down-regulation of micro-RNA genes miR15 and miR16 at 13q14 in chronic lymphocytic leukemia." *Proc Natl Acad Sci U S A* 99(24): 15524-9.

Canellos, G. P., J. R. Anderson, et al. (1992). "Chemotherapy of advanced Hodgkin's disease with MOPP, ABVD, or MOPP alternating with ABVD." *N Engl J Med* 327(21): 1478-84.

Casasnovas, R. O., N. Mounier, et al. (2007). "Plasma cytokine and soluble receptor signature predicts outcome of patients with classical Hodgkin's lymphoma: a study from the Groupe d'Etude des Lymphomes de l'Adulte." *J Clin Oncol* 25(13): 1732-40.

Chen, R. W., L. T. Bemis, et al. (2008). "Truncation in CCND1 mRNA alters miR-16-1 regulation in mantle cell lymphoma." *Blood* 112(3): 822-9.

Chetaille, B., F. Bertucci, et al. (2009). "Molecular profiling of classical Hodgkin lymphoma tissues uncovers variations in the tumor microenvironment and correlations with EBV infection and outcome." *Blood* 113(12): 2765-3775.

Dave, S. S., K. Fu, et al. (2006). "Molecular diagnosis of Burkitt's lymphoma." *N Engl J Med* 354(23): 2431-42.

Dave, S. S., G. Wright, et al. (2004). "Prediction of survival in follicular lymphoma based on molecular features of tumor-infiltrating immune cells." *N Engl J Med* 351(21): 2159-69.

Devilard, E., F. Bertucci, et al. (2002). "Gene expression profiling defines molecular subtypes of classical Hodgkin's disease." *Oncogene* 21(19): 3095-102.

Di Lisio, L., G. Gomez-Lopez, et al. (2010). "Mantle cell lymphoma: transcriptional regulation by microRNAs." *Leukemia* 24(7): 1335-42.

Esquela-Kerscher, A. and F. J. Slack (2006). "Oncomirs - microRNAs with a role in cancer." *Nat Rev Cancer* 6(4): 259-69.

Farinha, P., H. Masoudi, et al. (2005). "Analysis of multiple biomarkers shows that lymphoma-associated macrophage (LAM) content is an independent predictor of survival in follicular lymphoma (FL)." *Blood* 106(6): 2169-74.

Gibcus, J. H., L. P. Tan, et al. (2009). "Hodgkin lymphoma cell lines are characterized by a specific miRNA expression profile." *Neoplasia* 11(2): 167-76.

Gobbi, P. G., P. L. Zinzani, et al. (2001). "Comparison of prognostic models in patients with advanced Hodgkin disease. Promising results from integration of the best three systems." *Cancer* 91(8): 1467-78.

Hasenclever, D. and V. Diehl (1998). "A prognostic score for advanced Hodgkin's disease. International Prognostic Factors Project on Advanced Hodgkin's Disease." *N Engl J Med* 339(21): 1506-14.

Hayashita, Y., H. Osada, et al. (2005). "A polycistronic microRNA cluster, miR-17-92, is overexpressed in human lung cancers and enhances cell proliferation." *Cancer Res* 65(21): 9628-32.

He, L., J. M. Thomson, et al. (2005). "A microRNA polycistron as a potential human oncogene." *Nature* 435(7043): 828-33.

Herreros, B., A. Sanchez-Aguilera, et al. (2008). "Lymphoma microenvironment: culprit or innocent?" *Leukemia* 22(1): 49-58.

Hummel, M., S. Bentink, et al. (2006). "A biologic definition of Burkitt's lymphoma from transcriptional and genomic profiling." *N Engl J Med* 354(23): 2419-30.

Kamper, P., K. Bendix, et al. (2011). "Tumor-infiltrating macrophages correlate with adverse prognosis and Epstein-Barr virus status in classical Hodgkin's lymphoma." *Haematologica* 96(2): 269-76.

Kapatai, G. and P. Murray (2007). "Contribution of the Epstein Barr virus to the molecular pathogenesis of Hodgkin lymphoma." *J Clin Pathol* 60(12): 1342-9.

Kelley, T. W., B. Pohlman, et al. (2007). "The ratio of FOXP3+ regulatory T cells to granzyme B+ cytotoxic T/NK cells predicts prognosis in classical Hodgkin lymphoma and is independent of bcl-2 and MAL expression." *Am J Clin Pathol* 128(6): 958-65.

Khan, G. (2006). "Epstein-Barr virus, cytokines, and inflammation: a cocktail for the pathogenesis of Hodgkin's lymphoma?" *Exp Hematol* 34(4): 399-406.

Kluiver, J., B. J. Kroesen, et al. (2006). "The role of microRNAs in normal hematopoiesis and hematopoietic malignancies." *Leukemia* 20(11): 1931-6.

Kluiver, J., S. Poppema, et al. (2005). "BIC and miR-155 are highly expressed in Hodgkin, primary mediastinal and diffuse large B cell lymphomas." *J Pathol* 207(2): 243-9.

Kuppers, R. (2009). "The biology of Hodgkin's lymphoma." *Nat Rev Cancer* 9(1): 15-27.

Kuppers, R., U. Klein, et al. (2003). "Identification of Hodgkin and Reed-Sternberg cell-specific genes by gene expression profiling." *J Clin Invest* 111(4): 529-37.

Ma, M. M., J. W. Ding, et al. (2009). "Odd-even width effect on persistent current in zigzag hexagonal graphene rings." *Nanoscale* 1(3): 387-90.

Margalit, O., R. Somech, et al. (2005). "Microarray-based gene expression profiling of hematologic malignancies: basic concepts and clinical applications." *Blood Rev* 19(4): 223-34.

Monroy, C. M., A. C. Cortes, et al. (2011). "Hodgkin disease risk: role of genetic polymorphisms and gene-gene interactions in inflammation pathway genes." *Mol Carcinog* 50(1): 36-46.

Montalban, C., J. F. Garcia, et al. (2004). "Influence of biologic markers on the outcome of Hodgkin's lymphoma: a study by the Spanish Hodgkin's Lymphoma Study Group." *J Clin Oncol* 22(9): 1664-73.

Montes-Moreno, S., N. Martinez, et al. (2011). "miRNA expression in diffuse large B-cell lymphoma treated with chemoimmunotherapy." *Blood* 118(4): 1034-40.

Navarro, A., A. Gaya, et al. (2008). "MicroRNA expression profiling in classic Hodgkin lymphoma." *Blood* 111(5): 2825-32.

Ota, A., H. Tagawa, et al. (2004). "Identification and characterization of a novel gene, C13orf25, as a target for 13q31-q32 amplification in malignant lymphoma." *Cancer Res* 64(9): 3087-95.

Portlock, C. S., G. B. Donnelly, et al. (2004). "Adverse prognostic significance of CD20 positive Reed-Sternberg cells in classical Hodgkin's disease." *Br J Haematol* 125(6): 701-8.

Rassidakis, G. Z., L. J. Medeiros, et al. (2002). "BCL-2 expression in Hodgkin and Reed-Sternberg cells of classical Hodgkin disease predicts a poorer prognosis in patients treated with ABVD or equivalent regimens." *Blood* 100(12): 3935-41.

Rassidakis, G. Z., L. J. Medeiros, et al. (2002). "CD20 expression in Hodgkin and Reed-Sternberg cells of classical Hodgkin's disease: associations with presenting features and clinical outcome." *J Clin Oncol* 20(5): 1278-87.

Renna, S., F. Mocciaro, et al. (2009). "Is splenectomy a treatment option for aseptic abscesses in patients with Crohn's disease?" *Eur J Gastroenterol Hepatol* 21(11): 1314-6.

Rezaei, N., M. Hedayat, et al. (2011). "Primary immunodeficiency diseases associated with increased susceptibility to viral infections and malignancies." *J Allergy Clin Immunol* 127(6): 1329-41 e2; quiz 1342-3.

Rosenwald, A., G. Wright, et al. (2003). "Molecular diagnosis of primary mediastinal B cell lymphoma identifies a clinically favorable subgroup of diffuse large B cell lymphoma related to Hodgkin lymphoma." *J Exp Med* 198(6): 851-62.

Rosenwald, A., G. Wright, et al. (2003). "The proliferation gene expression signature is a quantitative integrator of oncogenic events that predicts survival in mantle cell lymphoma." *Cancer Cell* 3(2): 185-97.

Sanchez-Aguilera, A., C. Montalban, et al. (2006). "Tumor microenvironment and mitotic checkpoint are key factors in the outcome of classic Hodgkin lymphoma." *Blood* 108(2): 662-8.

Sánchez-Espiridión B, Figueroa V, et al. (2011). "MicroRNAS in advanced classical Hodgkin lymphoma:signatures with prognostic significance " *Ann Oncol* 22((Suppl 4)): iv179-iv182.

Sanchez-Espiridion, B., C. Montalban, et al. (2010). "A molecular risk score based on 4 functional pathways for advanced classical Hodgkin lymphoma." *Blood* 116(8): e12-7.

Sanchez-Espiridion, B., A. Sanchez-Aguilera, et al. (2009). "A TaqMan low-density array to predict outcome in advanced Hodgkin's lymphoma using paraffin-embedded samples." *Clin Cancer Res* 15(4): 1367-75.

Sinha, N., N. Adhikari, et al. (2001). "Effect of endosulfan during fetal gonadal differentiation on spermatogenesis in rats." *Environ Toxicol Pharmacol* 10(1-2): 29-32.

Skinnider, B. F. and T. W. Mak (2002). "The role of cytokines in classical Hodgkin lymphoma." *Blood* 99(12): 4283-97.

Slovak, M. L., V. Bedell, et al. (2011). "Molecular karyotypes of Hodgkin and Reed-Sternberg cells at disease onset reveal distinct copy number alterations in chemosensitive versus refractory Hodgkin lymphoma." *Clin Cancer Res* 17(10): 3443-54.

Steidl, C., T. Lee, et al. (2010). "Tumor-associated macrophages and survival in classic Hodgkin's lymphoma." *N Engl J Med* 362(10): 875-85.

Steidl, C., A. Telenius, et al. (2010). "Genome-wide copy number analysis of Hodgkin Reed-Sternberg cells identifies recurrent imbalances with correlations to treatment outcome." *Blood* 116(3): 418-27.

Stepensky, P., M. Weintraub, et al. (2011). "IL-2-inducible T-cell kinase deficiency: clinical presentation and therapeutic approach." *Haematologica* 96(3): 472-6.

Sup, S. J., C. A. Alemany, et al. (2005). "Expression of bcl-2 in classical Hodgkin's lymphoma: an independent predictor of poor outcome." *J Clin Oncol* 23(16): 3773-9.

ten Berge, R. L., J. J. Oudejans, et al. (2001). "Percentage of activated cytotoxic T-lymphocytes in anaplastic large cell lymphoma and Hodgkin's disease: an independent biological prognostic marker." *Leukemia* 15(3): 458-64.

Thai, T. H., D. P. Calado, et al. (2007). "Regulation of the germinal center response by microRNA-155." *Science* 316(5824): 604-8.

Tzankov, A., J. Krugmann, et al. (2003). "Prognostic significance of CD20 expression in classical Hodgkin lymphoma: a clinicopathological study of 119 cases." *Clin Cancer Res* 9(4): 1381-6.

Van Vlierberghe, P., A. De Weer, et al. (2009). "Comparison of miRNA profiles of microdissected Hodgkin/Reed-Sternberg cells and Hodgkin cell lines versus CD77+ B-cells reveals a distinct subset of differentially expressed miRNAs." *Br J Haematol* 147(5): 686-90.

Zanotti, R., A. Trolese, et al. (2002). "Serum levels of soluble CD30 improve International Prognostic Score in predicting the outcome of advanced Hodgkin's lymphoma." *Ann Oncol* 13(12): 1908-14.

Zhou, B., S. Wang, et al. (2007). "miR-150, a microRNA expressed in mature B and T cells, blocks early B cell development when expressed prematurely." *Proc Natl Acad Sci U S A* 104(17): 7080-5.

Part 3

Epidemiology of Hodgkin's Lymphoma

3

Epidemiology of Hodgkin's Lymphoma

Youssef Al-Tonbary
Mansoura University,
Egypt

1. Introduction

Hodgkin's lymphoma (HL), formerly called Hodgkin's disease, is a malignant tumor of the lymphatic system (Schnitzer, 2009). It was first recorded by Thomas Hodgkin in 1832, when he described seven patients suffering from enlargement of lymph nodes and spleen as a new disease entity (Thomas et al, 2002).

Understanding of its pathogenesis remains unclear (Mueller, 1991). The cellular origin of this lymphoma was failed to be clearly identified by molecular biology studies. The characteristic Reed Sternberg cell is thought to be derived from the histiocytes, granulocytes and reticulum cells (Lee et al, 1993). But other studies suggest that these cells represent immature lymphoid cells (Diehl et al, 1990).

Hodgkin's lymphoma was described microscopically for the first time by langhans in 1872 (Langhans, 1872). Jachson and Parker (1947) described the first histological classification of Hodgkin's lymphoma in 1947, later on this classification was revised at Rye in 1966 and in 1994 the Rye classification was incorporated into the revised European-American lymphoma classification (REAL). Accordingly, Hodgkin's lymphoma was classified into nodular lymphocyte predominant, nodular sclerosing, mixed cellularity, lymphocyte depletion and lymphocyte - rich classical disease (Cartwright and Watkins, 2004).

2. Incidence

The incidence of Hodgkin's lymphoma shows marked heterogeneity with respect to age, gender, race, geographic area, social class and histological subtype (Burke, 1992). Hodgkin's lymphoma is listed as a rare disease by the office of rare diseases (ORD) of the National Institutes of Health (NIH). This means that it affects less than 200.000 people in the US population. About 8000 new cases of Hodgkin's lymphoma occur each year in the United States. 1500 people in the US die from Hodgkin's lymphoma each year. It is more common in Caucasians (Lee et al, 1993). Asians have lower incidence than other races (Glaser and Hsu, 2002). The annual incidence of Hodgkin's lymphoma appears stable over the past several decades. Incidence in the United Kingdom is about 2.4 per 1000.000 per year. Worldwide prevalence rates vary, with more than 5.5 per 100.000 in Yemen and Lebanon and less than 1 per 100.000 in china and Japan. At least some of this variation appears to relate to the degree of industrialization (Hoffbrand et al, 2011).

3. Age

The incidence of Hodgkin's lymphoma has increased among adolescents and young adults in the Nordic countries in the past few decades, whereas it has decreased strikingly among those aged 40 years or more (Hjalgrim et al, 2001). In developing countries, Hodgkin's lymphoma appears more during childhood and its incidence decreases with age, while in developed countries, young children are rarely affected by Hodgkin's lymphoma in contrast with young adults where incidence increase with age (Thomas et al, 2002). It has a bimodal age distribution in both sexes, peaking in young adults (aged 15-34 y) and older individuals (>55years) (IARC, 1997). In the United States, Nodular sclerosing subtype predominates in young adults, while Mixed cellularity subtype is more common in children (aged 0-14 y) and older individuals (Grufferman and Delzell, 1984; IARC, 1997 & Muller and Grufferman, 1999). From 2004-2008, the median age at diagnosis for Hodgkin's lymphoma was 38 years of age and approximately 12.3% were diagnosed under age 20 years and 27.7% above 55 years of age.

There are two peaks in the age-specific incidence of Hodgkin's lymphoma. For males there is one in men aged 30-34 and another in older men aged 75-79 years. For women the two peaks occur in women aged 20-24 and 70-79 (Yung and Linch, 2003).

Hodgkin's lymphoma is the third most common cancer in people aged 15-29 years, and the sixth most commonly diagnosed cancer in children under 14 years (Yung and Linch, 2003 & Hoffbrand et al, 2011).

The bimodal incidence curve has been postulated to represent two etiology processes. The first hypothesis suggests an infectious cause of the disease in young adults and other environmental causes for older age groups (Cole et al, 1968).

Low childhood rates and high young adulthood rates were found in the USA and West Europe. The Baltic States and central and Eastern European countries had higher childhood rates than those seen in the United States and Europe, but had similar rates in young adults. The pattern in Latin America and other developed countries is more, whilst the rates in Asia remain low (Cartwright and Watkins, 2004).

A significant increase in the incidence of Hodgkin's lymphoma in adolescents and young adults was observed in Nordic countries (Langhans, 1872), India (Reed, 1902) and North America in the period between 1960 and 1997 (Cartwright and Watkins, 2004). Also, decrease rates has been reported in older adults.

Hodgkin's lymphoma is most common in children and young adults, between the ages of 15 and 40.

The mortality rates are low (0.4 per 100000 per year in the United Kingdom) due to the excellent response to treatment. Mortality increases with age and in Countries with less access to treatment (Hoffbrand et al, 2011).

4. Male : Female ratio

Overall male to female ratio is 1.4:1 (Hoffbrand et al, 2011). It is the third most commonly diagnosed cancer in people aged 15-29 years. There is a slight overall male predominance in the incidence of Hodgkin's lymphoma, which is most marked in the childhood form (Spitz et al, 1989). In adolescents, the incidence between males and females are roughly equal. Data from Norway showed that a sex ratio of 1:1 is seen in the 15-34 age group which increase to 2:1 in the 50 and over group (MacMahon, 1966). Hodgkin's lymphoma is nearly twice as common in males. It is higher in males than females and higher in whites than other races (Shenoy et al, 2011). Men are affected by Hodgkin's lymphoma slightly more than women among all subtypes except for the nodular sclerozing subtype (Thomas et al, 2002). The observed male predominance is particularly evident in children, in whom 85% of the cases are in males.

5. Season

May studies have revealed peaks in the early months of the years especially in February and March (Douglas, 1998; Neilly et al, 1995; & Newell et al, 1985).

6. Race

Both Blacks and Asians had lower incidence rates than whites, which may suggest genetic resistance possibly related to HLA type. Hodgkin's lymphoma is relatively rare in Japan (age-adjusted incidence of 0.3 per 100.000 males) and China (age-adjusted incidence of 0.2 per 100.000 males) in comparison to North America and Europe. Within the European Union the highest rates are in Austria and Greece and the lowest rates are in Spain and Slovakia, (Glaser and Hsu, 2002 & Shenoy et al, 2011).

7. Relation to infections

Hodgkin's lymphoma is a complex of related conditions that are part mediated by infectious diseases, immune deficits and genetic susceptibilities. The descriptive epidemiology of Hodgkin's lymphoma suggests an infectious disease process underlying its aetiology in children and young adults (MacMahon, 1966). There is a relationship between Hodgkin's lymphoma and Epstein-Barr virus (EBV) infection (Evans and Gutensohn, 1984; Mueller et al, 1989 & Swerdlow, 2003). The mechanisms underlying this association are unknown and the virus has never been isolated from or identified in most of Hodgkin's lymphoma tissue (Cartwright and Watkins, 2004 & Gruffeman and Delzell, 1984).

Patients with a history of infectious mononucleosis due to Epstein-Barr virus may have an increased risk of Hodgkin's lymphoma (Alexander et al, 2000; Hjalgrim et al, 2000 & Mueller and Grufferman, 1999).

EBV is the main candidate suggested as the infection causing Hodgkin's lymphoma for several years. However EBV genome has been found only within the tumor in about 20-40% of Hodgkin's lymphoma cases with a prior diagnosis of infectious mononucleosis (Landgren and Caporaso 2007). Several studies suggest that EBV may be a transforming agent in Hodgkin's lymphoma. Patients with a history of EBV infection are at a 2-3 fold higher risk for development of Hodgkin's lymphoma (Thomas et al, 2002). Mueller et al. (1989) analyzed EBV titers in pre-disease sera and found an enhanced level of EBV activation prior to onset of Hodgkin's lymphoma.

Many authors using novel molecular techniques found that EBV DNA is present in Hodgkin's lymphoma cases more frequently in developing countries than in developed countries (Glaser et al, 1997 & Zarate et al, 1995). In Western countries, about 50% of classical Hodgkin's lymphoma are EBV-positive (Brousset et al, 1991).

Reed-Sternberg cells in EBV positive patients show an expression pattern of EBV-encoded genes, termed type 2 latency, which resembles that found in endemic nasopharyngeal carcinoma or a subset of T-cell lymphomas (Thomas et al, 2002). Activated NFkB was found to be a characteristic feature of Reed-Sternberg cells (Bargou et al, 1996). This activation results in massive spontaneous apoptosis of Reed-Sternberg cells by downregulation of an antiapoptotic signaling network (Hinz et al, 2001). Many reports have noted geographic and familial clustering of Hodgkin's lymphoma (Smith et al, 1977; Vianna et al, 1971 & Vianna and Polan, 1973). Swedish investigators suggested that early exposure to viral infection may play a role in the pathogenesis of the disease (Chang et al, 2004).

EBV strain subtypes identified within Reed-Sternberg cells vary geographically. EBV type 1 is predominant in the United Kingdom, South America, Australia and Greece, whereas EBV type 2 is predominant in Egypt (Wrinreb et al, 1996). Mixed cellularity Hodgkin's lymphoma is more likely to be EBV-associated than nodular sclerosis subtype.

Many studies have found significant increase in risk of Hodgkin's lymphoma among patients with AIDS in the developed countries (Grulich et al, 1999 & Serraino et al, 2000). In contrast, these increased risk have not been observed in Africa (Chokunonga et al, 1999; Dolcetti et al, 2001 & lazzi et al, 1998). In addition, other studies have demonstrated an increased incidence in HIV-positive intravenous drug users (Andrieu et al, 1993; Roithmann et al, 1990 & Rubio, 1994).

Also, Human Herpes virus 6 (HHV-6), HHV-7, HHV-8 and cytomegalovirus infections were demonstrated in Hodgkin's lymphoma patients (Gompels et al, 1993; Josephs et al, 1988 & Salahuddin et al, 1986).

Patients with HIV infection have a 15- fold increase risk to develop Hodgkin's lymphoma than the general population (Biggar et al, 2006). They usually present at a more advanced age with associated extranodal involvement and B symptoms (Glaser et al, 2003).

8. Socio-economic status

The childhood form of Hodgkin's lymphoma tends to increase with increasing family size and decreasing socio-economic status. The young adult form is associated with a higher socioeconomic status in industrialized countries. The risk decreases significantly with increased sibship size and birth order (Westergard et al, 1997). It has been suggested that the risk of Hodgkin's lymphoma may be correlated to higher social classes in children and young adults (Alexander et al, 1991a & Alexander et al, 1991b). Reports regarding the socio-economic status in older adults are conflicting (DeLong et al, 1984; Glaser et al, 2001 & Gutensohn, 1982).

9. Occupational exposures

It is not possible to conclude that a causal relationship exists between the various occupational exposures and risk of Hodgkin's lymphoma. Although one study reported that the physicians had a risk 80% higher than that of controls (Vianna et al, 1974), yet other studies did not found this increased risk (Grufferman et al, 1976; Matanoski et al, 1975 & Smith et al, 1974). Some studies reported an increased risk of Hodgkin's lymphoma in white men employed in woodworking or wood-related industries (Fonte et al, 1982; Milham and Hesser, 1967; Olsen and Sabroe, 1979 & Petersen and Milham, 1974). Conflicting results were reported regarding the association between Hodgkin's lymphoma and benzene exposure, rubber and chemical industries (La Vecchia et al, 1989; Lagorio et al, 1994; Rushton and Alderson, 1983; Schnatter et al, 1993; Sorahan et al, 1989 & Vianna and Polan, 1979).

Smoking more than 14 cigarettes per day was associated with a 50% increased risk (Adami et al, 1998 & Paffenbarger et al, 1977).

10. Familial incidence and genetic susceptibility

There is 3 to 9 fold increased risk of developing Hodgkin's lymphoma in family members of these patients (Haim et al, 1982 & Mack et al, 1995). Razis et al. (1959) were the first to report a three fold risk in first-degree relatives of patients with Hodgkin's lymphoma.

Swedish Cancer registry reported that Hodgkin's lymphoma was the fourth in a list of cancers with high familial incidence (Lindeiof and Eklund, 2001). Many oncogenes and tumor–suppressor genes have been studied, but no consistent mutation pattern has been identified (Thomas et al, 2002). Translocation [t (2;14) (P13;q32.3)] involving the BcL 11 a gene was reported in classic Hodgkin's lymphoma (Martin-Subero et al, 2002).

Numerical and structural chromosomal alterations are frequent in Hodgkin's lymphoma patients but they lack any consistent pattern (Thomas et al, 2002). However, molecular clonal alterations such as gene amplifications or deletions reflect a distinct pattern of genetic instability.

Aggregation in families and persons with specific human leukocyte antigen (HLA) type indicates genetic susceptibility (Burke, 1992 & Maggioncalda et al, 2011). Several reports recorded aggregation and clustering of Hodgkin's lymphoma patients in the same families and races which may suggest a genetic predisposition or exposure to a certain etiologic agent.

The Antigens were found to be associated with Hodgkin's lymphoma: A1, B5 and B18 which might indicate that a disease susceptibility gene lies in or near the major histocompatibility region. These associations suggest that this disease is a result of genetic environmental interaction (Bodmer, 1973; Chakravarti et al, 1986; Robertson et al, 1987 & Svejgaard et al, 1975). Also, concordance of Hodgkin's lymphoma in first degree relatives and in parent-child pairs has been noted in many studies (Claser and Jarren, 1996) especially if they are of the same sex.

Familial Hodgkin's lymphoma lacked the classic bimodal age distribution and has a peak between 15 and 34 years. It represents about 4.5% of all new cases (Kerzin-Storrar et al, 1983).

Evidence of genetic susceptibility of this disease was supported by the finding that monozygotic twins have a 99-fold increased risk in contrast to dizygotic twins who have no increased risk to it (Mack et al, 1995). We found significant increase in the frequency of HLA DRB1*0403 and *1202 and DQ131*0604, *0201 and *0203 alleles which may confer suscepilibity (Al-Tonbary et al, 2004). Similar results were reported by Klitz et al. (1994) who reported a significant association of HLA class II alleles with Hodgkin's lymphoma and Harty et al. (2002) who reported that the DRB1*1501 allele is related to the development of familial Hodgkin's lymphoma particularly the familial nodular sclerosis type. The association of Hodgkin's lymphoma with different HLA-DRB1 and -DRQ1 alleles may be explained by three possibilities, first one implies that genes determining Hodgkin's lymphoma are located close to the major histocompatibility loci, and are thus transmitted along with whatever HLA haplotypes in the family (Hafez et al, 1985). Second one is the cross-tolerance to a self-component (Woda and Rappaport, 1981). The third possibility is that the immunogenic responsiveness to oncogenic viruses may be linked to genes coding for HLA antigens (Zimadahl et al, 1999). In conclusion, certain environmental factors in addition to HLA genotypes might play a role in the occurrence of Hodgkin's lymphoma indicating a genetic-environmental interaction.

		Age group of Hodgkin's Lymphoma							
Ethnic origin	**Country**	**0-14 years**		**15-34 years**		**35-59 years**		**Above 60 years**	
		M	**F**	**M**	**F**	**M**	**F**	**M**	**F**
European									
	Belarus	1.46	0.64	4.38	4.15	3.24	2.19	5.72	2.64
	Croatia	0.92	0.25	1.49	2.37	2.04	1.24	3.74	1.68
	Czech	0.94	0.52	3.83	4.26	3.40	1.92	5.92	3.79
	Denmark	0.53	0.21	4.00	2.88	3.58	1.40	4.43	2.41
	East Germany	0.56	0.51	3.59	3.58	2.67	1.58	5.24	3.15
	England and Wales	0.51	0.31	3.80	3.24	3.00	1.64	3.64	2.10
	Finland	0.43	0.50	3.11	2.73	2.96	1.73	4.42	2.56
	Netherlands	0.56	0.30	3.54	3.06	2.74	1.43	3.77	2.21
	Scotland	0.52	0.58	3.84	3.19	2.94	1.68	3.99	2.58
	Slovakia	0.89	0.71	2.58	2.95	2.58	1.53	4.29	1.76
North American/ Hispanic/ Australian	Australia-NSW	0.84	0.24	2.81	2.39	2.39	1.12	3.34	2.90
	Canada	0.69	0.47	4.24	4.38	3.35	1.89	3.95	2.71
	LA-Hispanic Whites	0.70	0.60	1.74	1.69	2.68	1.20	5.96	3.89
	LA-non-Hispanic Whites	0.42	0.15	5.17	4.88	4.10	2.34	4.15	2.91
	SEER-Whites	0.70	0.50	5.29	5.39	3.71	2.16	4.57	2.77
Asian	India - Bombay	0.82	0.19	0.76	0.39	1.51	0.94	3.48	1.96
	Hong Kong	042	0.03	0.47	0.39	0.67	0.24	1.77	0.62
	Japan-Osaka	0.09	0.10	0.27	0.35	0.52	0.17	2.25	0.61
	LA-Chinese	0.00	0.00	0.00	0.29	0.70	0.68	2.53	1.63
	LA-Filipino	0.78	0.78	1.25	1.22	2.34	0.62	2.49	1.45
	LA-Japanese	0.00	0.00	0.00	0.00	0.00	0.00	3.16	2.71
	LA-Korean	0.00	0.00	0.00	0.77	0.76	0.00	0.00	0.00
African	LA-Black	0.15	0.46	2.57	2.31	3.30	1.16	2.56	2.68
	SEER-Blacks	0.62	0.39	3.17	3.10	3.56	1.27	3.14	3.13
Israeli	Israel-all Jews	0.73	0.53	4.17	5.57	4.02	1.47	3.02	2.47
	Israel-non-Jews	1.40	0.56	3.02	1.57	3.27	0.20	1.20	6.01
	Israel-Jews born in America/Europe	0.91	0.00	4.16	6.51	4.12	1.55	2.62	3.11
	Israel-Jews born in Africa/Asia	0.00	0.00	0.87	1.38	4.04	1.98	3.81	0.88

Table 1. Age standardized (World) incidence rates /100 000/year for Hodgkin's lymphoma in males and females (IARC, 1997 and Cartwright & Watkins, 2004).

Region	Numbers per year	Incidence ASR	Deaths per year	Mortality ASR	Mortality to incidence ratio
WHO Africa region	5879	0.9	4893	0.8	0.9
WHO East Mediterranean region	7663	1.4	6004	1.2	0.9
Less developed regions	40137	0.7	23698	0.5	0.7
WHO South-East Asia region	11682	0.7	6276	0.4	0.6
WHO Western Pacific region	8476	0.4	3478	0.2	0.5
World	67887	1	30205	0.4	0.4
WHO Europe region	19342	2	5898	0.5	0.3
More developed regions	27750	2	6507	0.4	0.2
WHO Americas region	14802	1.5	3649	0.3	0.2

Table 2. Age-standardized incidence and mortality rates ranked by mortality to incidence ratio (case fatality ratio). Calculations are based on data from GLOBOCAN 2008.

11. Hormonal factors

Hormonal factors might have a role in the aetiology of this disease as evidenced by the male predominance in patients over 30 years and the higher risk in women aged less than 45 years at diagnosis (Cartwright and Watkins, 2004). In addition, prolonged use of human growth hormone was considered as a risk factor for Hodgkin's lymphoma.

12. Conclusion

Hodgkin's lymphoma is a malignant tumor of the lymphatic system. It arises from germinal center or post germinal center B cells. It has a unique cellular composition, containing a minority of neoplastic cell (Reed- Sternberg cells and their variants) in an inflammatory background. By 1902, the characteristic giant cells of Hodgkin's lymphoma were recognized by Sternberg and Reed.

The incidence of Hodgkin's lymphoma shows marked heterogeneity with respect to age, gender, race, geographic area, social class and histological subtype.

- About 3200 deaths were attributed to Hodgkin's lymphoma annually in the United States.
- About 8000 new cases of Hodgkin's lymphoma occur each year in the United States.
- It is nearly twice as common in males.
- It is more common in Caucasians
- There are 3 age periods: 0-14 years, 15-34 years and over 50 years.
- A significant peak in months of February and March were observed
- There is no direct person to person spread of Hodgkin's lymphoma

The descriptive epidemiology of Hodgkin's lymphoma suggests an infectious disease process underlying its aetiology in children and young adults. There is a relationship between Hodgkin's lymphoma and Epstein-Barr virus infection. The mechanisms underlying this association are unknown and the virus has never been isolated from or identified in Hodgkin's lymphoma tissue. Many studies have found significant increase in risk of Hodgkin's lymphoma among patients with AIDS. Also human herpes virus 6 (HHV-6), 7,8 and CMV infections were demonstrated in patients with Hodgkin's lymphoma than in controls. Mixed cellularity subtype is more likely to be EBV-associated than nodular sclerosis subtype.

The higher the socioeconomic status of person, the greater the risk in the young adult disease. It is not possible to conclude that a causal relationship exists between the occupational exposures and risk of Hodgkin's lymphoma. Smoking more than 14 cigarettes per day was associated with a 50% increased risk. Increased incidence in males may suggest hormonal background. Several reports record aggregation of Hodgkin's lymphoma patients within the same family.

Several studies of HLA typing showed that some AGs were associated with Hodgkin's lymphoma. This association might indicate that a disease susceptibility gene lies in or near the major histocompatibility region. These associations suggest that this disease is a result of genetic environmental interaction.

13. References

Adami J, Nyrén O, Bergström R, Ekbom A, Engholm G, et al. (1998). Smoking and the risk of leukemia, lymphoma, and multiple myeloma (Sweden). *Cancer Causes Control*, 9:46-56.

Alexander FE, Jarrett RF, Lawrence D, Armstrong AA, Freeland J, et al. (2000). Risk factors for Hodgkin's disease by Epstein-Barr virus (EBV) status: prior infection by EBV and other agents. *Br J Cancer*, 82:1117-1121.

Alexander FE, McKinney PA, Williams J, Ricketts TJ, Cartwright RA. (1991a). Epidemiological evidence for the 'two-disease hypothesis' in Hodgkin's disease. *Int J Epidemiol*, 20:354-361.

Alexander FE, Ricketts TJ, McKinney PA, Cartwright RA. (1991b). Community lifestyle characteristics and incidence of Hodgkin's disease in young people. *Int. J Cancer*, 48:10-14.

Al-Tonbary Y, Abdel-Razik N, Zaghloul H, Metwaly S, El-Deek B et al. (2004). HLA class II polymorphism in Egyptian children with lymphomas. *Hematology*, 9(2):139-145.

Andrieu JM, Roithmann S, Tourani JM, Levy R, Desablens B. et al. (1993). Hodgkin's disease during HIV1 infection: the French registry experience. French Registry of HIV-associated Tumors. *Ann Oncol*, 4:635-641.

Banerjee D, (2011). Recent advances in the pathobiology of Hodgkin's lymphoma: Potential impact on diagnostic, predictive, and therapeutic strategies. *Advances in Hematology*, Article ID 439456.

Bargou RC, Leng C, Krappmann D, Emmerich F, Mapara MY. et al. (1996). High-level nuclear NF-kB and Oct-2 is a common feature of cultured Hodgkin/Reed-Sternberg cells. *Blood*, 87:4340-4347.

Biggar RJ, Jaffe ES, Goedert JJ, Chaturvedi A, Pfeiffer R et al. (2006). Hodgkin lymphoma and immunodeficiency in persons with HIV/AIDS. *Blood*, 108(12):3786-3791.

Bodmer WF. (1973). Genetic factors in Hodgkin's disease association with a disease-susceptibility locus (DSA) in the HL-A region. *Natl Cancer Inst Monogr*, 36:127-134.

Brousset P, Chittal S, Schlaifer D, Icart J, Payen C, et al. (1991). Detection of Epstein-Barr virus in situ hybridization with biotinylated probes on specially processed modified acetone methyl benzoate xylene (ModAMeX) sections. *Blood*, 77:1781-1786.

Burke J. (1992). Hodgkin's disease: Histopathology and differential diagnosis, in Neoplastic Hematopathology, *D. Knowles, ED, Williams and Wilkins, Baltimore, MD, USA*, 497-533.
Cartwright RA and Watkins G. (2004). Epidemiology of Hodgkin's disease: A Review. *Hematolo Oncol*, 22:11-26.
Chakravarti A, Halloran SL, Bale SJ, Tucker MA. (1986). Etiological heterogeneity in Hodgkin's disease: HL-A linked and unlinked determinates of susceptibility independent of histological concordance. *Genet Epidemiol*, 3:407-415.
Chang ET, Montgomery SM, Richiardi L, Ehlin A, Ekbom A, et al. (2004). Number of siblings and risk of Hodgkin's lymphoma. *Cancer Epidemiol Biomarkers Prev*, 13:1236-1243.
Chokunonga E, Levy LM, Bassett MT, Borok MZ, Mauchaza BG, et al. (1999). AIDS and cancer in Africa: the evolving epidemic in Zimbabwe. *AIDS*, 13:2583-2588.
Claser SI, Jarren RJ. (1996). The epidemiology of Hodgkin's disease: cultivation in vitro. Homotransplantations and characterization as neoplastic macrophages. *Int J Cancer*, 19:511-523.
Cole P, MacMahon B, Aisenberg A. (1968). Mortality from Hodgkin's disease in the United States. Evidence for the multiple etiology hypothesis. *Lancet*, 2:1371-1376.
DeLong ER, Mail MC, Grufferman S. (1984). Climate, socioeconomic status and Hodgkin's disease mortality in the United States. *J Chronic Dis*, 37:209-213.
Diehl V, von Kalle C, Fonatsch C, Tesch H, Jüecker M, et al (1990). The cell of origin in Hodgkin's disease. *Semin Oncol* 17:660-672
Dolcetti R, Boiocchi M, Gloghini A, Carbone A.. (2001). Pathogenetic and histogenetic features of HIV-associated Hodgkin's disease. *EUR J Cancer*, 37:1276-1287.
Douglas S, Cortina–Borja M, Carturight RA. (1998) Seasonal variation in the incidence of Hodgkin's disease. *Br J Haematol*, 103:653-662.
Evans AS, Gutensohn NM. (1984). A population-based case-control study of EBV and other viral antibodies among persons with Hodgkin's disease and their siblings. Int J Cancer 34:149.
Fonte R, Grigis L, Grigis P, Franco G. (1982). Chemicals and Hodgkin's disease. *Lancet*, 3;2(8288):50.
Glaser SL, Hsu JL. (2002). Hodgkin's disease in Asians: incidence patterns and risk factors in population-based data. *Leukemia Research*, 26(3):261-269.
Glaser SL, Clarke CA, Gulley ML, Craig FE, DiGiuseppe JA et al. (2003). Population based patterns of human immunodeficiency virus-related Hodgkin lymphoma in the greater San Francisco bay area,1988-1998. *Cancer*, 89(2):300-309.
Glaser SL, Clarke CA, Stearns CB, Dorfman RF. (2001). Age variation in Hodgkin's risk factors in older women: evidence from a population-based case-control study. *Leuk Lymph*, 42:997-1004.
Glaser SL, Lin RJ, Stewart SL, Ambinder RF, Jarrett RF, et al. (1997). Epstein-Barr virus-associated Hodgkin's disease: epidemiologic characteristics in international data. *Int J Cancer*, 70:375-382.
Globocan (2008). International agency for research on cancer, 2008, http://globocan.iarc.fr/.
Gompels UA, Carrigan DR, Carss Al, Arno J.. (1993). Two groups of human herpes virus 6 identified by sequence analyses of laboratory strains and variants from Hodgkin's lymphoma and bone marrow transplant patients. *J Gen Virol*, 74(4):613-622.
Gruffeman S, Delzell E. (1984). Epidemiology of Hodgkin's disease. *Epidemiol Rev*, 6:76-106.
Grufferman S, Duong T, Cole P. (1976). Occupation and Hodgkin's disease. *J Natl Cancer Inst*, 57(5):1193-1195.

Grulich AE, Wan X, Law MG, Coates M, Kaldor JM. (1999). Risk of cancer in people with AIDS. *AIDS*, 13:839-843.

Gutensohn NM. (1982). Social class and age at diagnosis of Hodgkin's disease: new epidemiologic evidence for the 'two-disease hypothesis'. *Cancer Treat Rep*, 66:689-695.

Hafez M, EL-Tahan H, EL-Morsi Z, EL-Ziny M, AL-Tonbary Y, et al (1985). Genetic Susceptibility in Hodgkin's Lymphoma. Muller, Weber (eds), Familial cancer. 1st Int. Res. Conf., Basel, PP. 175-179.

Haim N, Cohen Y, Robinson E. (1982). Malignant lymphoma in first-degree blood relatives *Cancer*, 49:2197-2200.

Harty LC, Lin AY, Goldstein AM, Jaffe ES, Carrington M,, et al. (2002). HLA-DR, HLA-DQ and TAP genes in familial Hodgkin's disease. Blood, 15;99(2):690-693.

Hinz M, Löser P, Mathas S, Krappmann D, Dörken B,, et al. (2001). Constitutive NF-kappaB maintains high expression of a characteristic gene network, including CD40, CD86, and a set of antiapoptotic genes in Hodgkin/Reed-Sternberg cells.. *Blood*, 97:2798-2807.

Hjalgrim D, Askling J, Pukkala E, Hansen S, Munksgaard L and Frisch M. (2001). Incidence of Hodgkin's disease in Nordic countries. The Lancet, 358, 297-298.

Hjalgrim H, Askling J, Sørensen P, Madsen M, Rosdahl N, et al. (2000). Risk of Hodgkin's disease and other cancers after infectious mononucleosis. *J Nalt Cancer Inst*, 92:1522-1528.

Hodgkin T (1832). On some morbid appearance of the absorbent glands and spleen. *Ned-Chir Trans* 17:68

Hoffbrand AV, Catovsky D, Tuddenham EGD & Green AR. (2011). *Postgraduate Hematology, Wiley-Blackwell*, ISBN 978-4051-9180-7, Oxford.

IARC (1997). Cancer incidence in five continents. Vol. VII. IARC Scientific Publications (no. 143): Lyon.

Josephs SF, Buchbinder A, Streicher HZ, Ablashi DV, Salahuddin SZ, et al. (1988). Detection of human B-lymphotropic virus (human herpes-virus 6) sequences in B cell lymphoma tissues of three patients. *Leukemia*, 2:132-135.

Kerzin-Storrar L, Faed MJ, MacGillivray JB, Smith PG., et al. (1983). Incidence of familial Hodgkin's disease. *Br J Cancer*, 47:707-712.

Klitz W, Aldrich CL, Fildes N, et al. (1994). Localization of predisposing to Hodgkin's disease in the HLA-class II region. Am. J. Hum. Genet, 54(3):497-505.

La Vecchia C, Negri E, D'Avanzo B, Franceschi S. (1989). Occupation and lymphoid neoplasms. *Br J Cancer*, 60:385-388.

Lagorio S, Forastiere F, Iavarone I, Rapiti E, Vanacore N, et al. (1994). Mortality of filling station attendants. *Scand J Work Environ Health*, 20:331-338.

Landgren O, Caporaso, NE. (2007). New aspects in descriptive, etiology, and molecular epidemiology of Hodgkin's Disease. *Hematology/Oncology Clinics of North America*, 21(5):825-840.

Langhans T. (1872). Das malign lymphosarkon (Pseuddukanima). *Virchows Arch [A]* 54:509.

Lazzi S, Ferrari F, Nyongo A, Palummo N, de Milito A, et al. (1998). HIV-associated malignant lymphomas in Kenya (Equatorial Africa). *Hum Pathol*, 29:1285-1289.

Lee GR, Bithell TC, Foerster J, Athens JW & Lukens JN. (1993). *Wintrobes Clinical Hematology*, 9th edition, Lea & Febiger . ISBN 0-8121-1188-5, Philadelphia, London.

Lindelof B, Eklund G. (2001). Analysis of hereditary component of cancer by use of a familial index by site. *Lancet*, 358:1696-1698.

Mack TM, Cozen W, Shibata DK, Weiss LM, Nathwani BN, et al. (1995). Concordance for Hodgkin's disease in identical twins suggesting genetic susceptibility to the young-adult form of the disease. *N Engl J Med,* 332:413-418.

MacMahon B. (1966). Epidemilogy of Hodgkin's Disease. *Cancer Res,* 26:1189-1200.

Maggioncalda A, Malik N, Shenoy P, Smith M, Sinha R, and Flowers CR. (2011). Clinical, molecular, and environmental risk factors for Hodgkin lymphoma. *Advances in Hematology,* 2011, Article ID 736261, 10 pages.

Martín-Subero JI, Gesk S, Harder L, Sonoki T, Tucker PW, et al. (2002). Recurrent involvement of the REL and BCLIIA loci in classical Hodgkin's lymphoma. *Blood,* 99:1474-1477.

Matanoski GM, Sartwell PE, Elliott EA. (1975). Letter: Hodgkin's disease mortality among physicians. *Lancet,* I:926-927.

Milham S Jr, Hesser JE. (1967). Hodgkin's disease in woodworkers. *Lancet,* II:136-137.

Mueller N, Evans A, Harris NL, Comstock GW, Jellum E, et al. (1989). Hodgkin's disease and Epstein-Barr virus: altered antibody pattern before diagnosis. *N Engl J Med,* 320:689-695.

Mueller N, Grufferman S. (1999). Epidemiology. In Hodgkin's Disease, Mauch PM, Armitage J, Diehl V, Hopp R, Eiss LM (eds), Raven Press, Ltd.: New York.

Mueller N. (1991). An epidemiologist's view of the new molecular biology findings in Hodgkin's disease. *Ann Oncol,* 2(2):23-28.

Neilly IJ, Dawson AA, Bennett B Douglas S. (1995). Evidence for a seasonal variation in the presentation of Hodgkin's disease. *leuk lymph.* 18:325-328.

Newell GR, Lunch HK, Gibeau JM, Spitz MR. (1985). Seasonal diagnosis of Hodgkin's disease among young adults. *J Natl Cancer Inst,* 74:35-56.

Olsen J, Sabroe S. (1979). A follow-up study of non-retired and retired members of the Danish Carpenter/Cabinet Makers Trade Union. *Int J Epidemiol,* 8:375-382.

Paffenbarger RS Jr, Wing AL, Hyde RT. (1977). Characteristics in youth indicative of adult-onset Hodgkin's disease. *J Natl Cancer Inst,* 58:1489-1491.

Peter M, Armitage J, Diehl V, Hoppe R, Weiss L. (1999). Hodgkin's Disease. *Lippincott Williams & Wilkins.* 62-64, ISBN 0-781-1502-4.

Petersen GR, Milham S Jr. (1974). Hodgkin's disease mortality and occupational exposure to wood. *J Natl Cancer Inst,* 53:957-958.

Razis DV, Diamond HD, Craver LF. (1959). Familial Hodgkin's disease: its significance and implications. Ann Intern Med, 51:933-971.

Reed DM. (1902). On the pathological changes in Hodgkin's disease, with especial reference to its relation to tuberculosis. *Johns Hopkins Hosp Rev* 10:133.

Robertson SJ, Lowman JT, Grufferman S, Kostyu D, van der Horst CM et al. (1987). Familial Hodgkin's disease and laboratory investigation. *Cancer,* 59:1314-1319.

Roithmann S, Tourani JM, Andrieu JM. (1990). Hodgkin's disease in HIV-infected intravenous drug abusers. *New Engl J Med,* 323:275-276.

Rubio R. (1994). Hodgkin's disease associated with human immunodeficiency virus infection. A clinical study of 46 cases. Cooperative Study Group of Malignancies Associated with HIV Infection of Madrid. *Cancer,* 73:2400-2407.

Rushton L, Alderson MR. (1983). Epidemiological survey of oil distribution centers in Britain. *Br J Ind Med,* 40:330-339.

Salahuddin SZ, Ablashi DV, Markham PD, Josephs SF, Sturzenegger S, et al. (1986). Isolation of a new virus, HBLV, in patients with lympho-proliferative disorders. *Science,* 234:596-601.

Schnatter AR, Katz AM, Nicolich MJ, Thériault G.. (1993). A retrospective mortality study among Canadian petroleum marketing and distribution workers. *Environ Health Perspect*, 101(6):85-99.

Schnitzer B. (2009). Hodgkin lymphoma. *Hematology/Oncology Clinics of North America,* 23(4): 747-768.

Serraino D, Boschini A, Carrieri P, Pradier C, Dorrucci M, et al. (2000). Cancer risk among men with, or at risk of, HIV infection in southern Europe. *AIDS*, 14:553-559.

Shenoy P, Maggioncalda A, Malik N and Flowers CR. (2011). Incidence patterns and outcomes for Hodgkin's lymphoma patients in the United States. *Advances in Hematology*, 2011:725219.

Smith PG, Kinlen LJ, Doll R. (1974). Letter: Hodgkin's disease mortality among physicians. *Lancet*, 31;2(7879):525.

Smith PG, Pike MC, Kinlen LJ, Jones A, Harris R (1977). Contacts between young patients with Hodgkin's disease: A case control study. *Lancet*. 9;2(8028):59-62.

Sorahan T, Parkes HG, Veys CA, Waterhouse JA, Straughan JK,. (1989). Mortality in the British rubber industry 1946-85. *Br J Ind Med*, 46:1-10.

Spitz MR, Sider JG, Johnson CC, Butler JJ, Pollack ES, et al. (1989). Ethnic patterns of Hodgkin's disease incidence among children and adolescents in the United States 1973-82. *J Nath Cancer Inst*, 76:235-239.

Svejgaard A, Platz P, Ryder LP, Nielsen LS, Thomsen M (1975). HL-A and disease associations-a survey. *Transplant*, 22:3-43.

Swerdlow AJ. (2003). Epidemiology of Hodgkin's disease and non-Hodgkin's lymphoma. *Eur J Nucl Med Mol Imaging*, 30(1):3-12.

Thomas RK, Re D, Zander T, Wolf J and Diehl V. (2002). Epidemiology and etiology of Hodgkin's lymphoma. Ann Oncol. 13 (4):147-152.

Vianna JH, Polan AK. (1973). Epidemiological evidence for transmission of Hodgkin's disease. *N Engl J Med*, 289(10):499-502.

Vianna NJ, Greenwald P, Davies JNP. (1971). Extended epidemic of Hodgkin's disease in high school students. *Lancet*, 1(7711):1209-1211.

Vianna NJ, Polan A. (1979). Lymphomas and occupational benzene exposure. *Lancet*, 1:1394-1395.

Vianna NJ, Polan AK, Keogh MD, Greenwald P. (1974). Hodgkin's disease mortality among physicians. Lancet, 20:131-133.

Weinreb M, Day PJ, Niggli F, Powell JE, Raafat F et al. (1996). The role of Epstein-Barr virus in Hodgkin's disease from different geographical areas. *Arch Dis Child*, 74(1):27-31.

Westergaard T, Melbye M, Pedersen JB, Frisch M, Olsen JH et al. (1997). Birth order, sibship size and risk of Hodgkin's disease in children and young adults: a population-based study of 31 million preson-years. *Int J Cancer*, 72:977-981.

Woda BA, and Rappaport H. (1981). Altered expression of histocompatibility antigens on B large cell lymphomas. *Blood*, 57(4):802-804.

Yung L, Linch D. (2003). Hodgkin's lymphoma. Lancet. 15;361(9361): 943-951.

Zarate-Osorno A, Roman LN, Kingma DW, Meneses-Garcia A, Jaffe ES. (1995). Hodgkin's disease in Maxico. Prevalence of Epstein-Barr virus sequences and correlations with histologic subtypes. *Cancer*, 75(6):1360-1366.

Zimadahl A, Schifman M, Scott DR, et al. (1999). HLA-class I/II alleles and development of human papilloma virus- related B neoplasm: results from a case control study conducted in the United States. *Cancer Epidemiol, Biomark. Prev*, 7:1035.

Part 4

Hodgkin's Lymphoma: From Tumor Microenvironment to Immunotherapeutic Approach – Body's Own Power Protection Challenges

4

Hodgkin's Lymphoma: From Tumor Microenvironment to Immunotherapeutic Approach – Body's Own Power Protection Challenges

Marylène Lejeune[1], Luis de la Cruz-Merino[2] and Tomás Álvaro[3]
[1]*Molecular Biology and Research Section, Hospital de Tortosa Verge de la Cinta, IISPV, URV,*
[2]*Clinical Oncology Department, Hospital Universitario Virgen Macarena, Sevilla, Member of the Grupo Oncológico para el Tratamiento de las Enfermedades Linfoides (GOTEL),*
[3]*Pathology Department, Hospital de Tortosa Verge de la Cinta, IISPV, URV, Spain*

1. Introduction

Hodgkin's lymphoma (HL) is a highly curable disease and the reported results in last years relative to patient's survival were continuously improved. Cure rates > 90% for early HL and > 70% for those with advanced HL are expected. Nevertheless, there are high-risk patients (about 35%) refractory to initial treatment or relapse after achieving complete remission. The current approaches to identify these patients employ pathologic, clinical and classical biologic prognostic factors. The relative scarcity of markers that could reliably predict long-term survival generates excessive treatments with both radio- and chemotherapy for many patients. In this condition, the identification of innovative biologic markers that could help to design appropriately tailored treatment strategies for classic HL (cHL) patients at high risk of treatment failure and patients with low-risk disease remains a crucial challenge.

The presence of a characteristic inflammatory microenvironment in response to tumoral cells not only distinguishes HL from other lymphomas, but even more, this is the main characteristic that makes HL a separate entity itself allowing its diagnosis. However, the functional role of the microenvironment in the pathophysiology of HL remains a matter of debate. The ability of the immune system to act as a double-edge weapon, protective or stimulating, indicates that tumoral clearance requires the effective coordination of the different elements of the immune system in an appropriate balance in quantity and quality. Therefore, current cancer research in HL aims to develop methods to increase the effectiveness of host antitumoral immune response, or at least prevent that various cytokines and growth factors from different subpopulation of infiltrating reactive immune response do not contribute to real growth of the tumoral Hodgkin and Reed-Sternberg (H/RS) cells.

Biological therapy (also called immunotherapy, biotherapy or biological response modifier therapy) is one of the most promising strategies. These therapies use the body's immune system, either directly or indirectly, to fight HL or to help lessen the side effects of some cancer treatments for HL. Current biological therapy treatments for HL may be used either alone or in conjunction with other modalities such surgery, radiation and chemotherapy.

This chapter summarizes the data on clinical, histological, pathological and biological factors in HL, with special emphasis on the improvement of prognosis and their impact on therapeutical strategies. The recent advances in our understanding of HL biology and immunology seem indicate that infiltrated immune cells in the tumoral microenvironment may play different, even opposite, functions according to the signals it senses. Strategies aimed at interfering with the crosstalk between H/RS cells and their cellular partners have been taken into account in the development of new immunotherapy's that target different cell components of HL microenvironment. The current standard approaches with the use of combined modality therapy and systemic chemotherapy as well as the promising role of future response-adapted strategies is reviewed.

2. Histopathological diagnostic parameters

As classified by the World Health Organization (WHO), HL exists in 5 types (Swerdlow et al., 2008b). Four of these—nodular sclerosis (NSHL), mixed cellularity (MCHL), lymphocyte depleted (LDHL), and lymphocyte rich (LRHL)—are referred to as cHL. The fifth type, nodular lymphocyte predominant Hodgkin disease (NLPHL), accounts for 4–5% of all HL cases and is a distinct entity with unique clinical features and a different treatment paradigm. Regarding cHL, NSHL represents the most common histological type in European countries, accounting for 40–70% of cases whereas MCHL account for about 30%.

Histologically, cHL is characterized by a minority of neoplastic cells (1-2%) named H/RS cells embedded in a rich background composed of a variety of reactive, mixed inflammatory cells consisting of lymphocytes, plasma cells, neutrophils, eosinophils, and histiocytes (Figure 1A). Thus, the presence of an appropriate cellular background—along with the results of immunophenotyping—is basic for the diagnosis. Evidence has accumulated that H/RS cells harbor clonally rearranged and somatically mutated immunoglobulin genes, indicating their derivation, in most cases, from germinal center (GC) B-cells (Kuppers, 2002; Kuppers et al., 2003; Staudt, 2000; Thomas et al., 2004). Some HL cases have been identified in which the H/RS is of T-cell origin but these are rare, accounting for 1-2% of cHL. Under normal conditions, GC B-cells, that lack a functional high affinity antibody, undergo apoptosis in the germinal center. H/RS cells show a characteristically defective B-cell differentiation program, lose the capacity to express immunoglobulin and, therefore, should die. However, H/RS cells escape apoptosis and instead proliferate, giving rise to the tumor and the immune response that characterizes (Kuppers, 2002; Kuppers et al., 2003; Staudt, 2000; Thomas et al., 2004). Gray zones between cHL and some types of diffuse B-cell lymphoma, especially primary mediastinal large B-cell lymphoma have been appreciated during these last 20 years (Campo et al., 2011). Both share a close biologic relationship and similar profiling at the epigenetic level (Eberle et al., 2011).

Concerning the phenotypic findings, expression of the CD30 molecule by H/RS cells is seen in more than 98% of cHLs although the intensity of the immunostaining can vary from one case to another, and even within the same case. CD30 molecule appears also to be a possible target for specific antibodies conjugated with toxins and administered to patients with cHL

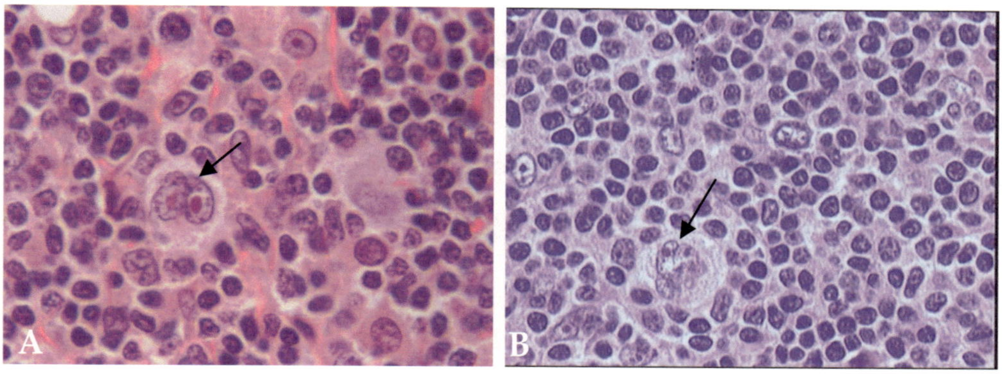

Fig. 1. Reed-Sternberg cell (A: black arrow) seen in a cellular background rich in lymphocytes of a classical Hodgkin lymphoma. Popcorn cell (B: black arrow) with typically lobated nuclei seen in a Nodular lymphocyte predominant Hodgkin lymphoma.

for therapeutic purposes. Preliminary studies have shown that these immunotoxins have remarkable cytotoxic activity (Falini et al., 1992; Foyil & Bartlett, 2010; Tazzari et al., 1992). CD15, characteristic but not specific for H/RS, is detected in about 80% of cHL patients (Ascani et al., 1997; Foyil & Bartlett, 2010; Pileri et al., 1991; Pileri et al., 1995). H/RS cells usually lack CD45 (Falini et al., 1990; Filippa et al., 1996; Korkolopoulou et al., 1994), whereas B and, to lesser extent, T cell markers are seen in a proportion of cases. In particular, CD20 is found in 30%–40% of cHL cases (usually EBV negative) (Filippa et al., 1996), and CD79a is found even less often (Tzankov et al., 2003a; Tzankov et al., 2003c; Watanabe et al., 2000). Positivity (usually weak) for one or more T cell marker is detected in a minority of cases in H/RS cells (Casey et al., 1989; Falini et al., 1987). Under these circumstances, single cell PCR studies have shown T-cell receptor (TCR) gene rearrangement in only three instances, with clonal Ig gene rearrangements occurring in most cHL cases with T-cell marker expression (Marafioti et al., 2000; Muschen et al., 2000). In contrast to that seen in NLPHL, the elements of cHL show variable expression of the BCL6 molecule (Stein et al., 2008b). Antibodies against the nuclear-associated antigens Ki-67 and proliferating cell nuclear antigen (PCNA) stain most H/RS cells, suggesting that a large number of neoplastic cells enter the cell cycle (Gerdes et al., 1987; Sabattini et al., 1993).

NLPHL differs greatly from the common type in terms of morphology, phenotype, genotype, and clinical behavior (Piccaluga et al., 2011). The only feature shared by NLPHL and cHL is the low number of neoplastic cells. The neoplastic population consists of large elements called lymphocytic/histiocytic or popcorn cells (Figure 1B) (Mason et al., 1994). However, these neoplastic cells have a characteristic profile, which differs greatly from that of cHL (Anagnostopoulos et al., 2000; Harris et al., 2000; Harris et al., 1994). In particular, they are $CD45^{+}$, $CD20^{+}$, $CD22^{+}$, $CD79a^{+}$, J $chain^{+/-}$, $EMA^{+/-}$, and $CD15^{-}$. CD30 positivity is rare and, when detected, weak. Popcorn cells regularly express the transcription factor OCT2 and its coactivator BOB.1 (Stein et al., 2001). Although NLPHL is characterized by a more preserved B-cell phenotype compared to the classical variant, a certain degree of defectivity was also described since a downregulation of several markers associated with the B-cell lineage (CD19, CD37, CD79b, and LYN) and with the germinal center maturation stage (CD10, LCK, and PAG) have been observed (Tedoldi et al., 2007). In comparison to cHL, NLPHL has a higher age of onset (30-40 years), a higher incidence in males, a tendency for peripheral distribution, lack of B symptoms in the majority of cases, and mostly early-stage disease (Diehl et al., 1999; Nogova et al., 2008).

3. Clinicobiological prognostic parameters

The high curability rates of HL coupled with increasing awareness of late treatment related morbidity, especially in young population, has highlighted the importance of some clinicobiological risk factors that might guide the therapeutical strategies. Although these factors are probably the clinical translation of some alterations at the molecular level, to date there exist global consensus based upon these clinicobiological characteristics in order to decide the total amount of treatment to administer to every single patient, especially with respect to the type and number of cycles of chemotherapy, and thus to apply more intensive treatments to those cases with higher risk of relapse and, on the contrary, to avoid unnecessary treatment in patients with good prognosis.

3.1 Staging and clinical risk categories

Selection of treatments depends on initial risk stratification. In this sense, stage remains the most important factor in the initial approach for treatment of HL, being the Ann Arbor system with Cotswolds modifications the current staging system used for patients with HL (Table 1) (Diehl et al., 2004).

Stage I – Involvement of a single lymph node region (I) or of a single extralymphatic organ or site (Ie).
Stage II – Involvement of two or more lymph node regions on the same side of the diaphragm alone (II) or with involvement of limited, contiguous extralymphatic organ or tissue (IIe). The number of anatomic regions should be indicated by a subscript
Stage III – Involvement of lymph node regions or lymphoid structures on both sides of the diaphragm (III) which may include the spleen (IIIs) or limited, a contiguous extralymphatic organ or site (IIIe) or both (IIIes). This may be subdivided into stage III-1 or III-2: stage III-1 is used for patients with involvement of the spleen or splenic hilar, celiac or portal nodes; and stage III-2 is used for patients with involvement of the paraaortic, iliac, inguinal, or mesenteric nodes.
Stage IV – Diffuse or disseminated foci of involvement of one or more extralymphatic organs or tissues, with or without associated lymphatic involvement.

Table 1. Ann-Arbor/Costwolds staging system.

In clinical practice, HL is classified in early and advanced disease (Connors, 2005). Early disease includes stages I-II and it is generally divided into favorable and unfavorable categories based upon the presence or absence of certain clinical features, such as age, erythrocyte sedimentation rate (ESR), B symptoms, and large mediastinal adenopathy. Cooperative research groups have used diverse definitions of favorable and unfavorable prognosis disease (Table 2) (Specht & Hasenclever, 1999).

However, probably the most commonly used definition of favorable/unfavorable disease is the one proposed by the European Organization for the Research and Treatment of Cancer

(EORTC). Patients with one of the risk factors mentioned above are considered to have unfavorable prognosis early stage HL. This stratification is highly pertinent and useful since patients with favorable prognosis disease may have acceptable outcomes with less intensive therapy than that required for those with unfavorable prognosis early stage or advanced stage disease (Engert et al., 2010).

EORTC: age 50 or older; large mediastinal adenopathy; with an ESR of more than 50/h and B symptoms (or with an ESR of more than 30 mm/h in those who have B symptoms); and disease with four or more regions of involvement
GHSG: Three or more sites of disease; extranodal extension; mediastinal mass measuring one-third the maximum thoracic diameter or greater; and ESR more than 50 mm/h (more than 30 mm/h if B symptoms present)
NCCN: large mediastinal adenopathy; bulky disease lager than 10 cm; B symptoms; ESR more than 50 mm/h; and disease with four or more regions of involvement
NCI-C: age 40 or older; ESR more than 50 mm/h; and disease with four or more regions of involvement

Table 2. Definitions of unfavorable disease by different cooperative research groups.

Among patients with advanced stage HL (stage III/IV, and for some groups stage II plus bulky nodal disease), prognosis is largely determined by the International Prognostic Score (IPS) (Hasenclever & Diehl, 1998). The IPS was created by the IPS Project on Advanced Hodgkin's Disease based upon the total number of seven potential unfavorable features at diagnosis: serum albumin less than 4 g/dL, hemoglobin less than 10.5 g/dL, male gender, age over 45 years, stage IV disease, white blood cell count ≥15,000/microL, and lymphocyte count less than 600/microL and/or less than 8 percent of the white blood cell count.

In this system, one point is given for each of the above characteristics present in the patient, for a total score ranging from zero to seven, representing increasing degrees of risk. When applied to an initial group of 5141 patients with HL treated with combination chemotherapy ABVD-like with or without radiotherapy, event-free survival rates at five years correlated well with IPS (Table 3) (Hasenclever & Diehl, 1998).

No factors —84% (7 percent of patients)
One factor — 77% (22 percent of patients)
Two factors — 67% (29 percent of patients)
Three factors — 60% (23 percent of patients)
Four factors — 51% (12 percent of patients)
Five or more factors — 42% (7 percent of patients)

Table 3. Event free survival correlated with IPS.

Consequently, different treatment policies are indicated upon the presence of these clinicobiological parameters, with application of more aggressive approaches when more risk factors are present.

3.2 Positron Emission Tomography (PET) and correlation with clinical outcomes

In the last years, F fluoro-2-deoxy-D-glucose positron emission tomography (FDG-PET) has been established as a potent tool that can provide early information about disease control in the course of antineoplastic therapy. Monitoring clinical evolution with PET is emerging as a new powerful predictor of outcome that can eventually diminish the amount of treatment to administer, sparing unnecessary cycles of chemotherapy or radiotherapy, or, on the contrary, making advisable the indication of more intensified treatments.

Some trials have revealed that interim PET scans after one to three cycles of chemotherapy may predict long term outcomes in HL (Hutchings et al., 2005). In a prospective trial including 260 patients with advanced HL treated with ABVD, PET scans were made per protocol after 2 cycles of treatment (Gallamini A et al, 2007). This study demonstrated that patients with an interim negative PET scan had excellent prognosis, with two year event free survival rates of 95%, compared with 13% in those cases with PET positive. On multivariate analysis, interim PET status was the only significant prognostic factor, showing superiority over the classical IPS model (Gallamini et al., 2007).

After these findings, next question is how to incorporate the interim PET results in the global management of treatment of HL in order to tailor a risk-adapted treatment strategy to the individual patient. There are several prospective trials ongoing in the United States and in Europe in early and advanced disease, testing different therapeutic approaches depending on PET scan findings. Their results are eagerly awaited to definitely establish finer tune therapeutic strategies in this disease.

4. Role of virus in HL

A negative association has been observed between HL and repeated early common infections (Rudant et al., 2010). Viruses are etiologically associated with a significant number of human leukaemia/lymphomas. Recognition of virus involvement in these malignancies is important as prevention of infection can lead to a reduction in the number of individuals at risk of disease. Early epidemiologic data suggested that HL develops among persons with a delayed exposure to a ubiquitous infectious agent such as Epstein-Barr virus (EBV) or among persons with acquired less common new infections such as human deficiency virus (HIV). The role of mediators of immunity genes may be important in the lack of adequate immune control of infectious agents. Several cytokines and interleukins are produced by neoplastic cells in lymphomas.

EBV, a γ herpesvirus with a worldwide distribution, is present in H/RS cells of 40%–60% of cHL lesions and contributes to their pathogenesis (Kapatai & Murray, 2007; Khan, 2006). EBV positivity is higher with MCHL (60-70%) than with NSHL (15-30%). EBV+ H/RS cells express the latent membrane proteins 1, 2A y 2B (LMP1, LMP2A, LMP2B), the EBV nuclear antigens 1 (EBNA1), and the EBER RNAs, but consistently lack EBNA2 (latency II) (Jarrett, 2002, 2006). LMP1 is likely to contribute to survival and proliferation of H/RS cells through activation of NF-κB and AP-1 (Kilger et al., 1998; Lam & Sugden, 2003). The role of LMP2A is more difficult to predict. Although LMP2A can deliver a survival signal in B-cells, H/RS cells have down-regulated many B-cell specific molecules including intracellular components involved in this signaling pathway (Kilger et al., 1998; Schwering et al., 2003). LMP2A may indeed contribute to this 'loss of B-cell signature', since cDNA microarray analysis of LMP2A expressing B-cells reveals a similar pattern of downregulated genes (Portis et al., 2003). It is also possible that EBNA1 and the EBERs contribute to the rescue of H/RS cells from apoptosis (Kennedy et al., 2003; Young & Rickinson, 2004).

Immunologic reactions (cytotoxic responses) against EBV can occur in the peripheral blood of some cHL patients (Khan, 2006). It has been estimated that EBV-specific T-cells might constitute up to 5% of circulating $CD8^+$ T-cells (Hislop et al., 2002; Rickinson & Kieff, 2001). The intratumoral immunological alterations induced by EBV^+ H/RS cells remain unclear. The abnormal network of cytokines/chemokines and/or their receptors in H/RS cells is involved in the attraction of many of the microenvironmental cells into the lymphoma background. There is increasing evidence suggesting a change in the balance between Th1 and Th2 cells in the pathogenesis of HL and that this change induces reactivation of latent viral infections, including EBV. For example, interleukin like IL-1 β is produced by H/RS cells in culture (Hsu et al., 1989) and IL-3 have demonstrated to present significant biological activity as growth and antiapoptotic factor for H/RS cells (Aldinucci et al., 2005). Serum levels of the receptor antagonist IL-1 (IL-1r α) are elevated in HL patients, patients with B symptoms have significantly lower levels of IL-1rα than those without symptoms (Gruss et al., 1992). IL-10 is a pleiotropic cytokine that protects hematopoietic cells from apoptosis induced by glucocorticoids and doxorubicin. H/RS cells express functional IL-10 receptors and elevated IL-10 levels may inhibit apoptosis of H/RS cells. Elevated serum IL-10 levels have been found in up to 50% of HL patients and have been associated with inferior failure free survival (FFS) and overall survival (OS) in patients treated with ABVD or BEACOPP chemotherapy (Rautert et al., 2008; Sarris et al., 1999; Vassilakopoulos et al., 2001; Viviani et al., 2000). Elevated serum IL-10 levels confer a poor survival and may add to the prognostic value of the IPS in prediction of outcomes in HL (Axdorph et al., 2000). CCL17/TARC is a chemokine secreted by H/RS cells and its chemotactic properties may explain the infiltration of reactive T lymphocytes in HL (Niens et al., 2008; Peh et al., 2001; van den Berg et al., 1999). Elevated CCL7/TARC levels have been seen in the majority of patients with HL (Niens et al., 2008). Persistent elevation of TARC after completion of treatment has been associated with poorer survival and could be important for treatment monitoring (Hnatkova et al., 2009; Weihrauch et al., 2005). EBV-infected H/RS cells were shown to stimulate also the stromal production of particular chemokines such as the interferon-inducible chemokine IP-10 (CXCL10) (Teichmann et al., 2005), Rantes/CCL5 (Aldinucci et al., 2008; Fischer et al., 2003), the ligand CCL28 (Hanamoto et al., 2004), CCL20 that is capable of attracting regulatory T cells (Baumforth et al., 2008) and the macrophage-derived chemoattractant (MDC)/CCL22 (Niens et al., 2008). It has been also suggested that immunologic reactions against EBV can occur in the peripheral blood of some cHL patients (Khan, 2006). However, no comprehensive characterization of intratumoral immunologic alterations induced by EBV+ H/RS cells has been described so far. EBV was shown to contribute to HL patients survival (Kapatai & Murray, 2007). The observation of Th1/antiviral response in EBV^+ cHL tissues provides a basis for novel treatment strategies (Chetaille et al., 2009; Skinnider & Mak, 2002).

Although HL is not considered an acquired immunodeficiency syndrome (AIDS)-defining neoplasm, HIV-infected patients treated with highly active antiretroviral therapy (HAART) present a higher incidence of HL compared with the population without HIV infection (Powles & Bower, 2000; Powles et al., 2009). Almost 100% of HIV-associated cases are EBV-positive and, in these patients, EBV is found more frequently in H/RS cells (Powles & Bower, 2000). HIV-HL exhibits pathological features that are different from those of HL in "general population"(Carbone et al., 2009; Grogg et al., 2007) while is characterized by the predominance of unfavorable histological subtypes (MCHL and LDHL) (Carbone et al., 2009; Grogg et al., 2007; Tirelli et al., 1995). One of the peculiar clinical features of HIV-cHL is the widespread extent of the disease at presentation and the frequency of systemic B-symptoms. At the time of diagnosis, 70–96% of the patients have B-symptoms, and 74–92% have advanced stages of disease with frequent involvement of extranodal sites, the most common being bone marrow (40–50%), liver (15–40%), and spleen (around 20%) (Tirelli et al., 1995). The widespread use of HAART has resulted in substantial improvement in the survival of patients with HIV infection and lymphomas because of the reduction of the incidence of opportunistic infections and the opportunity to allow more aggressive chemotherapy. Moreover, the less-aggressive presentation of lymphoma in patients treated with HAART compared with untreated patients may also favorably change the outcome for HIV-infected patients with lymphomas (Vaccher et al., 2003). In fact, compared with patients who never received HAART, patients in HAART before the onset of cHL generally are older, have less B-symptoms, and a higher leukocyte and neutrophil counts and hemoglobin level (Chimienti et al., 2008).

5. Antitumoral immunity

Tumors are more than an accumulation of neoplastic cells; they might be more properly considered as a functional tissue immunologically mediated and formed by a complex tissue network in which neoangiogenesis, infiltrating immune competent cells, stromal cells, and a differentiated and specific extracellular matrix constitute the tumor microenvironment with the capacity of regulating cancer development (Alvaro et al., 2010; Tlsty & Coussens, 2006). The interplay between the host immune system, malignant cells, and all other components of tumoral stroma determine proliferation, invasion, angiogenesis, and remodelling of extracellular matrix and metastasis.

The hypothesis of immunesurveillance postulates that one of the principal functions of the immune system would be recognizing neoplastic cells and eliminating them before they form tumors (Burns & Leventhal, 2000). In these conditions, the absence of an effective immune system increases the risk of developing cancer. If the immune system is a complex system of different types of cells and molecules whose primary function is to act as an effective tumor suppressor, it is certain that the system may behave inefficiently, as indicated by the fact of tumors in immunocompetent individuals. Thus, in addition to the concept of immunosurveillance arises of immunostimulation (Ichim, 2005). Although various mechanisms could induce immunosuppression (virus, transplant ..), the increasing likelihood of cancer (Burnet, 1957) in immunologically intact individuals suggests that the immune response might not only be ineffective but may itself contribute to tumor progression (Prehn, 1972). That is, the immune system has the ability to act as a double-edged sword, indicating that tumor elimination requires a good coordination of the various elements of the immune system.

The products of mutated or deregulated genes of tumoral cells contribute to the growth and invasion of tumoral cells, as well as to the expression of proteins with the ability to stimulate the immune response. The immunogenic capacity of the tumor can be evaluated by means of the study of the reactive infiltration, which is mainly composed by innate immune cells. The nature, function and specificity of the effector cells that drive the antitumoral immune response have been widely studied. Innate immunity is represented essentially by dendritic cells (DCs), macrophages, natural killer (NK), NK/T cells, neutrophils, cytokines and complement proteins, whereas adaptive immune cells are represented by B lymphocytes, $CD4^+$ T-helper lymphocytes and $CD8^+$ cytotoxic lymphocytes (CTL). The general mechanisms for tumor suppression have been principally attributed to $CD4^+$ T helper lymphocytes. Cytokines and lymphokines from $CD4^+$ T cells can also activate $CD8^+$ CTL, NK cells and macrophages, which have all been shown to be involved in tumor immunity (Adam et al., 2003; Gonthier et al., 2004; Ikeda et al., 2002; Peipp & Valerius, 2002; Smyth et al., 2002). Immunoregulatory cytokines such as IL-10 and TGF-β play an important role in immune tolerance, and it seems that suppressor effect of regulatory T cells ($CD4^+CD25^+$) on the development of tumor associated antigen-reactive lymphocytes is independent of cytokines (Aldinucci et al., 2005). Contributing to the complexity of the interactions between the reactive background and malignant cells, immune cells present in the local infiltrate have proved capable of modulating apoptosis and of inducing proliferation of tumoral cells via death receptors, cytotoxic granule liberation, and withdrawal of growth factors or production of immunosuppressive cytokines (Atkinson & Bleackley, 1995; Berke, 1995; de Visser & Kast, 1999; Skinnider & Mak, 2002). The efficacy of tumoral–immune cells interactions depends on several factors, such as the expression of MHC class I molecules and immunogenic epitopes in tumoral cells, the type of immune cell and the accessibility of tumor cells.

Tumor antigens recognized by T cells (generally $CD8^+$ lymphocytes) represent the principal target of antitumoral immunity and are presented by MHC class I molecules; that is to say, that tumoral cells behave as antigen presenting cells (APC), presenting their own antigens to T cells. Naturally, professional APC can also present antigens to $CD4^+$ lymphocytes through MHC class II molecules (Quezada et al., 2010). Dendritic cells (DC) and other APC are dispersed between tissues as sentinels or alarm systems ready to detect the presence of foreign antigens. While in the tumor microenvironment IL-12 production tends to be suppressed, resulting in a decrease in Th1 activity, DCs represent probably the most important regulators of naïve T cells, with a great capacity to produce and release IL-12. In their process of polarization, DCs are under the influence of inflammatory mediators such as prostaglandins produced by macrophages, fibroblasts, and tumor cells. A new route of junction between innate and adaptive immunity through the interaction between DC and NK cells has been suggested (Adam et al., 2005). Actually, at least four distinct CD4 T cells subsets have been described: Th1, Th2, Th17, and regulatory T cells, each one with a unique cytokine secretion pattern and function (Zhu & Paul, 2008). Their primary roles is providing cytokines for the development of CTL, in addition to being able to secrete tumor necrosis factor (TNF) and interferon (IFN)-gamma, which can increase the expression of MHC class I by the tumor cell and therefore increase its sensitivity to CTL lysis. Among natural CTL, natural killer cells (NK cells) can be activated directly by contact with the tumor or as a result of the stimulus provided by cytokines. In addition, lymphokine-activated killer cells (LAK) are a group of NK cells derived from peripheral blood cells or tumor infiltrating lymphocytes (TIL) in patients with high concentrations of IL-2 and show a high capacity, nonspecific in this case, to lyse tumor cells. Others cellular mediators such as the macrophages are also capable of lysing tumor cells by releasing a large amount of lysosomal enzymes and reactive oxygen metabolites. Once activated they also produce cytokines such as TNF that exerts its cytotoxic activity triggering apoptosis in a similar way to that mediated by Fas.

6. Molecular markers

In HL, a striking feature of both NLPHL and cHL entities is that the malignant cells account for only around 1% of the tumor mass (Stein et al., 2008a). However, notable significant differences exist between these entities in terms of natural history, relation to EBV, cell morphology, phenotype, molecular characteristics, and clinical behavior (Farrell & Jarrett, 2011; Maggioncalda et al., 2011).

There is compelling evidence that H/RS cells are clonal B cells that have lost their B cell phenotype. Effectively, H/RS cells, from nearly all cHL cases, and malignant popcorn cells from NLPHL have detectable rearrangements of Ig heavy and/or light chain genes, confirming a B cell origin (Kuppers et al., 1996; Kuppers et al., 1994) and, in any given case, the rearrangements are identical, proving the clonal nature of the disease (Kanzler et al., 1996; Kuppers et al., 1994; Marafioti et al., 2000). Furthermore, the Ig variable (IgV) gene regions show evidence of somatic hypermutation, revealing a GC or post-GC origin (Kuppers, 2002). It was also suggested that cHL and B cell non-Hodgkin lymphoma (BNHL) arisen from a common precursor (pre-GC or GC B cell) since both generally harbor identical IgV gene rearrangements but have distinct somatic Ig gene mutations (Brauninger et al., 2006). Intraclonal IgV gene diversity is observed in popcorn cells, indicating ongoing somatic hypermutation, whereas identical somatic hypermutations were observed in H/RS cells indicating a later stage of B cell differentiation (Kanzler et al., 1996; Kuppers et al., 1994; Marafioti et al., 2000). Around 25% of cHL cases present non-functional Ig genes due to "crippling" mutations (Brauninger et al., 2006; Kanzler et al., 1996; Kuppers et al., 1994; Kuppers et al., 2001). H/RS cells harbor uncommonly rearranged T cell receptor genes (<2%), suggesting a T cell origin in a small minority of cases (Muschen et al., 2001; Muschen et al., 2000; Seitz et al., 2000). At phenotypic level, markers of B lineage (CD20, CD19, CD79, surface Ig) and transcription factors (OCT2, BOB1 and PU1) are generally down-regulated in H/RS cells (Hertel et al., 2002; Schwering et al., 2003), and expression of the B cell-specific transcription factor PAX5 is usually retained (Foss et al., 1999). In contrast, popcorn cells express B cell markers including CD20, CD79, PAX5, OCT2 and BOB1. The global suppression of the B cell signature results from transcriptional reprogramming (Kuppers et al., 2003; Mathas et al., 2006; Nie et al., 2003; Renne et al., 2006; Smith et al., 2005; Ushmorov et al., 2006; Ushmorov et al., 2004).

Mature B cells lacking B cell receptors would normally die by apoptosis, and therefore H/RS cells must have developed mechanisms to facilitate survival. The escape from apoptosis and transcriptional reprogramming of H/RS cells are interlinked and seem important to disease pathogenesis. EBV gene products appear to contribute to H/RS cell survival, proliferation and reprogramming through dysregulation of several signaling networks and transcription factors such as intrinsic overexpression of CD30 (Horie et al., 2002), deleterious mutations of the genes encoding IκB proteins (IκBα) (Emmerich et al., 1999; Emmerich et al., 2003; Jungnickel et al., 2000; Lake et al., 2009; Wood et al., 1998) and amplification of the chromosomal region including the c-Rel gene (Barth et al., 2003; Joos et al., 2002; Martin-Subero et al., 2002). In cHL EBV-associated cases, the virus can contribute directly to activation of NF-κB though its protein latent membrane protein 1 (LMP-1), which mimics CD40 signaling. Mutations of genes encoding inhibitors and regulators of NF-κB such as inactivating mutations of the TNF-α induced protein 3 (TNFAIP3) gene have been detected in a large proportion of EBV-negative cases (Kato et al., 2009; Schmitz et al., 2009). Others genomic lesions affecting different signaling pathways in H/RS cells (JAK-STAT, PI3K-Akt-mTOR, MAPK-MEK-ERK and AP1-Jun/Fos) have also been demonstrated (Dutton et al., 2005; Emmerich et al., 1999; Joos et al., 2003; Juszczynski et al., 2007; Kube et al., 2001; Skinnider et al., 2002; Weniger et al., 2006; Zheng et al., 2003). In cHL and primary mediastinal B-cell lymphoma, genomic breaks of the major major histocompatibility complex (MHC) class II transactivator CIITA have been demonstrated to be highly recurrent (15% and 38% respectively) (Steidl et al., 2011b). The functional consequences of CIITA gen fusions is the downregulation of surface HLA class II expression and overexpression of ligands of the receptor molecule programmed cell death 1 (CD274/PDL1 and CD273/PDL2). These receptor-ligand interactions have been shown to impact anti-tumour immune responses in several cancers, whereas decreased MHC class II expression has been linked to reduced tumour cell immunogenicity.

Several of these recurring genetic lesions appear correlated with disease outcome (Slovak et al., 2011). Nonrandom DNA copy number alterations in cHL (H/RS cells CD30^{+}) have been identified in the molecular karyotypes of cHL as comparing with the genomic profiles of GC B cells. Frequent gains (>65%) were associated with growth and proliferation, NF-κB activation, cell-cycle control, apoptosis, and immune and lymphoid development. Frequent losses (>40%) observed encompassed tumor suppressor genes, transcriptional repressors and SKP2 (Slovak et al., 2011).

Thus, multiple transcriptional and signaling pathways are disrupted in HL, and are thought to cooperate to increase H/RS cell proliferation, reduce apoptosis and promote a favorable cellular microenvironment through the release of multiple cytokines and chemokines. These findings may be useful prognostic markers in the counselling and management of patients and for the development of novel therapeutic approaches in primary refractory HL.

7. Biological factors: Immune response in HL

The tumor microenvironment consists of a specific mixture of immune cells that express a distinctive profile for each tumor type, from which the efficacy of the immune response against the tumor is eventually derived (Alvaro et al., 2009). Exist increasing evidence of the importance of the microenvironment in the molecular pathogenesis of HL (Steidl et al., 2011a), and a promising therapeutic target has been raised focused on this approach. The presence of a characteristically rich inflammatory background particularly distinguishes HL from other lymphoproliferative syndromes. Differences in gene expression profiles of malignant cells in lymphoproliferative syndromes do not always determine the aggressiveness of the lymphoma, while recent contributions determine that HL represents the prototypical tumor in which the interplay between H/RS and the reactive microenvironment determines not only the histological morphology and classification but also the clinicopathological features and prognosis of these patients. Quantitative analysis of infiltrating immune cells reveals undisclosed relationships between the relative proportion of these cells and HL clinical outcome, illustrating how factors other than tumoral cellularity, or the immunophenotype and molecular anomalies present in the H/RS cells, can play a role in tumoral behaviour.

7.1 Patterns of immune response in HL and prognosis

An abnormal pattern with overexpression of cytokines and their receptors is characteristic in H/RS cells. This pattern explains the abundant mixture of inflammatory cells, stromal changes and the predominance of Th2 cells between the various subpopulations of lymphoid cells in the tumoral microenvironment of HL (Swerdlow et al., 2008b). A predominance of $CD4^+$ T lymphocytes in the background of tumoral cells in addition to a high number of cytotoxic cells (CD8, CD57, TIA-1) has been observed in the majority of HL-tissues (Figure 2) (Alvaro-Naranjo et al., 2005; Oudejans et al., 1997; Poppema et al., 1998).

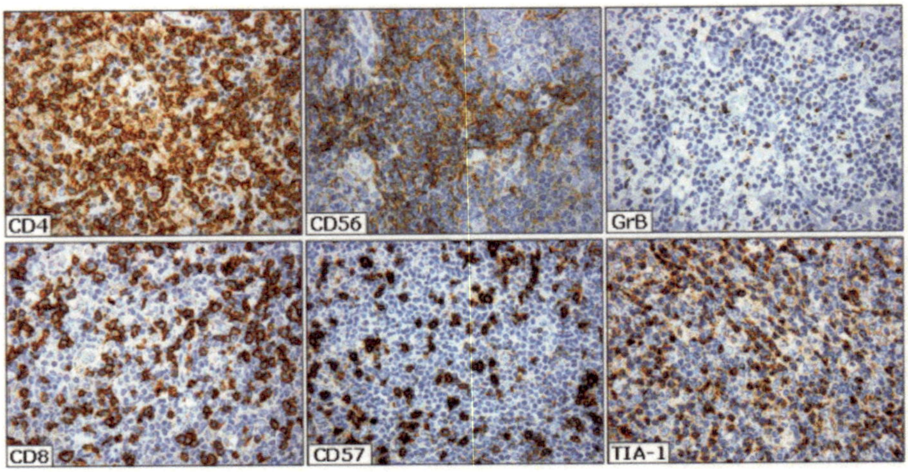

Fig. 2. Immunohistochemical staining of inflammatory background in HL: T lymphocytes (CD4 and CD8), NK cells (CD56 and CD57) and cytotoxic cells (GrB and TIA-1).

Regardless of the classic clinical and pathological features, a high proportion of infiltrating $CD8^+$ and $CD57^+$ cells as well as a low number of infiltrating CTL (evaluated by the presence of Granzyme B and TIA-1) appear to be associated with a favorable outcome for HL patients (without B symptoms and lower clinical stages) and better response to treatment (Alvaro-Naranjo et al., 2005; Alvaro et al., 2005; Ansell et al., 2001). It is unclear to date whether the presence of $CD8^+$ T cells correlates with the antitumor cytotoxic response. Nevertheless, it has been suspected that $CD8^+$ T cells may be recruited in an antigen-non-specific mode in HL (Willenbrock et al., 2000).

Although the activation status of infiltrating cells have been demonstrated to be independent of the degree of malignancy in HL (Bosshart, 2002), others studies have shown that the presence of activated cytotoxic T cells (granzyme B^+) is associated with unfavorable follow-up in these patients (Kanavaros et al., 1999; Oudejans et al., 1997; ten Berge et al., 2001). A higher level of not activated cytotoxic cells ($TIA\text{-}1^+$) has been observed in advanced-stage cHL without prognostic value (Camilleri-Broet et al., 2004). However, $TIA\text{-}1^+$ CTL associated with the presence of regulatory T cells $FOXP3^+$ appears to play an important role in monitoring HL patients (Alvaro et al., 2005). Variations in the level ofcytotoxic $TIA\text{-}1^+$ and regulatory T cells observed during the course of the disease could be implicated in the progression of HL (Alvaro et al., 2005).

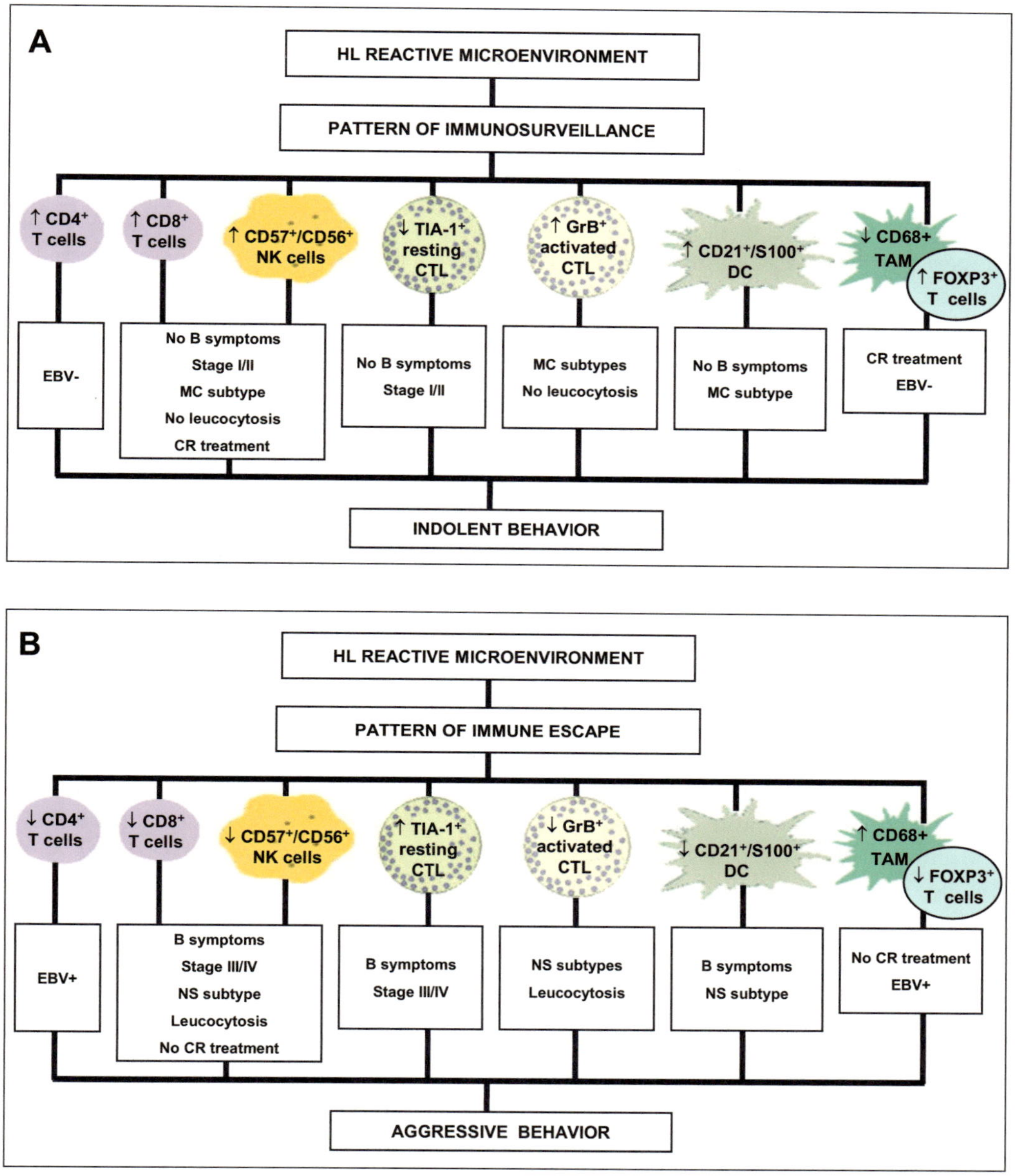

Fig. 3. Representation of the two immune patterns observed in HL significantly associated with their clinicopathological features. The immunesurveillance pattern (A) with a high proportion of infiltrating T lymphocytes, NK cells, DCs, activated CTL but low proportion of resting CTL and TAM is associated with a favorable outcome. The immune escape pattern (B) with a high proportion of infiltrating resting CTL and TAM, but low proportion of T lymphocytes, NK cells, DCs and activated CTL is associated with an unfavorable outcome. MC, mixed celularity; NS, nodular sclerosis; CR, complete response.

Association of tumor-associated macrophages (TAM) $CD68^+$ with adverse clinical outcomes has been confirmed in several studies in hematologic and solid tumors (Pages et al., 2010).

Recently, a gene expression profile analysis performed on 130 biopsy samples from patients with HL identified a signature of TAM and monocytes that was predictive of treatment failure (Steidl et al., 2010). In this study the sensitivity and specificity of this GEP signature for outcome in this cohort was greater than that of the International Prognostic Score (IPS). After these findings, biopsy samples from an independent cohort of 166 patients were evaluated with immunohistochemistry for the presence of CD68 expressing macrophages using a score from 1 to 3, from lower to higher infiltration (Steidl et al., 2010). When compared with those with low CD68 expression, patients with tumors that demonstrated an increased number of CD68 expressing macrophages had shorter median progression-free survival (PFS), lower rate of 10-year disease-specific survival (60 versus 89%), and higher failure rate of secondary treatment with curative intent (63 versus 13%). It has been also recently demonstrated that high level of CD68 correlated with poorer survival, event-free survival (EFS) and with the presence of EBV in the tumor cell population (Kamper et al., 2011). These results suggest a new pathological prognostic factor to be considered, however it is unclear at this time how CD68 status should affect patient management.

A plausible explanation for the extensive inflammatory infiltrate present in HL secretion could be a variety of cytokines produced by both tumor cells and surrounding stromal tissue. $CD4^+$ T cells produce Th2 cytokines that could contribute to local suppression of the cellular immune response mediated by Th1. However, the categorization of $CD4^+$ T cells in Th1 and/or Th2 is an oversimplification (Marshall et al., 2004) as regulatory T cells with $CD4^+CD25^+$ phenotype not only play a regulatory role of autoimmunity, but also have suppressive effects on the development of antigen-reactive lymphocytes associated with the tumor (Wei et al., 2004). The H/RS cells secrete high amounts of chemokine, thymus and activation-regulated chemokine (TARC) and macrophages-derived chemokine (MDC) in particular, which attract lymphocytes expressing CCR4 receptor, such as Th2 (Skinnider & Mak, 2002). These cytokines may contribute to the pathogenesis of the disease initiated and sustained the presence of the reactive infiltrate. Alternatively, immune cells can produce cytokines responsible for proliferation and survival of tumor, producing a positive feedback between the tumoral cells and immune system. The composition of the infiltrate may also differ depending on the state of immunosuppression of HL patients. Moreover, HIV infection affects, for direct or indirect mechanisms, both reactive changes as neoplastic lymphoid tissue. Recently we have seen a significant loss of intratumoral T cells $CD4^+$ (CD4/CD8 ratio reversal) and a decrease in intratumoral activated CTL in patients with HIV-infected HL (Bosch Princep et al., 2005). A low proportion of $CD4^+$ cells appears also to be significantly related to EBV status, probably due to the relation with the local tumor-associated suppression of EBV-specific T-cell responses observed in EBV^+ HL cases (Frisan et al., 1995).

7.2 Immune response regulation in HL

Tumors employ a plethora of immunosuppressive mechanisms, which may act in concert to counteract effective immune responses. Different mechanisms have been suggested to account for the CTL-mediated apoptosis resistance of H/RS cells, such as the downregulation of MHC class I molecules of the H/RS cells, prevention of recognition of tumor-associated antigens by CTLs (Poppema & Visser, 1994), or the local secretion of both IL-10 and transforming growth factor-b by H/RS cells (Newcom et al., 1988; Ohshima et al., 1995), which are able to inhibit CTL function. In this respect, it appears that the blockage of the Granzyme B pathway of apoptosis through the overexpression of serine protease inhibitor PI-9/SPI-6 is an important additional mechanism for immune escape by tumors (Medema et al., 2001). The expression of PI9 tends to be associated with a high percentage of activated CTLs, especially in HL (Bladergroen et al., 2002), suggesting that PI9 may play a role in protecting against Granzyme B-induced apoptosis, and partially explaining why tumors expressing high levels of PI9 have a particularly poor clinical outcome, irrespective of the number of Granzyme B^+ cells in the inflammatory infiltrate.

Different subsets of immune cells contribute also to this immunosuppressive network, including $CD4^+CD25^+$ regulatory T cells. In HL, it has been initially proposed that $CD4^+$ T cells produce cytokines of Th2 type that could contribute to local suppression of the cellular immune response mediated by Th1 cells (Bladergroen et al., 2002; Poppema et al., 1999). However, the categorization of $CD4^+$ T cells in Th1 and/or Th2 constitutes an oversimplification and it has been shown that regulatory T cells with $CD4^+CD25^+$ phenotype not only play a role in controlling autoimmunity, but also have suppressive effects on lymphocyte development tumor associated antigen reagents (Curiel et al., 2004; Fontenot et al., 2003; Suri-Payer et al., 1998). Functional and molecular characterization of these cells has been facilitated by the identification of markers such as FOXP3 and others (Shimizu et al., 2002; Sutmuller et al., 2001; Takahashi et al., 2000). FOXP3 encodes a transcription factor known as Scurfina, specifically expressed by T cells $CD4^+CD25^+$(Karube et al., 2004), that acts converting naïve regulatory T cells $CD4^+CD25^-$ phenotype to $CD25^+$ (Hori et al., 2003). More recently, it was suggested that regulatory T cells and $PD1^+$ T cells interact with H/RS cells (Alvaro et al., 2005; Teichmann et al., 2005; Yamamoto et al., 2008), which produce the T regulatory attractant galectin-1 and the PD-1 ligand, PDL-1 (Yamamoto et al., 2008). On the other hand, the observation of numerous $CXCR3^+$ lymphocytes in some HL tumors has raised the possibility of an occasional Th1-predominant immune response (Alvaro-Naranjo et al., 2005).

The regulatory T cells can inhibit the production of both IL-2 to regulate the high expression of IL-2Rα (CD25), ie, delay or block the activation of $CD8^+$ cells and natural killer (NK) cells against tumor antigens (Azuma et al., 2003; Wolf et al., 2003). The immunosuppressive properties of regulatory T cells appear to be particularly important because of its large effect on cellular cytotoxicity represented by CTLs and NK cells. The presence of low numbers of $FOXP3^+$ cells and a consequent high rate of TIA-1^+ cells in the infiltrate represents an independent prognostic factor negatively affecting the survival of the disease. Furthermore, when the disease relapses and progresses, larger number of TIA-1^+ cells and lower proportion of $FOXP3^+$ on the reactive background of the tumor are also prone to be seen (Alvaro et al., 2005).

8. Apoptotic and cell cycle pathways in HL

The aberrant expression of proteins involved in regulation and execution of apoptosis and cell cycle of lymphocytes has been demonstrated in several types of lymphoma and the importance of the level of apoptosis and proliferation in clinically aggressive lymphoproliferative syndromes (Bai et al., 2005; Bai et al., 2003; Garcia et al., 2003; Sanchez-Beato et al., 2003). These anomalies are probably not sufficient to explain the development of lymphomas, even if the effectiveness of therapy is presumed to be mediated by activation of apoptosis (Messineo et al., 1998). In HL, different studies have described alterations in genes controlling apoptosis and proliferation of H/RS cells and biological factors such as EBV detection, which influence the clinical aggressiveness of the disease (Bargou et al., 1997; Garcia et al., 1999; Hinz et al., 2002; Hinz et al., 2001; Izban et al., 2001; Kupper et al., 2001; Leoncini et al., 1997; Mathas et al., 2002; Montesinos-Rongen et al., 1999; Morente et al., 1997; Sanchez-Beato et al., 1996). These studies have demonstrated alterations of the p53, Rb and p27 tumor suppressor pathways (Bai et al., 2005; Garcia et al., 1999; Guenova et al., 1999; Hinz et al., 2001; Lauritzen et al., 1999; Montesinos-Rongen et al., 1999; Morente et al., 1997; Sanchez-Beato et al., 1996; Sanchez-Beato et al., 2003; Tzardi et al., 1996), overexpression of cyclins involved in the G1/S and G2/M transition such as cyclins E, D2, D3, A and B1 (Garcia et al., 2003; Kolar et al., 2000; Leoncini et al., 1997; Ohshima et al., 1999; Teramoto et al., 1999; Tzankov et al., 2003b), overexpression of cyclin-dependent kinases such as CDK1, 2 and 6 (Garcia et al., 2003) and overexpression of the anti-apoptotic proteins c-FLIP, bcl-xl, c-IAP2 and surviving (Brink et al., 1998; Garcia et al., 2003; Kanavaros et al., 2000; Kuppers, 2002; Kuppers et al., 2003; Staudt, 2000; Thomas et al., 2004).

These findings raised the questions of how H/RS cells escape apoptosis, acquire self-sufficiency in growth signals and proliferate (Kuppers, 2002; Kuppers et al., 2003; Staudt, 2000; Thomas et al., 2004). The physiologic relevance of the deregulation of the cell cycle and apoptosis regulators in cHL could be related to the different probabilities of survival of HL patients. Many studies have analyzed the clinical relevance of the expression of cell cycle and apoptosis regulators in cHL using IHC or gene expression profiling (Brink et al., 1998; Devilard et al., 2002; Garcia et al., 2003; Montalban et al., 2000; Morente et al., 1997; Smolewski et al., 2000). Shorter survival was significantly associated with high proliferation index (Ki67), high expression of bcl2, bcl-xl, bax and p53, low expression of Rb and caspase 3 and high apoptotic index (Montalban et al., 2004; Rassidakis et al., 2002a; Rassidakis et al., 2002b; Sup et al., 2005; Abele et al., 1997; Brink et al., 1998; Garcia et al., 2003; Montalban et al., 2004; Morente et al., 1997; Smolewski et al., 2000). Evidence has accumulated that the constitutive activation of the NF-κB pathway in H/RS cells is of particular importance for explaining the apoptosis deregulation in cHL by up-regulating an anti-apoptotic gene expression program (Bai et al., 2005; Hinz et al., 2002; Hinz et al., 2001; Mathas et al., 2002). By gene expression profiling, the good outcome cHL were characterized by up-regulation of genes involved in apoptosis induction (APAF, bax, bid, caspase 8, p53, TRAIL) and cell signaling, including cytokines and transduction molecules (IL-10, IL-18, STAT3), while the bad outcome cHL were characterized by upregulation of genes involved in cell proliferation (Ki67) and by down-regulation of tumor suppressor genes PTEN (Phospatase and Tensin homolog deleted on chromosome 10) and DCC (Deleted in Colorectal Cancer) (Devilard et al., 2002).

Within the complexity of the interactions between the reactive substance and tumor cells, immune cells present in the infiltrate have been shown to modulate the apoptosis and proliferation of tumor cells via apoptotic receptors, cytotoxic granule release, growth factors or immunosuppressive cytokines (Atkinson & Bleackley, 1995; Berke, 1995; de Visser & Kast, 1999; Famularo et al., 1994; Hahne et al., 1996). IHC study has demonstrated that the antiapoptotic profile observed in H/RS cells is associated with a general increase in $CD4^+$ T cells infiltrating (related to Bcl-XL and Mcl-1) and an overall decline $CD8^+$ T lymphocytes infiltrating, NK cells and dendritic cells (related to Bcl-XL and Bax) (Alvaro et al., 2008). Alterations observed in the G1-S checkpoint of H/RS cell cycle, in the principal tumor suppressor pathways Rb-p16INK4a and p27KIP1, and the high rate of proliferation (MIB1, BCL6) are also strongly associated with higher infiltration of the overall immune response against the tumor (Alvaro et al., 2008). These results point to the regulation of proteins involved in apoptosis and proliferation of tumor cells by direct interactions between these cells and the surrounding inflammatory microenvironment.

These infiltrated cells are able to activate apoptotic caspase proteolytic cascade through TNF receptor superfamily interactions (FasL/Fas and CD40/CD40L). The different members of this superfamily share common cell signaling pathways that mediate the activation of nuclear factor NF-κB and mitogen-activated protein kinases. In this case, CD40/CD40L interactions are known to induce the upregulation of Bcl-XL and Mcl1 expression and to mediate the activation of NF-κB (Hinz et al., 2001; Hong et al., 2000; Inoue et al., 2000; Kater et al., 2004; Lee et al., 1999; Metkar et al., 2001). CTLs are also able to trigger a second proapoptotic pathway through the protease granzyme B, which, once released from CTLs, is translocated into the target cell by perforin, where it activates the effector caspase cascade (Thome & Tschopp, 2001). On the other hand, the wide variety of cytokines and chemokines present in HL tumoral tissue (IL-2, IL-4, IL-6, and IL-13), responsible for the massive influx of activated immune cells (Poppema et al., 1999), has been shown to regulate the expression of the various members of Bcl2 family, such as the antiapoptotic Bcl2 homologues Bcl-XL and Mcl1 and the proapoptotic Bax (Akbar et al., 1996; Jourdan et al., 2000; Puthier et al., 1999; Song et al., 2002; Tang et al., 2002).

Likewise for the apoptotic markers, the physiologic signals present in the reactive microenvironment also interfere with components of the G1-CDK checkpoint (cyclin D3, CDK6, and p27) (Malumbres & Barbacid, 2001; Wagner et al., 1998). The constitutively activated NF-κB has also been shown to induce changes in the expression of a set of proteins regulating cell cycle progression and gene transcription, including cyclin D1, p53, p16 INK4a, and p27KIP1 (Hinz et al., 2001; Sanchez-Beato et al., 2003). Cytotoxic cells are able to induce directly the permanent down-regulation of p27KIP1, probably as a consequence of increased degradation mediated by SKP2, a ubiquitin ligase for p27KIP1 (Blanchard et al., 1997; Ren et al., 2005; Wagner et al., 1998). Related with the heightened proliferative state in these tumors is the high level of expression of Bcl6, a multifunctional regulator that is able not only to down-regulate cyclin D2 and p27KIP1 expression (Shaffer et al., 2000) but also to repress Bcl-XL (Tang et al., 2002).

The presence of EBV was significantly associated with the overexpression of STAT1 and STAT3. STAT3 was found to be associated with a low infiltration of CD4 T lymphocytes and a high infiltration of activated cytotoxic cells. Although STAT1 is considered to be a potential tumor suppressor (promoting apoptosis), STAT3 is thought to be an oncogene because it leads to the activation of cyclin D1 and Bcl-XL expression and is involved in promoting cell cycle progression and cellular transformation and in preventing apoptosis (Calo et al., 2003).

The physiologic relevance of these relationships could be related to the different probabilities of survival of HL patients. Different sets of deregulated immune and tumoral genes have shown to be associated with a therapeutically unfavorable response in HL patients (Sanchez-Aguilera et al., 2006). For example, altered expression of bcl-2 and the bcl-2 family of proteins (e.g., bcl-Xl, BAX) in H/RS cells may prevent apoptosis and explain resistance to treatment-induced apoptosis. Under these conditions, the concomitant analysis of the immune infiltrate and the apoptotic/proliferative pathways of tumoral cells should provide more accurate information about the specific molecular pathways critical for cancer cell growth. Possible molecules that interfere with these molecular links, particularly some enzymes representative of the immune metabolic state or tumoral cell cycle (Sanchez-Aguilera et al., 2006), might be pharmaceutically manipulated and could be candidates for new therapeutic targets pertinent to patient care.

9. HL in immunosuppressed patients

Epidemiologic and molecular findings suggest that cHL is not a single disease but consists of more than one entity and may occur in different clinical settings. According to the acknowledged international literature (Swerdlow et al., 2008a), cHL arises either in the general population (Stein et al., 2008a) but also in the immunosuppressed host, specifically in HIV-infected individuals (Raphael et al., 2008), and in post-transplant patients, most often in renal post-transplant patients (Swerdlow et al., 2008c).

From a clinical perspective, HIV-infected HLs have some peculiarities. Firstly, it must be distinguished two eras, before and after the widespread use of highly active antiretroviral therapy (HAART) (Powles et al., 2009). Before HAART, HIV-HL patients were generally diagnosed with an aggressive presentation. Advanced stages were the rule at diagnosis with frequent involvement of extranodal sites, particularly bone marrow, liver and spleen. In addition, up to 95% of patients had systemic B symptoms when diagnosed, and consequently survival rates were extremely disappointing (Tirelli et al., 1995). Nevertheless, introduction of HAART have led to forms of presentation less aggressive, a dramatic reduction in the incidence of opportunistic infections, and finally it have allowed to complete curative treatment with chemotherapy in most of the patients (Carbone et al., 2009). Regarding chemotherapy, optimal treatment for HIV-HL has not been definitely established due to the relatively low incidence of this disease. However, little phase II studies with few patients have found that, in this modern HAART era, standard ABVD treatment may be safely administered with or without growth-colony stimulating factors (G-CSF) support (Xicoy et al., 2007), although some groups argue in favor of G-CSF introduction from the beginning to minimize risks. Prophylaxis against Pneumocystis jiroveci infection with trimethoprim-sulfamethoxazole is also strongly recommended in all these patients. Other more intensive regimens like BEACOPP or Stanford V with consolidation radiotherapy have been tested with acceptable results in terms of complete responses (100% and 81%, respectively), although a higher incidence of opportunistic infections and hematologic toxicity were registered. Finally, even the use of high dose chemotherapy and autologous stem cell transplantation have been demonstrated feasible in HL-HIV relapsed patients with curative purposes (Carbone et al., 2009). To conclude, it must be said that clinical outcomes of patients with HIV-HL has improved after HAART introduction, with higher curability rates when a combined antineoplastic and antiretroviral strategy is followed and completed.

Post-transplant lymphoproliferative disorders (PTLDs) are a heterogeneous group of monoclonal or polyclonal lymphoproliferative lesions that occur in immunosuppressed recipients after solid-organ or bone marrow transplantation. cHL occurs in the post-transplant setting, most often in renal transplant patients, is almost always EBV-positive and should complete the diagnostic criteria for cHL (Adams et al., 2009; Knight et al., 2009; Rohr et al., 2008; Swerdlow et al., 2008c). All patients received post-transplant immunosuppression and/or antiviral agents (Dharnidharka et al., 2004; Goyal et al., 1996; Krishnamurthy et al., 2010). Clinically, the majority of patients are men and all ages are affected. Generally, the time from transplant to the onset of the disease ranges from few months (4–6 months) to several years, with a median time of 113 months. Half cases presented as extranodal masses, especially in the liver or in the lung even if other extranodal sites (especially tonsil) can be involved. The best therapeutic approach is not well defined yet. Recently, rituximab has gained favor in the treatment of PTLD because of its targeting of CD20-positive B cells, with fairly promising results (Pham et al., 2002).

The iatrogenic lymphoproliferative disorders are lymphoid proliferations or lymphomas that arise in patients treated with immunosuppressive drugs. Among iatrogenic lymphoproliferative disorders, other than PTLD, there is an increase in frequency of cHL and lymphoid proliferations with Hodgkin-like features. Thus, lesions containing RS-like cells but do not fulfill the criteria of CHL, the so-called Hodgkin-like lesions, have been included in this setting (Gaulard et al., 2008). Because cHL has only recently been recognized as an iatrogenic complication, few cases have been reported in the medical literature (Gaulard et al., 2008).

10. Antineoplastic therapy in HL: From classical to biological therapies

Chemotherapy and radiotherapy remain the cornerstone of HL treatment. Especially, polychemotherapy schedules have increased the survival rates in these patients along the last decades. Nevertheless, up to 30% and 10% of patients will recur and die of HL in advanced and early disease respectively, and unlike what happened in non Hodgkin lymphomas, newer active compounds against HL have not been introduced in clinic since the early 1970s. In addition, patients exposed to chemotherapy and radiation fields are at highest risk of lethal second malignancies (Friedberg, 2011). Therefore it would be more than desirable having new therapeutic drugs and strategies for a better control of the disease and minimizing toxicity of therapy, especially when relapses occur.

10.1 Conventional treatment

Nowadays HL is considered one of the most oncological curable diseases, as a matter of fact of its extremely chemo and radiosensitivity. Among chemotherapy options, ABVD (doxorubicin, bleomycin, vinblastine and dacarbazine) represent the standard schedule for HL treatment in the majority of centers worldwide. However the management of advanced-stage cHL is often predicated on the IPS, and thus escalated BEACOPP (bleomycin, etoposide, doxorubicin, cyclophosphamide, vincristine, procarbazine, prednisone) is another schedule to consider, especially in high-risk patients with IPS scores of 4 or greater (Diehl et al., 2003). Therefore, an apparently more effective initial treatment may be unattractive because of increased toxic effects (Connors, 2011) and highest risk of second malignancies, especially in relation with large radiation fields (Ng et al., 2002).

Canellos et al showed in 1992 that ABVD was equally effective and less toxic than MOPP (mechlorethamine, vincristine, procarbazine, prednisone) or MOPP alternating with ABVD, and this has subsequently become the chemotherapy of choice worldwide (Canellos et al., 1992). Although standard ABVD can cure most of HL, advanced stage- high risk patients based on IPS still represent a major concern with EFS rates of 50% or less (Hasenclever &

Diehl, 1998). The HD9 trial conducted by Diehl et al showed that among patients with advanced-stage cHL, ABVD is insufficient for patients with an IPS of 4 or more (Diehl A et at, 2003). In this trial of the German Hodgkin Study Group (GHSG), 1,195 patients with advanced-stage HL were recruited and randomized between COPP-ABVD, standard BEACOPP, and escalated BEACOPP. For patients with an IPS of 4 or greater, the more intensive regimen improved the freedom from treatment failure from 59% to 82% and OS from 67% to 82%. It is important to underscore that there was no significant difference for the more favorable groups. A 10-year update of this study confirms superiority of escalated BEACOPP over COPP-ABVD for the high-risk patients (Diehl et al., 2003). However, there is increased late toxicity with escalated BEACOPP, with more risk of sterility, infections and secondary leukaemia's, and thus universal application of this schedule for advanced-stage disease remain difficult to implement.

In addition of chemotherapy, radiotherapy is another treatment modality frequently used in HL. It is generally indicated in early disease, regardless of the favorable/unfavorable stratification, and when bulky disease is present, or there remain residual foci of disease after chemotherapy in advanced HL.

10.2 Impact of chemotherapy and radiotherapy on tumoral microenvironment

In the last few years, many interesting data have emerged about the enormous impact of the antineoplastic treatments into the immune microenvironment of the tumors, which demonstrate a sort of cancer vaccination effect (Haynes et al., 2008). In this sense, chemotherapeutics like anthracyclines (included in all of the upfront standard treatments of HL) and radiotherapy seem to induce a type of apoptotic death via calreticulin exposure and release of the pro-inflammatory factor High Mobility Group Box-1 (HMGB1) with well known immune stimulating properties (Tesniere et al., 2008).

Anthracyclines can induce a highly potent immune response by increasing antigen (neoantigens) threshold and presentation (via antigen presenting cells), with enhancement of T-cell response and generation of memory T cells (Obeid et al., 2007a). Other chemotherapeutics like cyclophosphamide, etoposide and taxanes have also proved to have an immunogenic effect in preclinical models (Tsavaris et al., 2002), however evidence is scarce and further investigation is required.

These new concepts might serve to consider chemotherapeutics like anthracyclines as less empirical and more specific drugs, and thus it would be desirable to customize chemotherapies taking into account their potential effects on microenvironment. In this sense, there is an interesting field of clinical research to discover that may combine classical CT agents with immunogenic effects with boosting costimulators molecules like cytokines (GM-CSF, IL2) (de la Cruz-Merino et al., 2008). Specifically in the case of the anthracycline´s effect on cancer cells, the calreticulin exposure do not induce DC maturation which is, on the contrary, one of the main effects of cytokines like GM-CSF that induce selective DC maturation and activation, giving a strong rationale to combine these two therapeutic modalities (anthracyclines and GM-CSF). These combinatorial strategies may eventually sustain immunogenic effect of tumoral cell death. Regarding to this, biomarkers of immune activity should be of the greatest interest, in order to serve as proof of principle of efficacy with an earlier detection of the eventual benefits of oncological treatments in patients.

Furthermore, monitoring changes detected during oncological treatments in blood samples, especially in immunophenotype, regulatory T cells amount and TCD8/regulatory T cells ratio, may represent interesting biomarkers to analyze and validate in the future.

As happen with chemotherapy, the intrinsic radiosensitivity of malignant lymphocytes is extremely high. Although the underlying mechanisms which explain it are not fully elucidated, recently new evidence is emerging about some changes induced by radiation at a molecular level, which may provoke a type of cell death highly immunogenic (Formenti & Demaria, 2009). Ionising radiation has different immune effects regarding the dose administered, and while in the case of low doses the final effect is mostly protumorigenic, at higher doses with cytotoxic activity, cell death may induce tumoral neoantigens which can be embraced by DC, and thus activate an effective adaptive immune response (Apetoh et al., 2007). As with anthracyclines, the two critical mediators of this process seem to be translocation of calreticulin to the cell surface and release of HMGB1 by the dying cells (Formenti & Demaria, 2009). Both of them trigger danger signals which activate immune mechanisms. In addition, surviving cancer cells after radiation show increased expression of death receptors, adhesion molecules (ICAM-1) and major histocompatibility complex class I (MHC-I), which activate APCs (Obeid et al., 2007b).

To conclude, some groups argue that these immune effects are the major determinants of the therapeutical success of the antineoplastic treatments in oncological diseases, including HL.

10.3 Modern therapeutic approaches targeting the tumor microenvironment

Apart from chemotherapy and radiotherapy, other biological compounds with significant effects upon tumor microenvironment like unconjugated and conjugated monoclonal antibodies, radioimmunconjugates, immunotoxins and novel immunomodulatory compounds like lenalidomide are under clinical investigation, and at this moment they represent the most promising therapeutical strategies in HL. Recently, Kasamon et al revised this topic (Kasamon & Ambinder, 2008) and pointed out three major HL therapeutic targets: EBV, CD20 and CD30.

As previously cited, up to 40-60% of cHL might be associated with EBV and thus some EBV antigens expressed on HL cells like latent membrane protein 1 and 2 (LMP1 and LMP2) have been postulated as eventual immunotherapeutic targets. Some interesting results have been obtained with the use of adoptive cellular immunotherapy with EBV-specific CTL among patients with EBV-associated posttransplant lymphoproliferative diseases (Haque T et al., 2007), rendering a proof of principle of activity for this approach. In a small study of 16 patients with relapsed or high risk EBV^+ lymphoproliferative diseases that included cases of HL, infusions of autologous LMP2- specific CTL induced clinical responses with tumor regression in 5 of 6 patients with previously detectable tumor (Lucas et al., 2004).

After elucidation of the B cell origin of H/RS in classical HL, targeting B cell antigens on HL has gained renewed interest. Specifically in classical HL, the monoclonal antibody anti-CD20 Rituximab has shown activity as single agent or combined with chemotherapies like ABVD and gemcitabine in different clinical settings (Kasamon & Ambinder, 2008). Impact of rituximab on tumor microenviroment by depleting benign $CD20^+$ cells, is postulated as the main antineoplastic mechanism of action of this drug in HL, independently of CD20 expresssion on the H/RS cells. Rituximab has also been tested in the uncommon nodular lymphocyte predominant Hodgkin lymphoma, with impressive clinical results (Rehwald et al., 2003; Ekstrand et al., 2003) that merit further investigation.

Among new molecular targets in HL, the member of the tumor necrosis factor (TNF)-receptor family CD30 merits special consideration. CD30 is expressed abundantly on RS cells of HL, and in other numerous lymphoid malignancies of B-, T-, and natural killer (NK)-cell origin (Deutsch et al., 2011). Regarding its biological activity CD30 has pleiotropic biologic functions, being capable of promoting cell proliferation and survival as well as inducing antiproliferative responses and cell death. Final effects of CD30 activation seem largely dependent on the microenvironment context (Deutsch et al., 2011). Unconjugated anti-CD30 antibodies have been tested in phase I and II studies showing limited clinical activity (Kasamon & Ambinder, 2008). On the contrary, another attractive approach as it is the use of antibody–drug conjugates (ADCs) have rendered better results.

Brentuximab vedotin (SGN-35) is an ADC consisting of chimeric anti-CD30 antibody cAC10 (SGN-30) conjugated to the tubulin destabilizer monomethylauristatin E (MMAE) (Okeley et al., 2010). In an initial phase I dose escalation study, brentuximab vedotin was administered at a dose of 0.1–3.6 mg/kg every 3 weeks to 45 patients with relapsed or refractory CD30-positive lymphomas, primarily HL and ALCL (Younes et al., 2010). Brentuximab vedotin was well tolerated and associated mainly with grade 1 or 2 adverse events including neutropenia and peripheral neuropathy. Objective response was observed in 17 (38%) patients, including 11 (24%) complete remissions, with a median duration of response of 9.7 months. Tumor regression was observed in 86% of patients. The maximum tolerated dose was 1.8 mg/kg, and of 12 patients who received this dose, six patients (50%) had an objective response (Younes A et al, 2010). A second phase I study, with weekly brentuximab vedotin resulted in an objective response rate of 59% and rapid median time to response. Anti-tumor activity was similar to that observed for dosing once every 3 weeks. However, significant peripheral neuropathy was observed with continued weekly dosing, so the administration every 3 weeks was preferred for phase II studies (Deutsch et al., 2011).

Clearly, brentuximab vedotin is an exciting new agent in the setting of relapsed HL and other lymphoid neoplasms $CD30^+$. Multiple clinical trials are ongoing including different clinical settings and combinations with chemotherapy, in order to find the safer and more successful way of administering this drug.

11. Body's own power protection challenges in HL

Evidences in the literature suggest that targeting elements of the tumor microenvironment, or signaling pathways in tumor cells activated as a consequence of stromal interactions, may prove a useful therapeutic strategy to prevent tumor development and progression. However, given the tumor cells' ability to circumvent various therapeutic agents when given as monotherapy, the success of these agents is likely to be seen when used in combination with existing treatments.

Apart from the infiltrating immune competent cells, the complex tissue network of the tumor microenvironment is also formed by neoangiogenesis, stromal cells, and a differentiated and specific extracellular matrix. Among stromal cells, there are macrophages—derived from hematopoietic stem cells, fibroblasts, adipocytes, and osteoblasts. In order to delay or circumvent tumor progression, a number of strategies are being developed to disrupt tumor-stroma interactions (Hiscox et al., 2011). Macrophages and fibroblasts within the tumor microenvironment present an important point for therapeutic intervention by using agents which reverse their phenotype or block key growth factor receptors (Allavena et al., 2005; Banciu et al., 2008; Hagemann et al., 2008; Hiscox et al., 2011; Karin & Greten, 2005). On the other hand, the regulation of adhesion between cancer cells and the surrounding matrix by different kind of integrins activates tumor cell signaling pathways that result in growth progression, invasion and migration (Green et al., 2009; Hiscox et al., 2011; Inoki et al., 2002; Kim et al., 2009; Parsons et al., 2008; Stupp & Ruegg, 2007).

The different immunotherapeutic models that have been tested for the treatment of HL include unconjugated monoclonal antibodies (Ansell et al., 2007; Bartlett et al., 2008; Klimm et al., 2005), immunotoxins (Falini et al., 1992; Kreitman et al., 2000), radioimmunoconjugates (Klimm et al., 2005; Schnell et al., 2005) and, most recently, immunomodulatory compounds (Bollard et al., 2004; Borchmann et al., 2002; Davies et al., 2001; Hartmann et al., 2001; Hartmann et al., 1997; Maier & Hammond, 2006; Roskrow et al., 1998). Some strategies, in particular radioimmunotherapeutic approaches and immunotoxins have already shown significant effectivity (Friedberg, 2011). First experiences with relatively non-toxic immunomodulatory compounds have implemented a whole new kind of immunotherapy in NLPHL where the anti-CD20-antibody Rituximab might be the future effective but less toxic treatment (Ekstrand et al., 2003; Schulz et al., 2008).

The integration of the new biologic markers evaluated in HL, that clearly driving force for an abnormal local and systemic antitumor immunity in HL, make of HL an ideal candidate for immunotherapeutic strategies (Rathore & Kadin, 2010; Younes, 2009). The pro-survival and pro-death receptors expressed by tumoral cells are currently being explored for novel treatment strategies by using a variety of naked and conjugated monoclonal antibodies. Furthermore, signaling pathways triggered by these receptors and other intracellular proteins can now be therapeutically inhibited by a variety of small molecules. Nowadays, the present challenge remains to know the best way to implement immunotherapeutic concepts into the current treatment concepts of HL in order to conserve or even improve the good long term survival in these patients and to reduce toxicity and long-term side-effects.

12. Conclusion

Although the relatively good prognosis and high current overall cure rate of cHL, it is important to underscore that clinicobiological factors still remain the main information to guide treatment policies in HL. Due to the fact that this disease is commonly diagnosed in young population, and antineoplastic treatments may induce worrying iatrogenic consequences in terms of secondary tumors (solid and hematologic malignancies), cardiopathies or respiratory long-term morbidities among others, it is indispensable to administer always the minimum effective and curative therapy. In this sense, beyond the well known clinical risk factors, interim information in the course of chemotherapy of PET scans will probably aid in the next future to apply a less empiric and more tailored and personalized treatment. Since early 90´s ABVD schedule represent the standard treatment of HL for curative purposes worldwide and little has changed in clinical practice in the last two decades. However there is room for improvement since a significant percentage of patients will ultimately relapse after successful treatment.

The recent research activities led to a better understanding of the phenotype, molecular characteristics, histogenesis, and possible mechanisms of HL lymphomagenesis. There is complete consensus on the B-cell derivation of the tumor in most cases, and on the relevance of EBV infection and defective cytokinesis in at least a proportion of patients. The influence of the cellular components of the microenvironment and that of the elaborate network of interactions they produce, on the clinical course of HL, has progressively emerged over the past decades. The expression of a variety of cytokines and chemokines by the tumoral cells is believed to drive an abnormal immune response and additional factors secreted by reactive cells in the microenvironment help to maintain the inflammatory milieu. In these conditions, tumoral cells manipulate microenvironment, permitting them to develop their malignant phenotype fully and evade host immune response attack. The interplay between tumoral cells and the reactive microenvironment determines not only the histological morphology and classification but also the clinicopathological features and prognosis of these patients. Genes and proteins expression signatures derived from immune cells have demonstrated to correlate well with response to treatments the outcome of HL patients respectively. This could be critical to the development of adoptive T-cell therapies that target the virus or different cell components of HL microenvironment. In aggressive HL, the development of prognostic systems modelled on the integration of biologic prognostic markers appears essential for more appropriate risk stratification.

New knowledge about impact of chemotherapy upon microenvironment has changed old paradigms, conferring to some cytotoxic agents like anthracyclines immunogenic properties that can explain the final mechanism of action of these drugs. These discoveries are extremely important since give a strong rationale to exploit this activity in the context of combinatorial strategies that might include other immunogenic agents like cytokines and monoclonal antibodies, among others. Therefore, it is conceivable to hypothesize that chemotherapy can still improve its efficacy in HL in the next future. Furthermore, recently new molecules have shown impressive clinical activity in HL. It is the case of the antibody-drug conjugate anti-CD30 brentuximab vedotin that have obtained very promising results in relapsed $CD30^{+}$ lymphomas, and thus has given place to ongoing phase III confirmatory studies.

To summarize, the incorporation of PET scans in HL diagnostic and follow-up algorithms, the widespread use of the new prognostic molecular and biological factors at diagnosis, the new highly effective molecules and the recent knowledge regarding chemotherapy effects on microenviroment, permit forsee a different and customized therapeutical approach to HL in the next future.

13. References

Abele, M.C.; Valente, G.; Kerim, S.; Navone, R.; Onesti, P.; Chiusa, L.; Resegotti, L. & Palestro, G. (1997). Significance of cell proliferation index in assessing histological prognostic categories in Hodgkin's disease. An immunohistochemical study with Ki67 and MIB-1 monoclonal antibodies. *Haematologica,* Vol.82, No.3, pp. 281-285, 0390-6078

Adam, C.; King, S.; Allgeier, T.; Braumuller, H.; Luking, C.; Mysliwietz, J.; Kriegeskorte, A.; Busch, D.H.; Rocken, M. & Mocikat, R. (2005). DC-NK cell cross talk as a novel

CD4+ T-cell-independent pathway for antitumor CTL induction. *Blood,* Vol.106, No.1, pp. 338-344, 0006-4971

Adam, J.K.; Odhav, B. & Bhoola, K.D. (2003). Immune responses in cancer. *Pharmacol Ther,* Vol.99, No.1, pp. 113-132, 0163-7258

Adams, H.; Campidelli, C.; Dirnhofer, S.; Pileri, S.A. & Tzankov, A. (2009). Clinical, phenotypic and genetic similarities and disparities between post-transplant and classical Hodgkin lymphomas with respect to therapeutic targets. *Expert Opin Ther Targets,* Vol.13, No.10, pp. 1137-1145, 1744-7631

Akbar, A.N.; Borthwick, N.J.; Wickremasinghe, R.G.; Panayoitidis, P.; Pilling, D.; Bofill, M.; Krajewski, S.; Reed, J.C. & Salmon, M. (1996). Interleukin-2 receptor common gamma-chain signaling cytokines regulate activated T cell apoptosis in response to growth factor withdrawal: selective induction of anti-apoptotic (bcl-2, bcl-xL) but not pro-apoptotic (bax, bcl-xS) gene expression. *Eur J Immunol,* Vol.26, No.2, pp. 294-299, 0014-2980

Aldinucci, D.; Lorenzon, D.; Cattaruzza, L.; Pinto, A.; Gloghini, A.; Carbone, A. & Colombatti, A. (2008). Expression of CCR5 receptors on Reed-Sternberg cells and Hodgkin lymphoma cell lines: involvement of CCL5/Rantes in tumor cell growth and microenvironmental interactions. *Int J Cancer,* Vol.122, No.4, pp. 769-776, 1097-0215

Aldinucci, D.; Olivo, K.; Lorenzon, D.; Poletto, D.; Gloghini, A.; Carbone, A. & Pinto, A. (2005). The role of interleukin-3 in classical Hodgkin's disease. *Leuk Lymphoma,* Vol.46, No.3, pp. 303-311, 1042-8194

Allavena, P.; Signorelli, M.; Chieppa, M.; Erba, E.; Bianchi, G.; Marchesi, F.; Olimpio, C.O.; Bonardi, C.; Garbi, A.; Lissoni, A.; de Braud, F.; Jimeno, J. & D'Incalci, M. (2005). Anti-inflammatory properties of the novel antitumor agent yondelis (trabectedin): inhibition of macrophage differentiation and cytokine production. *Cancer Res,* Vol.65, No.7, pp. 2964-2971, 0008-5472

Alvaro-Naranjo, T.; Lejeune, M.; Salvado-Usach, M.T.; Bosch-Princep, R.; Reverter-Branchat, G.; Jaen-Martinez, J. & Pons-Ferre, L.E. (2005). Tumor-infiltrating cells as a prognostic factor in Hodgkin's lymphoma: a quantitative tissue microarray study in a large retrospective cohort of 267 patients. *Leuk Lymphoma,* Vol.46, No.11, pp. 1581-1591, 1042-8194

Alvaro, T.; de la Cruz-Merino, L.; Henao-Carrasco, F.; Villar Rodriguez, J.L.; Vicente Baz, D.; Codes Manuel de Villena, M. & Provencio, M. (2010). Tumor microenvironment and immune effects of antineoplastic therapy in lymphoproliferative syndromes. *J Biomed Biotechnol,* Vol.2010, pp. , 1110-7251

Alvaro, T.; Lejeune, M.; Escriva, P.; Pons, L.E.; Bosch, R.; Jaen, J.; Lopez, C.; Salvado, M.T. & de Sanjose, S. (2009). Appraisal of immune response in lymphoproliferative syndromes: a systematic review. *Crit Rev Oncol Hematol,* Vol.70, No.2, pp. 103-113, 1879-0461

Alvaro, T.; Lejeune, M.; Garcia, J.F.; Salvado, M.T.; Lopez, C.; Bosch, R.; Jaen, J.; Escriva, P. & Pons, L.E. (2008). Tumor-infiltrated immune response correlates with alterations in the apoptotic and cell cycle pathways in Hodgkin and Reed-Sternberg cells. *Clin Cancer Res,* Vol.14, No.3, pp. 685-691, 1078-0432

Alvaro, T.; Lejeune, M.; Salvado, M.T.; Bosch, R.; Garcia, J.F.; Jaen, J.; Banham, A.H.; Roncador, G.; Montalban, C. & Piris, M.A. (2005). Outcome in Hodgkin's lymphoma can be predicted from the presence of accompanying cytotoxic and regulatory T cells. *Clin Cancer Res,* Vol.11, No.4, pp. 1467-1473, 1078-0432

Anagnostopoulos, I.; Hansmann, M.L.; Franssila, K.; Harris, M.; Harris, N.L.; Jaffe, E.S.; Han, J.; van Krieken, J.M.; Poppema, S.; Marafioti, T.; Franklin, J.; Sextro, M.; Diehl, V. & Stein, H. (2000). European Task Force on Lymphoma project on lymphocyte predominance Hodgkin disease: histologic and immunohistologic analysis of submitted cases reveals 2 types of Hodgkin disease with a nodular growth pattern and abundant lymphocytes. *Blood,* Vol.96, No.5, pp. 1889-1899, 0006-4971

Ansell, S.M.; Horwitz, S.M.; Engert, A.; Khan, K.D.; Lin, T.; Strair, R.; Keler, T.; Graziano, R.; Blanset, D.; Yellin, M.; Fischkoff, S.; Assad, A. & Borchmann, P. (2007). Phase I/II study of an anti-CD30 monoclonal antibody (MDX-060) in Hodgkin's lymphoma and anaplastic large-cell lymphoma. *J Clin Oncol,* Vol.25, No.19, pp. 2764-2769, 1527-7755

Ansell, S.M.; Stenson, M.; Habermann, T.M.; Jelinek, D.F. & Witzig, T.E. (2001). Cd4+ T-cell immune response to large B-cell non-Hodgkin's lymphoma predicts patient outcome. *J Clin Oncol,* Vol.19, No.3, pp. 720-726, 0732-183X

Apetoh, L.; Ghiringhelli, F.; Tesniere, A.; Obeid, M.; Ortiz, C.; Criollo, A.; Mignot, G.; Maiuri, M.C.; Ullrich, E.; Saulnier, P.; Yang, H.; Amigorena, S.; Ryffel, B.; Barrat, F.J.; Saftig, P.; Levi, F.; Lidereau, R.; Nogues, C.; Mira, J.P.; Chompret, A.; Joulin, V.; Clavel-Chapelon, F.; Bourhis, J.; Andre, F.; Delaloge, S.; Tursz, T.; Kroemer, G. & Zitvogel, L. (2007). Toll-like receptor 4-dependent contribution of the immune system to anticancer chemotherapy and radiotherapy. *Nat Med,* Vol.13, No.9, pp. 1050-1059, 1078-8956

Ascani, S.; Zinzani, P.L.; Gherlinzoni, F.; Sabattini, E.; Briskomatis, A.; de Vivo, A.; Piccioli, M.; Fraternali Orcioni, G.; Pieri, F.; Goldoni, A.; Piccaluga, P.P.; Zallocco, D.; Burnelli, R.; Leoncini, L.; Falini, B.; Tura, S. & Pileri, S.A. (1997). Peripheral T-cell lymphomas. Clinico-pathologic study of 168 cases diagnosed according to the R.E.A.L. Classification. *Ann Oncol,* Vol.8, No.6, pp. 583-592, 0923-7534

Atkinson, E.A. & Bleackley, R.C. (1995). Mechanisms of lysis by cytotoxic T cells. *Crit Rev Immunol,* Vol.15, No.3-4, pp. 359-384, 1040-8401

Axdorph, U.; Sjoberg, J.; Grimfors, G.; Landgren, O.; Porwit-MacDonald, A. & Bjorkholm, M. (2000). Biological markers may add to prediction of outcome achieved by the International Prognostic Score in Hodgkin's disease. *Ann Oncol,* Vol.11, No.11, pp. 1405-1411, 0923-7534

Azuma, T.; Takahashi, T.; Kunisato, A.; Kitamura, T. & Hirai, H. (2003). Human CD4+ CD25+ regulatory T cells suppress NKT cell functions. *Cancer Res,* Vol.63, No.15, pp. 4516-4520, 0008-5472

Bai, M.; Papoudou-Bai, A.; Kitsoulis, P.; Horianopoulos, N.; Kamina, S.; Agnantis, N.J. & Kanavaros, P. (2005). Cell cycle and apoptosis deregulation in classical Hodgkin lymphomas. *In Vivo,* Vol.19, No.2, pp. 439-453, 0258-851X

Bai, M.; Tsanou, E.; Agnantis, N.J.; Chaidos, A.; Dimou, D.; Skyrlas, A.; Dimou, S.; Vlychou, M.; Galani, V. & Kanavaros, P. (2003). Expression of cyclin D3 and cyclin E and identification of distinct clusters of proliferation and apoptosis in diffuse large B-cell lymphomas. *Histol Histopathol,* Vol.18, No.2, pp. 449-457, 0213-3911

Banciu, M.; Metselaar, J.M.; Schiffelers, R.M. & Storm, G. (2008). Antitumor activity of liposomal prednisolone phosphate depends on the presence of functional tumor-associated macrophages in tumor tissue. *Neoplasia,* Vol.10, No.2, pp. 108-117, 1476-5586

Bargou, R.C.; Emmerich, F.; Krappmann, D.; Bommert, K.; Mapara, M.Y.; Arnold, W.; Royer, H.D.; Grinstein, E.; Greiner, A.; Scheidereit, C. & Dorken, B. (1997). Constitutive nuclear factor-kappaB-RelA activation is required for proliferation and survival of Hodgkin's disease tumor cells. *J Clin Invest,* Vol.100, No.12, pp. 2961-2969, 0021-9738

Barth, T.F.; Martin-Subero, J.I.; Joos, S.; Menz, C.K.; Hasel, C.; Mechtersheimer, G.; Parwaresch, R.M.; Lichter, P.; Siebert, R. & Mooller, P. (2003). Gains of 2p involving the REL locus correlate with nuclear c-Rel protein accumulation in neoplastic cells of classical Hodgkin lymphoma. *Blood,* Vol.101, No.9, pp. 3681-3686, 0006-4971

Bartlett, N.L.; Younes, A.; Carabasi, M.H.; Forero, A.; Rosenblatt, J.D.; Leonard, J.P.; Bernstein, S.H.; Bociek, R.G.; Lorenz, J.M.; Hart, B.W. & Barton, J. (2008). A phase 1 multidose study of SGN-30 immunotherapy in patients with refractory or recurrent CD30+ hematologic malignancies. *Blood,* Vol.111, No.4, pp. 1848-1854, 0006-4971, 0006-4971

Baumforth, K.R.; Birgersdotter, A.; Reynolds, G.M.; Wei, W.; Kapatai, G.; Flavell, J.R.; Kalk, E.; Piper, K.; Lee, S.; Machado, L.; Hadley, K.; Sundblad, A.; Sjoberg, J.; Bjorkholm, M.; Porwit, A.A.; Yap, L.F.; Teo, S.; Grundy, R.G.; Young, L.S.; Ernberg, I.; Woodman, C.B. & Murray, P.G. (2008). Expression of the Epstein-Barr virus-encoded Epstein-Barr virus nuclear antigen 1 in Hodgkin's lymphoma cells mediates Up-regulation of CCL20 and the migration of regulatory T cells. *Am J Pathol,* Vol.173, No.1, pp. 195-204, 1525-2191

Berke, G. (1995). The CTL's kiss of death. *Cell,* Vol.81, No.1, pp. 9-12, 0092-8674

Bladergroen, B.A.; Meijer, C.J.; ten Berge, R.L.; Hack, C.E.; Muris, J.J.; Dukers, D.F.; Chott, A.; Kazama, Y.; Oudejans, J.J.; van Berkum, O. & Kummer, J.A. (2002). Expression of the granzyme B inhibitor, protease inhibitor 9, by tumor cells in patients with non-Hodgkin and Hodgkin lymphoma: a novel protective mechanism for tumor cells to circumvent the immune system? *Blood,* Vol.99, No.1, pp. 232-237.

Blanchard, D.A.; Affredou, M.T. & Vazquez, A. (1997). Modulation of the p27kip1 cyclin-dependent kinase inhibitor expression during IL-4-mediated human B cell activation. *J Immunol,* Vol.158, No.7, pp. 3054-3061, 0022-1767

Bollard, C.M.; Aguilar, L.; Straathof, K.C.; Gahn, B.; Huls, M.H.; Rousseau, A.; Sixbey, J.; Gresik, M.V.; Carrum, G.; Hudson, M.; Dilloo, D.; Gee, A.; Brenner, M.K.; Rooney, C.M. & Heslop, H.E. (2004). Cytotoxic T lymphocyte therapy for Epstein-Barr virus+ Hodgkin's disease. *J Exp Med,* Vol.200, No.12, pp. 1623-1633, 0022-1007

Borchmann, P.; Schnell, R.; Fuss, I.; Manzke, O.; Davis, T.; Lewis, L.D.; Behnke, D.; Wickenhauser, C.; Schiller, P.; Diehl, V. & Engert, A. (2002). Phase 1 trial of the novel bispecific molecule H22xKi-4 in patients with refractory Hodgkin lymphoma. *Blood,* Vol.100, No.9, pp. 3101-3107, 0006-4971

Bosch Princep, R.; Lejeune, M.; Salvado Usach, M.T.; Jaen Martinez, J.; Pons Ferre, L.E. & Alvaro Naranjo, T. (2005). Decreased number of granzyme B+ activated CD8+ cytotoxic T lymphocytes in the inflammatory background of HIV-associated Hodgkin's lymphoma. *Ann Hematol,* Vol.84, No.10, pp. 661-666, 0939-5555

Bosshart, H. (2002). T helper cell activation in B-cell lymphomas. *J Clin Oncol,* Vol.20, No.12, pp. 2904-2905; author reply 2905, 0732-183X

Brauninger, A.; Schmitz, R.; Bechtel, D.; Renne, C.; Hansmann, M.L. & Kuppers, R. (2006). Molecular biology of Hodgkin's and Reed/Sternberg cells in Hodgkin's lymphoma *Int J Cancer,* Vol.118, No.8, pp. 1853-1861, 0020-7136

Brink, A.A.; Oudejans, J.J.; van den Brule, A.J.; Kluin, P.M.; Horstman, A.; Ossenkoppele, G.J.; van Heerde, P.; Jiwa, M. & Meijer, C.J. (1998). Low p53 and high bcl-2 expression in Reed-Sternberg cells predicts poor clinical outcome for Hodgkin's disease: involvement of apoptosis resistance? *Mod Pathol,* Vol.11, No.4, pp. 376-383, 0893-3952

Burnet, M. (1957). Cancer: a biological approach. III. Viruses associated with neoplastic conditions. IV. Practical applications. *Br Med J,* Vol.1, No.5023, pp. 841-847, 0007-1447

Burns, E.A. & Leventhal, E.A. (2000). Aging, immunity, and cancer. *Cancer Control,* Vol.7, No.6, pp. 513-522, 1073-2748

Calo, V.; Migliavacca, M.; Bazan, V.; Macaluso, M.; Buscemi, M.; Gebbia, N. & Russo, A. (2003). STAT proteins: from normal control of cellular events to tumorigenesis. *J Cell Physiol,* Vol.197, No.2, pp. 157-168, 0021-9541

Camilleri-Broet, S.; Ferme, C.; Berger, F.; Lepage, E.; Bain, S.; Briere, J.; Marmey, B.; Gaulard, P. & Audouin, J. (2004). TiA1 in advanced-stage classical Hodgkin's lymphoma: no prognostic impact for positive tumour cells or number of cytotoxic cells. *Virchows Arch,* Vol.445,N°4, pp. 344-346, 0945-6317

Campo, E.; Swerdlow, S.H.; Harris, N.L.; Pileri, S.; Stein, H. & Jaffe, E.S. (2011). The 2008 WHO classification of lymphoid neoplasms and beyond: evolving concepts and practical applications. *Blood,* Vol.117, No.19, pp. 5019-5032, 1528-0020

Canellos, G.P.; Anderson, J.R.; Propert, K.J.; Nissen, N.; Cooper, M.R.; Henderson, E.S.; Green, M.R.; Gottlieb, A. & Peterson, B.A. (1992). Chemotherapy of advanced Hodgkin's disease with MOPP, ABVD, or MOPP alternating with ABVD. *N Engl J Med,* Vol.327, No.21, pp. 1478-1484, 0028-4793

Carbone, A.; Gloghini, A.; Serraino, D. & Spina, M. (2009). HIV-associated Hodgkin lymphoma. *Curr Opin HIV AIDS,* Vol.4, No.1, pp. 3-10, 1746-6318

Casey, T.T.; Olson, S.J.; Cousar, J.B. & Collins, R.D. (1989). Immunophenotypes of Reed-Sternberg cells: a study of 19 cases of Hodgkin's disease in plastic-embedded sections. *Blood,* Vol.74, No.8, pp. 2624-2628, 0006-4971

Chetaille, B.; Bertucci, F.; Finetti, P.; Esterni, B.; Stamatoullas, A.; Picquenot, J.M.; Copin, M.C.; Morschhauser, F.; Casasnovas, O.; Petrella, T.; Molina, T.; Vekhoff, A.; Feugier, P.; Bouabdallah, R.; Birnbaum, D.; Olive, D. & Xerri, L. (2009). Molecular profiling of classical Hodgkin lymphoma tissues uncovers variations in the tumor microenvironment and correlations with EBV infection and outcome. *Blood,* Vol.113, No.12, pp. 2765-3775, 1528-0020

Chimienti, E.; Spina, M. & Gastaldi, R. (2008). Clinical characteristics and outcome of 290 patients (pts) with Hodgkin's disease and HIV infection (HD-HIV) in pre and HAART (highly active antiretroviral therapy) era. . *Ann Oncol* Vol.9 pp. iv136

Connors, J.M. (2005). State-of-the-art therapeutics: Hodgkin's lymphoma. *J Clin Oncol,* Vol.23, No.26, pp. 6400-6408, 0732-183X

Connors, J.M. (2011). Hodgkin's lymphoma--the great teacher. *N Engl J Med,* Vol.365, No.3, pp. 264-265, 1533-4406

Curiel, T.J.; Coukos, G.; Zou, L.; Alvarez, X.; Cheng, P.; Mottram, P.; Evdemon-Hogan, M.; Conejo-Garcia, J.R.; Zhang, L.; Burow, M.; Zhu, Y.; Wei, S.; Kryczek, I.; Daniel, B.; Gordon, A.; Myers, L.; Lackner, A.; Disis, M.L.; Knutson, K.L.; Chen, L. & Zou, W. (2004). Specific recruitment of regulatory T cells in ovarian carcinoma fosters immune privilege and predicts reduced survival. *Nat Med,* Vol.10, No.9, pp. 942-949, 1078-8956

Davies, F.E.; Raje, N.; Hideshima, T.; Lentzsch, S.; Young, G.; Tai, Y.T.; Lin, B.; Podar, K.; Gupta, D.; Chauhan, D.; Treon, S.P.; Richardson, P.G.; Schlossman, R.L.; Morgan, G.J.; Muller, G.W.; Stirling, D.I. & Anderson, K.C. (2001). Thalidomide and immunomodulatory derivatives augment natural killer cell cytotoxicity in multiple myeloma. *Blood,* Vol.98, No.1, pp. 210-216, 0006-4971

de la Cruz-Merino, L.; Grande-Pulido, E.; Albero-Tamarit, A. & Codes-Manuel de Villena, M.E. (2008). Cancer and immune response: old and new evidence for future challenges. *Oncologist,* Vol.13, No.12, pp. 1246-1254, 1549-490X

de Visser, K.E. & Kast, W.M. (1999). Effects of TGF-beta on the immune system: implications for cancer immunotherapy. *Leukemia,* Vol.13, No.8, pp. 1188-1199, 0887-6924

Deutsch, Y.E.; Tadmor, T.; Podack, E.R. & Rosenblatt, J.D. (2011). CD30: an important new target in hematologic malignancies. *Leuk Lymphoma,* Vol.52, No.9, pp. 1641-1654, 1029-2403

Devilard, E.; Bertucci, F.; Trempat, P.; Bouabdallah, R.; Loriod, B.; Giaconia, A.; Brousset, P.; Granjeaud, S.; Nguyen, C.; Birnbaum, D.; Birg, F.; Houlgatte, R. & Xerri, L. (2002). Gene expression profiling defines molecular subtypes of classical Hodgkin's disease. *Oncogene,* Vol.21, No.19, pp. 3095-3102, 0950-9232

Dharnidharka, V.R.; Douglas, V.K.; Hunger, S.P. & Fennell, R.S. (2004). Hodgkin's lymphoma after post-transplant lymphoproliferative disease in a renal transplant recipient. *Pediatr Transplant,* Vol.8, No.1, pp. 87-90, 1397-3142

Diehl, V.; Franklin, J.; Pfreundschuh, M.; Lathan, B.; Paulus, U.; Hasenclever, D.; Tesch, H.; Herrmann, R.; Dorken, B.; Muller-Hermelink, H.K.; Duhmke, E. & Loeffler, M. (2003). Standard and increased-dose BEACOPP chemotherapy compared with COPP-ABVD for advanced Hodgkin's disease. *N Engl J Med,* Vol.348, No.24, pp. 2386-2395, 1533-4406

Diehl, V.; Sextro, M.; Franklin, J.; Hansmann, M.L.; Harris, N.; Jaffe, E.; Poppema, S.; Harris, M.; Franssila, K.; van Krieken, J.; Marafioti, T.; Anagnostopoulos, I. & Stein, H. (1999). Clinical presentation, course, and prognostic factors in lymphocyte-predominant Hodgkin's disease and lymphocyte-rich classical Hodgkin's disease: report from the European Task Force on Lymphoma Project on Lymphocyte-Predominant Hodgkin's Disease. *J Clin Oncol,* Vol.17, No.3, pp. 776-783, 0732-183X

Diehl, V.; Thomas, R.K. & Re, D. (2004). Part II: Hodgkin's lymphoma--diagnosis and treatment. *Lancet Oncol,* Vol.5, No.1, pp. 19-26, 1470-2045

Dutton, A.; Reynolds, G.M.; Dawson, C.W.; Young, L.S. & Murray, P.G. (2005). Constitutive activation of phosphatidyl-inositide 3 kinase contributes to the survival of Hodgkin's lymphoma cells through a mechanism involving Akt kinase and mTOR. *J Pathol,* Vol.205, No.4, pp. 498-506, 0022-3417

Eberle, F.C.; Rodriguez-Canales, J.; Wei, L.; Hanson, J.C.; Killian, J.K.; Sun, H.W.; Adams, L.G.; Hewitt, S.M.; Wilson, W.H.; Pittaluga, S.; Meltzer, P.S.; Staudt, L.M.; Emmert-Buck, M.R. & Jaffe, E.S. (2011). Methylation profiling of mediastinal gray zone lymphoma reveals a distinctive signature with elements shared by classical Hodgkin's lymphoma and primary mediastinal large B-cell lymphoma. *Haematologica,* Vol.96, No.4, pp. 558-566, 1592-8721

Ekstrand, B.C.; Lucas, J.B.; Horwitz, S.M.; Fan, Z.; Breslin, S.; Hoppe, R.T.; Natkunam, Y.; Bartlett, N.L. & Horning, S.J. (2003). Rituximab in lymphocyte-predominant Hodgkin disease: results of a phase 2 trial. *Blood,* Vol.101, No.11, pp. 4285-4289, 0006-4971

Emmerich, F.; Meiser, M.; Hummel, M.; Demel, G.; Foss, H.D.; Jundt, F.; Mathas, S.; Krappmann, D.; Scheidereit, C.; Stein, H. & Dorken, B. (1999). Overexpression of I kappa B alpha without inhibition of NF-kappaB activity and mutations in the I kappa B alpha gene in Reed-Sternberg cells. *Blood,* Vol.94, No.9, pp. 3129-3134, 0006-4971

Emmerich, F.; Theurich, S.; Hummel, M.; Haeffker, A.; Vry, M.S.; Dohner, K.; Bommert, K.; Stein, H. & Dorken, B. (2003). Inactivating I kappa B epsilon mutations in Hodgkin/Reed-Sternberg cells. *J Pathol,* Vol.201, No.3, pp. 413-420, 0022-3417

Engert, A.; Plutschow, A.; Eich, H.T.; Lohri, A.; Dorken, B.; Borchmann, P.; Berger, B.; Greil, R.; Willborn, K.C.; Wilhelm, M.; Debus, J.; Eble, M.J.; Sokler, M.; Ho, A.; Rank, A.; Ganser, A.; Trumper, L.; Bokemeyer, C.; Kirchner, H.; Schubert, J.; Kral, Z.; Fuchs, M.; Muller-Hermelink, H.K.; Muller, R.P. & Diehl, V. (2010). Reduced treatment intensity in patients with early-stage Hodgkin's lymphoma. *N Engl J Med,* Vol.363, No.7, pp. 640-652, 1533-4406

Falini, B.; Bolognesi, A.; Flenghi, L.; Tazzari, P.L.; Broe, M.K.; Stein, H.; Durkop, H.; Aversa, F.; Corneli, P.; Pizzolo, G. & et al. (1992). Response of refractory Hodgkin's disease to monoclonal anti-CD30 immunotoxin. *Lancet,* Vol.339, No.8803, pp. 1195-1196, 0140-6736

Falini, B.; Pileri, S.; Stein, H.; Dieneman, D.; Dallenbach, F.; Delsol, G.; Minelli, O.; Poggi, S.; Martelli, M.F.; Pallesen, G. & et al. (1990). Variable expression of leucocyte-common (CD45) antigen in CD30 (Ki1)-positive anaplastic large-cell lymphoma: implications for the differential diagnosis between lymphoid and nonlymphoid malignancies. *Hum Pathol,* Vol.21, No.6, pp. 624-629, 0046-8177

Falini, B.; Stein, H.; Pileri, S.; Canino, S.; Farabbi, R.; Martelli, M.F.; Grignani, F.; Fagioli, M.; Minelli, O.; Ciani, C. & et al. (1987). Expression of lymphoid-associated antigens on Hodgkin's and Reed-Sternberg cells of Hodgkin's disease. An immunocytochemical study on lymph node cytospins using monoclonal antibodies. *Histopathology,* Vol.11, No.12, pp. 1229-1242, 0309-0167

Famularo, G.; De Simone, C.; Tzantzoglou, S. & Trinchieri, V. (1994). Apoptosis, anti-apoptotic compounds and TNF-alpha release. *Immunol Today,* Vol.15, No.10, pp. 495-496, 0167-5699

Farrell, K. & Jarrett, R.F. (2011). The molecular pathogenesis of Hodgkin lymphoma. *Histopathology,* Vol.58, No.1, pp. 15-25, 1365-2559

Filippa, D.A.; Ladanyi, M.; Wollner, N.; Straus, D.J.; O'Brien, J.P.; Portlock, C.; Gangi, M. & Sun, M. (1996). CD30 (Ki-1)-positive malignant lymphomas: clinical, immunophenotypic, histologic, and genetic characteristics and differences with Hodgkin's disease. *Blood,* Vol.87, No.7, pp. 2905-2917, 0006-4971

Fischer, M.; Juremalm, M.; Olsson, N.; Backlin, C.; Sundstrom, C.; Nilsson, K.; Enblad, G. & Nilsson, G. (2003). Expression of CCL5/RANTES by Hodgkin and Reed-Sternberg cells and its possible role in the recruitment of mast cells into lymphomatous tissue. *Int J Cancer,* Vol.107, No.2, pp. 197-201, 0020-7136

Fontenot, J.D.; Gavin, M.A. & Rudensky, A.Y. (2003). Foxp3 programs the development and function of CD4+CD25+ regulatory T cells. *Nat Immunol,* Vol.4, No.4, pp. 330-336,

Formenti, S.C. & Demaria, S. (2009). Systemic effects of local radiotherapy. *Lancet Oncol,* Vol.10, No.7, pp. 718-726, 1474-5488

Foss, H.D.; Reusch, R.; Demel, G.; Lenz, G.; Anagnostopoulos, I.; Hummel, M. & Stein, H. (1999). Frequent expression of the B-cell-specific activator protein in Reed-Sternberg cells of classical Hodgkin's disease provides further evidence for its B-cell origin. *Blood,* Vol.94, No.9, pp. 3108-3113, 0006-4971

Foyil, K.V. & Bartlett, N.L. (2010). Anti-CD30 Antibodies for Hodgkin lymphoma. *Curr Hematol Malig Rep,* Vol.5, No.3, pp. 140-147, 1558-822X

Friedberg, J.W. (2011). Hodgkin lymphoma: answers take time! *Blood,* Vol.117, No.20, pp. 5274-5276, 1528-0020

Frisan, T.; Sjoberg, J.; Dolcetti, R.; Boiocchi, M.; De Re, V.; Carbone, A.; Brautbar, C.; Battat, S.; Biberfeld, P.; Eckman, M. & et al. (1995). Local suppression of Epstein-Barr virus (EBV)-specific cytotoxicity in biopsies of EBV-positive Hodgkin's disease. *Blood,* Vol.86, No.4, pp. 1493-1501, 0006-4971

Gallamini, A.; Hutchings, M.; Rigacci, L.; Specht, L.; Merli, F.; Hansen, M.; Patti, C.; Loft, A.; Di Raimondo, F.; D'Amore, F.; Biggi, A.; Vitolo, U.; Stelitano, C.; Sancetta, R.; Trentin, L.; Luminari, S.; Iannitto, E.; Viviani, S.; Pierri, I. & Levis, A. (2007). Early interim 2-[18F]fluoro-2-deoxy-D-glucose positron emission tomography is prognostically superior to international prognostic score in advanced-stage Hodgkin's lymphoma: a report from a joint Italian-Danish study. *J Clin Oncol,* Vol.25, No.24, pp. 3746-3752, 1527-7755

Garcia, J.F.; Camacho, F.I.; Morente, M.; Fraga, M.; Montalban, C.; Alvaro, T.; Bellas, C.; Castano, A.; Diez, A.; Flores, T.; Martin, C.; Martinez, M.A.; Mazorra, F.; Menarguez, J.; Mestre, M.J.; Mollejo, M.; Saez, A.I.; Sanchez, L. & Piris, M.A. (2003). Hodgkin and Reed-Sternberg cells harbor alterations in the major tumor suppressor pathways and cell-cycle checkpoints: analyses using tissue microarrays. *Blood,* Vol.101, No.2, pp. 681-689, 0006-4971

Garcia, J.F.; Villuendas, R.; Algara, P.; Saez, A.I.; Sanchez-Verde, L.; Martinez-Montero, J.C.; Martinez, P. & Piris, M.A. (1999). Loss of p16 protein expression associated with methylation of the p16INK4A gene is a frequent finding in Hodgkin's disease. *Lab Invest,* Vol.79, No.12, pp. 1453-1459, 0023-6837

Gaulard, P.; Swerdlow, S.; Harris, S. & al., e. (2008). Other iatrogenic immunodeficiencyassociated lymphoproliferative disorders. In: *World Health Organization Classification of Tumours, Pathology and Genetics of Tumours of Haematopoietic and Lymphoid Tissues.,* Swerdlow SH C.E., Harris NL, et al. (eds) (eds),350-351. IARC Press Lyon

Gerdes, J.; Van Baarlen, J.; Pileri, S.; Schwarting, R.; Van Unnik, J.A. & Stein, H. (1987). Tumor cell growth fraction in Hodgkin's disease. *Am J Pathol,* Vol.128, No.3, pp. 390-393, 0002-9440

Gonthier, M.; Llobera, R.; Arnaud, J. & Rubin, B. (2004). Self-reactive T cell receptor-reactive CD8+ T cells inhibit T cell lymphoma growth in vivo. *J Immunol,* Vol.173, No.11, pp. 7062-7069, 0022-1767

Goyal, R.K.; McEvoy, L. & Wilson, D.B. (1996). Hodgkin disease after renal transplantation in childhood. *J Pediatr Hematol Oncol,* Vol.18, No.4, pp. 392-395, 1077-4114

Green, T.P.; Fennell, M.; Whittaker, R.; Curwen, J.; Jacobs, V.; Allen, J.; Logie, A.; Hargreaves, J.; Hickinson, D.M.; Wilkinson, R.W.; Elvin, P.; Boyer, B.; Carragher, N.; Ple, P.A.; Bermingham, A.; Holdgate, G.A.; Ward, W.H.; Hennequin, L.F.; Davies, B.R. & Costello, G.F. (2009). Preclinical anticancer activity of the potent, oral Src inhibitor AZD0530. *Mol Oncol,* Vol.3, No.3, pp. 248-261, 1574-7891

Grogg, K.L.; Miller, R.F. & Dogan, A. (2007). HIV infection and lymphoma. *J Clin Pathol,* Vol.60, No.12, pp. 1365-1372, 1472-4146

Gruss, H.J.; Brach, M.A.; Drexler, H.G.; Bonifer, R.; Mertelsmann, R.H. & Herrmann, F. (1992). Expression of cytokine genes, cytokine receptor genes, and transcription factors in cultured Hodgkin and Reed-Sternberg cells. *Cancer Res,* Vol.52, No.12, pp. 3353-3360, 0008-5472

Guenova, M.; Rassidakis, G.Z.; Gorgoulis, V.G.; Angelopoulou, M.K.; Siakantaris, M.R.; Kanavaros, P.; Pangalis, G.A. & Kittas, C. (1999). p16INK4A is regularly expressed in Hodgkin's disease: comparison with retinoblastoma, p53 and MDM2 protein status, and the presence of Epstein-Barr virus. *Mod Pathol,* Vol.12, No.11, pp. 1062-1071, 0893-3952

Hagemann, T.; Lawrence, T.; McNeish, I.; Charles, K.A.; Kulbe, H.; Thompson, R.G.; Robinson, S.C. & Balkwill, F.R. (2008). "Re-educating" tumor-associated macrophages by targeting NF-kappaB. *J Exp Med,* Vol.205, No.6, pp. 1261-1268, 1540-9538

Hahne, M.; Renno, T.; Schroeter, M.; Irmler, M.; French, L.; Bornard, T.; MacDonald, H.R. & Tschopp, J. (1996). Activated B cells express functional Fas ligand. *Eur J Immunol,* Vol.26, No.3, pp. 721-724, 0014-2980

Hanamoto, H.; Nakayama, T.; Miyazato, H.; Takegawa, S.; Hieshima, K.; Tatsumi, Y.; Kanamaru, A. & Yoshie, O. (2004). Expression of CCL28 by Reed-Sternberg cells defines a major subtype of classical Hodgkin's disease with frequent infiltration of eosinophils and/or plasma cells. *Am J Pathol,* Vol.164, No.3, pp. 997-1006, 0002-9440

Haque, T.; Wilkie, G.M.; Jones, M.M.; Higgins, C.D.; Urquhart, G.; Wingate, P.; Burns, D.; McAulay, K.; Turner, M.; Bellamy, C.; Amlot, P.L.; Kelly, D.; MacGilchrist, A.; Gandhi, M.K.; Swerdlow, A.J.; Crawford, D.H. (2007). Allogeneic cytotoxic T cell therapy for EBV-positive posttransplantation lymphoproliferative disease: results of a phase 2 multicenter clinical trial. *Blood,* Vol. 110, No.4, pp 1123-31, 0006-4971

Harris, N.L.; Jaffe, E.S.; Diebold, J.; Flandrin, G.; Muller-Hermelink, H.K.; Vardiman, J.; Lister, T.A. & Bloomfield, C.D. (2000). The World Health Organization classification of neoplastic diseases of the haematopoietic and lymphoid tissues: Report of the Clinical Advisory Committee Meeting, Airlie House, Virginia, November 1997. *Histopathology,* Vol.36, No.1, pp. 69-86, 0309-0167

Harris, N.L.; Jaffe, E.S.; Stein, H.; Banks, P.M.; Chan, J.K.; Cleary, M.L.; Delsol, G.; De Wolf-Peeters, C.; Falini, B.; Gatter, K.C. & et al. (1994). A revised European-American classification of lymphoid neoplasms: a proposal from the International Lymphoma Study Group. *Blood,* Vol.84, No.5, pp. 1361-1392, 0006-4971

Hartmann, F.; Renner, C.; Jung, W.; da Costa, L.; Tembrink, S.; Held, G.; Sek, A.; Konig, J.; Bauer, S.; Kloft, M. & Pfreundschuh, M. (2001). Anti-CD16/CD30 bispecific antibody treatment for Hodgkin's disease: role of infusion schedule and costimulation with cytokines. *Clin Cancer Res,* Vol.7, No.7, pp. 1873-1881, 1078-0432

Hartmann, F.; Renner, C.; Jung, W.; Deisting, C.; Juwana, M.; Eichentopf, B.; Kloft, M. & Pfreundschuh, M. (1997). Treatment of refractory Hodgkin's disease with an anti-CD16/CD30 bispecific antibody. *Blood,* Vol.89, No.6, pp. 2042-2047, 0006-4971

Hasenclever, D. & Diehl, V. (1998). A prognostic score for advanced Hodgkin's disease. International Prognostic Factors Project on Advanced Hodgkin's Disease. *N Engl J Med,* Vol.339, No.21, pp. 1506-1514, 0028-4793

Haynes, N.M.; van der Most, R.G.; Lake, R.A. & Smyth, M.J. (2008). Immunogenic anti-cancer chemotherapy as an emerging concept. *Curr Opin Immunol,* Vol.20, No.5, pp. 545-557, 0952-7915

Hertel, C.B.; Zhou, X.G.; Hamilton-Dutoit, S.J. & Junker, S. (2002). Loss of B cell identity correlates with loss of B cell-specific transcription factors in Hodgkin/Reed-Sternberg cells of classical Hodgkin lymphoma. *Oncogene,* Vol.21, No.32, pp. 4908-4920, 0950-9232

Hinz, M.; Lemke, P.; Anagnostopoulos, I.; Hacker, C.; Krappmann, D.; Mathas, S.; Dorken, B.; Zenke, M.; Stein, H. & Scheidereit, C. (2002). Nuclear factor kappaB-dependent gene expression profiling of Hodgkin's disease tumor cells, pathogenetic significance, and link to constitutive signal transducer and activator of transcription 5a activity. *J Exp Med,* Vol.196, No.5, pp. 605-617, 0022-1007

Hinz, M.; Loser, P.; Mathas, S.; Krappmann, D.; Dorken, B. & Scheidereit, C. (2001). Constitutive NF-kappaB maintains high expression of a characteristic gene network, including CD40, CD86, and a set of antiapoptotic genes in Hodgkin/Reed-Sternberg cells. *Blood,* Vol.97, No.9, pp. 2798-2807, 0006-4971

Hiscox, S.; Barrett-Lee, P. & Nicholson, R.I. (2011). Therapeutic targeting of tumor-stroma interactions. *Expert Opin Ther Targets,* Vol.15, No.5, pp. 609-621, 1744-7631

Hislop, A.D.; Annels, N.E.; Gudgeon, N.H.; Leese, A.M. & Rickinson, A.B. (2002). Epitope-specific evolution of human CD8(+) T cell responses from primary to persistent phases of Epstein-Barr virus infection. *J Exp Med,* Vol.195, No.7, pp. 893-905, 0022-1007

Hnatkova, M.; Mocikova, H.; Trneny, M. & Zivny, J. (2009). The biological environment of Hodgkin's lymphoma and the role of the chemokine CCL17/TARC. *Prague Med Rep,* Vol.110, No.1, pp. 35-41, 1214-6994

Hong, S.Y.; Yoon, W.H.; Park, J.H.; Kang, S.G.; Ahn, J.H. & Lee, T.H. (2000). Involvement of two NF-kappa B binding elements in tumor necrosis factor alpha -, CD40-, and epstein-barr virus latent membrane protein 1-mediated induction of the cellular inhibitor of apoptosis protein 2 gene. *J Biol Chem,* Vol.275, No.24, pp. 18022-18028, 0021-9258

Hori, S.; Nomura, T. & Sakaguchi, S. (2003). Control of regulatory T cell development by the transcription factor Foxp3. *Science,* Vol.299, No.5609, pp. 1057-1061, 0036-8075

Horie, R.; Watanabe, T.; Morishita, Y.; Ito, K.; Ishida, T.; Kanegae, Y.; Saito, I.; Higashihara, M.; Mori, S.; Kadin, M.E. & Watanabe, T. (2002). Ligand-independent signaling by overexpressed CD30 drives NF-kappaB activation in Hodgkin-Reed-Sternberg cells. *Oncogene,* Vol.21, No.16, pp. 2493-2503, 0950-9232

Hsu, S.M.; Krupen, K. & Lachman, L.B. (1989). Heterogeneity of interleukin 1 production in cultured Reed-Sternberg cell lines HDLM-1, HDLM-1d, and KM-H2. *Am J Pathol*, Vol.135, No.1, pp. 33-38, 0002-9440

Hutchings, M.; Mikhaeel, N.G.; Fields, P.A.; Nunan, T. & Timothy, A.R. (2005). Prognostic value of interim FDG-PET after two or three cycles of chemotherapy in Hodgkin lymphoma. *Ann Oncol*, Vol.16, No.7, pp. 1160-1168, 0923-7534

Ichim, C.V. (2005). Revisiting immunosurveillance and immunostimulation: Implications for cancer immunotherapy. *J Transl Med*, Vol.3, No.1, pp. 8, 1479-5876, 1479-5876

Ikeda, H.; Old, L.J. & Schreiber, R.D. (2002). The roles of IFN gamma in protection against tumor development and cancer immunoediting. *Cytokine Growth Factor Rev*, Vol.13, No.2, pp. 95-109, 1359-6101

Inoki, K.; Li, Y.; Zhu, T.; Wu, J. & Guan, K.L. (2002). TSC2 is phosphorylated and inhibited by Akt and suppresses mTOR signalling. *Nat Cell Biol*, Vol.4, No.9, pp. 648-657, 1465-7392

Inoue, J.; Ishida, T.; Tsukamoto, N.; Kobayashi, N.; Naito, A.; Azuma, S. & Yamamoto, T. (2000). Tumor necrosis factor receptor-associated factor (TRAF) family: adapter proteins that mediate cytokine signaling. *Exp Cell Res*, Vol.254, No.1, pp. 14-24, 0014-4827

Izban, K.F.; Ergin, M.; Huang, Q.; Qin, J.Z.; Martinez, R.L.; Schnitzer, B.; Ni, H.; Nickoloff, B.J. & Alkan, S. (2001). Characterization of NF-kappaB expression in Hodgkin's disease: inhibition of constitutively expressed NF-kappaB results in spontaneous caspase-independent apoptosis in Hodgkin and Reed-Sternberg cells. *Mod Pathol*, Vol.14, No.4, pp. 297-310, 0893-3952

Jarrett, R.F. (2002). Viruses and Hodgkin's lymphoma. *Ann Oncol*, Vol.13 Suppl 1, pp. 23-29, 0923-7534

Jarrett, R.F. (2006). Viruses and lymphoma/leukaemia. *J Pathol*, Vol.208, No.2, pp. 176-186, 0022-3417

Joos, S.; Granzow, M.; Holtgreve-Grez, H.; Siebert, R.; Harder, L.; Martin-Subero, J.I.; Wolf, J.; Adamowicz, M.; Barth, T.F.; Lichter, P. & Jauch, A. (2003). Hodgkin's lymphoma cell lines are characterized by frequent aberrations on chromosomes 2p and 9p including REL and JAK2. *Int J Cancer*, Vol.103, No.4, pp. 489-495, 0020-7136

Joos, S.; Menz, C.K.; Wrobel, G.; Siebert, R.; Gesk, S.; Ohl, S.; Mechtersheimer, G.; Trumper, L.; Moller, P.; Lichter, P. & Barth, T.F. (2002). Classical Hodgkin lymphoma is characterized by recurrent copy number gains of the short arm of chromosome 2. *Blood*, Vol.99, No.4, pp. 1381-1387, 0006-4971

Jourdan, M.; De Vos, J.; Mechti, N. & Klein, B. (2000). Regulation of Bcl-2-family proteins in myeloma cells by three myeloma survival factors: interleukin-6, interferon-alpha and insulin-like growth factor 1. *Cell Death Differ*, Vol.7, No.12, pp. 1244-1252, 1350-9047

Jungnickel, B.; Staratschek-Jox, A.; Brauninger, A.; Spieker, T.; Wolf, J.; Diehl, V.; Hansmann, M.L.; Rajewsky, K. & Kuppers, R. (2000). Clonal deleterious mutations in the IkappaBalpha gene in the malignant cells in Hodgkin's lymphoma. *J Exp Med*, Vol.191, No.2, pp. 395-402, 0022-1007

Juszczynski, P.; Ouyang, J.; Monti, S.; Rodig, S.J.; Takeyama, K.; Abramson, J.; Chen, W.; Kutok, J.L.; Rabinovich, G.A. & Shipp, M.A. (2007). The AP1-dependent secretion of galectin-1 by Reed Sternberg cells fosters immune privilege in classical Hodgkin lymphoma. *Proc Natl Acad Sci U S A,* Vol.104, No.32, pp. 13134-13139, 0027-8424

Kamper, P.; Bendix, K.; Hamilton-Dutoit, S.; Honore, B.; Nyengaard, J.R. & d'Amore, F. (2011). Tumor-infiltrating macrophages correlate with adverse prognosis and Epstein-Barr virus status in classical Hodgkin's lymphoma. *Haematologica,* Vol.96, No.2, pp. 269-276, 1592-8721

Kanavaros, P.; Stefanaki, K.; Vlachonikolis, J.; Eliopoulos, G.; Kakolyris, S.; Rontogianni, D.; Gorgoulis, V. & Georgoulias, V. (2000). Expression of p53, p21/waf1, bcl-2, bax, Rb and Ki67 proteins in Hodgkin's lymphomas. *Histol Histopathol,* Vol.15, No.2, pp. 445-453, 0213-3911

Kanavaros, P.; Vlychou, M.; Stefanaki, K.; Rontogianni, D.; Gaulard, P.; Pantelidaki, E.; Zois, M.; Darivianaki, K.; Georgoulias, V.; Boulland, M.L.; Gorgoulis, V. & Kittas, C. (1999). Cytotoxic protein expression in non-Hodgkin's lymphomas and Hodgkin's disease. *Anticancer Res,* Vol.19, No.2A, pp. 1209-1216, 0250-7005

Kanzler, H.; Kuppers, R.; Hansmann, M.L. & Rajewsky, K. (1996). Hodgkin and Reed-Sternberg cells in Hodgkin's disease represent the outgrowth of a dominant tumor clone derived from (crippled) germinal center B cells. *J Exp Med,* Vol.184, No.4, pp. 1495-1505, 0022-1007

Kapatai, G. & Murray, P. (2007). Contribution of the Epstein Barr virus to the molecular pathogenesis of Hodgkin lymphoma. *J Clin Pathol,* Vol.60, No.12, pp. 1342-1349, 1472-4146

Karin, M. & Greten, F.R. (2005). NF-kappaB: linking inflammation and immunity to cancer development and progression. *Nat Rev Immunol,* Vol.5, No.10, pp. 749-759, 1474-1733

Karube, K.; Ohshima, K.; Tsuchiya, T.; Yamaguchi, T.; Kawano, R.; Suzumiya, J.; Utsunomiya, A.; Harada, M. & Kikuchi, M. (2004). Expression of FoxP3, a key molecule in CD4CD25 regulatory T cells, in adult T-cell leukaemia/lymphoma cells. *Br J Haematol,* Vol.126, No.1, pp. 81-84, 0007-1048

Kasamon, Y.L.; Ambinder, R.F. (2008). Immunotherapies for Hodgkin´s lymphoma. *Crit Rev Oncol Hematol,* Vol. 66, No.2, pp 135-144, 1040-8428

Kater, A.P.; Evers, L.M.; Remmerswaal, E.B.; Jaspers, A.; Oosterwijk, M.F.; van Lier, R.A.; van Oers, M.H. & Eldering, E. (2004). CD40 stimulation of B-cell chronic lymphocytic leukaemia cells enhances the anti-apoptotic profile, but also Bid expression and cells remain susceptible to autologous cytotoxic T-lymphocyte attack. *Br J Haematol,* Vol.127, No.4, pp. 404-415, 0007-1048

Kato, M.; Sanada, M.; Kato, I.; Sato, Y.; Takita, J.; Takeuchi, K.; Niwa, A.; Chen, Y.; Nakazaki, K.; Nomoto, J.; Asakura, Y.; Muto, S.; Tamura, A.; Iio, M.; Akatsuka, Y.; Hayashi, Y.; Mori, H.; Igarashi, T.; Kurokawa, M.; Chiba, S.; Mori, S.; Ishikawa, Y.; Okamoto, K.; Tobinai, K.; Nakagama, H.; Nakahata, T.; Yoshino, T.; Kobayashi, Y. & Ogawa, S. (2009). Frequent inactivation of A20 in B-cell lymphomas. *Nature,* Vol.459, No.7247, pp. 712-716, 1476-4687

Kennedy, G.; Komano, J. & Sugden, B. (2003). Epstein-Barr virus provides a survival factor to Burkitt's lymphomas. *Proc Natl Acad Sci U S A,* Vol.100, No.24, pp. 14269-14274, 0027-8424

Khan, G. (2006). Epstein-Barr virus, cytokines, and inflammation: a cocktail for the pathogenesis of Hodgkin's lymphoma? *Exp Hematol,* Vol.34, No.4, pp. 399-406, 0301-472X

Kilger, E.; Kieser, A.; Baumann, M. & Hammerschmidt, W. (1998). Epstein-Barr virus-mediated B-cell proliferation is dependent upon latent membrane protein 1, which simulates an activated CD40 receptor. *Embo J,* Vol.17, No.6, pp. 1700-1709, 0261-4189

Kim, T.H.; Kim, H.I.; Soung, Y.H.; Shaw, L.A. & Chung, J. (2009). Integrin (alpha6beta4) signals through Src to increase expression of S100A4, a metastasis-promoting factor: implications for cancer cell invasion. *Mol Cancer Res,* Vol.7, No.10, pp. 1605-1612, 1557-3125

Klimm, B.; Schnell, R.; Diehl, V. & Engert, A. (2005). Current treatment and immunotherapy of Hodgkin's lymphoma. *Haematologica,* Vol.90, No.12, pp. 1680-1692, 1592-8721

Knight, J.S.; Tsodikov, A.; Cibrik, D.M.; Ross, C.W.; Kaminski, M.S. & Blayney, D.W. (2009). Lymphoma after solid organ transplantation: risk, response to therapy, and survival at a transplantation center. *J Clin Oncol,* Vol.27, No.20, pp. 3354-3362, 1527-7755

Kolar, Z.; Flavell, J.R.; Ehrmann, J., Jr.; Rihakova, P.; Macak, J.; Lowe, D.; Crocker, J.; Vojtesek, B.; Young, L.S. & Murray, P.G. (2000). Apoptosis of malignant cells in Hodgkin's disease is related to expression of the cdk inhibitor p27KIP1. *J Pathol,* Vol.190, No.5, pp. 604-612, 0022-3417

Korkolopoulou, P.; Cordell, J.; Jones, M.; Kaklamanis, L.; Tsenga, A.; Gatter, K.C. & Mason, D.Y. (1994). The expression of the B-cell marker mb-1 (CD79a) in Hodgkin's disease. *Histopathology,* Vol.24, No.6, pp. 511-515, 0309-0167

Kreitman, R.J.; Wilson, W.H.; White, J.D.; Stetler-Stevenson, M.; Jaffe, E.S.; Giardina, S.; Waldmann, T.A. & Pastan, I. (2000). Phase I trial of recombinant immunotoxin anti-Tac(Fv)-PE38 (LMB-2) in patients with hematologic malignancies. *J Clin Oncol,* Vol.18, No.8, pp. 1622-1636, 0732-183X

Krishnamurthy, S.; Hassan, A.; Frater, J.L.; Paessler, M.E. & Kreisel, F.H. (2010). Pathologic and clinical features of Hodgkin lymphoma--like posttransplant lymphoproliferative disease. *Int J Surg Pathol,* Vol.18, No.4, pp. 278-285, 1940-2465

Kube, D.; Holtick, U.; Vockerodt, M.; Ahmadi, T.; Haier, B.; Behrmann, I.; Heinrich, P.C.; Diehl, V. & Tesch, H. (2001). STAT3 is constitutively activated in Hodgkin cell lines. *Blood,* Vol.98, No.3, pp. 762-770, 0006-4971

Kupper, M.; Joos, S.; von Bonin, F.; Daus, H.; Pfreundschuh, M.; Lichter, P. & Trumper, L. (2001). MDM2 gene amplification and lack of p53 point mutations in Hodgkin and Reed-Sternberg cells: results from single-cell polymerase chain reaction and molecular cytogenetic studies. *Br J Haematol,* Vol.112, No.3, pp. 768-775, 0007-1048

Kuppers, R. (2002). Molecular biology of Hodgkin's lymphoma. *Adv Cancer Res,* Vol.84, pp. 277-312, 0065-230X

Kuppers, R.; Hajadi, M.; Plank, L.; Rajewsky, K. & Hansmann, M.L. (1996). Molecular Ig gene analysis reveals that monocytoid B cell lymphoma is a malignancy of mature B cells carrying somatically mutated V region genes and suggests that rearrangement of the kappa-deleting element (resulting in deletion of the Ig kappa enhancers) abolishes somatic hypermutation in the human. *Eur J Immunol,* Vol.26, No.8, pp. 1794-1800, 0014-2980

Kuppers, R.; Klein, U.; Schwering, I.; Distler, V.; Brauninger, A.; Cattoretti, G.; Tu, Y.; Stolovitzky, G.A.; Califano, A.; Hansmann, M.L. & Dalla-Favera, R. (2003). Identification of Hodgkin and Reed-Sternberg cell-specific genes by gene expression profiling. *J Clin Invest,* Vol.111, No.4, pp. 529-537, 0021-9738

Kuppers, R.; Rajewsky, K.; Zhao, M.; Simons, G.; Laumann, R.; Fischer, R. & Hansmann, M.L. (1994). Hodgkin disease: Hodgkin and Reed-Sternberg cells picked from histological sections show clonal immunoglobulin gene rearrangements and appear to be derived from B cells at various stages of development. *Proc Natl Acad Sci U S A,* Vol.91, No.23, pp. 10962-10966, 0027-8424

Kuppers, R.; Sousa, A.B.; Baur, A.S.; Strickler, J.G.; Rajewsky, K. & Hansmann, M.L. (2001). Common germinal-center B-cell origin of the malignant cells in two composite lymphomas, involving classical Hodgkin's disease and either follicular lymphoma or B-CLL. *Mol Med,* Vol.7, No.5, pp. 285-292, 1076-1551

Lake, A.; Shield, L.A.; Cordano, P.; Chui, D.T.; Osborne, J.; Crae, S.; Wilson, K.S.; Tosi, S.; Knight, S.J.; Gesk, S.; Siebert, R.; Hay, R.T. & Jarrett, R.F. (2009). Mutations of NFKBIA, encoding IkappaB alpha, are a recurrent finding in classical Hodgkin lymphoma but are not a unifying feature of non-EBV-associated cases. *Int J Cancer,* Vol.125, No.6, pp. 1334-1342, 1097-0215

Lam, N. & Sugden, B. (2003). CD40 and its viral mimic, LMP1: similar means to different ends. *Cell Signal,* Vol.15, No.1, pp. 9-16, 0898-6568

Lauritzen, A.F.; Moller, P.H.; Nedergaard, T.; Guldberg, P.; Hou-Jensen, K. & Ralfkiaer, E. (1999). Apoptosis-related genes and proteins in Hodgkin's disease. *Apmis,* Vol.107, No.7, pp. 636-644, 0903-4641

Lee, H.H.; Dadgostar, H.; Cheng, Q.; Shu, J. & Cheng, G. (1999). NF-kappaB-mediated up-regulation of Bcl-x and Bfl-1/A1 is required for CD40 survival signaling in B lymphocytes. *Proc Natl Acad Sci U S A,* Vol.96, No.16, pp. 9136-9141, 0027-8424

Leoncini, L.; Spina, D.; Megha, T.; Gallorini, M.; Tosi, P.; Hummel, M.; Stein, H.; Pileri, S.; Kraft, R.; Laissue, J.A. & Cottier, H. (1997). Cell kinetics, morphology, and molecular IgVH gene rearrangements in Hodgkin's disease. *Leuk Lymphoma,* Vol.26, No.3-4, pp. 307-316, 1042-8194

Lucas, K.G.; Salzman, D.; García, A.; Sun, Q. (2004). Adoptive immunotherapy with allogeneic Epstein-Barr virus (EBV)-specific cytotoxic T-lymphocytes for recurrent EBV-positive Hodgkin disease. *Cancer,* Vol. 100, No 9, pp 1892-901, 0008-543X

Maggioncalda, A.; Malik, N.; Shenoy, P.; Smith, M.; Sinha, R. & Flowers, C.R. (2011). Clinical, molecular, and environmental risk factors for hodgkin lymphoma. *Adv Hematol,* Vol.2011, pp. 736261, 1687-9112

Maier, S.K. & Hammond, J.M. (2006). Role of lenalidomide in the treatment of multiple myeloma and myelodysplastic syndrome. *Ann Pharmacother,* Vol.40, No.2, pp. 286-289, 1060-0280

Malumbres, M. & Barbacid, M. (2001). To cycle or not to cycle: a critical decision in cancer. *Nat Rev Cancer,* Vol.1, No.3, pp. 222-231, 1474-175X

Marafioti, T.; Hummel, M.; Foss, H.D.; Laumen, H.; Korbjuhn, P.; Anagnostopoulos, I.; Lammert, H.; Demel, G.; Theil, J.; Wirth, T. & Stein, H. (2000). Hodgkin and reed-sternberg cells represent an expansion of a single clone originating from a germinal center B-cell with functional immunoglobulin gene rearrangements but defective immunoglobulin transcription. *Blood,* Vol.95, No.4, pp. 1443-1450, 0006-4971

Marshall, N.A.; Christie, L.E.; Munro, L.R.; Culligan, D.J.; Johnston, P.W.; Barker, R.N. & Vickers, M.A. (2004). Immunosuppressive regulatory T cells are abundant in the reactive lymphocytes of Hodgkin lymphoma. *Blood*, Vol.103, No.5, pp. 1755-1762, 0006-4971

Martin-Subero, J.I.; Gesk, S.; Harder, L.; Sonoki, T.; Tucker, P.W.; Schlegelberger, B.; Grote, W.; Novo, F.J.; Calasanz, M.J.; Hansmann, M.L.; Dyer, M.J. & Siebert, R. (2002). Recurrent involvement of the REL and BCL11A loci in classical Hodgkin lymphoma. *Blood*, Vol.99, No.4, pp. 1474-1477, 0006-4971

Mason, D.Y.; Banks, P.M.; Chan, J.; Cleary, M.L.; Delsol, G.; de Wolf Peeters, C.; Falini, B.; Gatter, K.; Grogan, T.M.; Harris, N.L. & et al. (1994). Nodular lymphocyte predominance Hodgkin's disease. A distinct clinicopathological entity. *Am J Surg Pathol*, Vol.18, No.5, pp. 526-530, 0147-5185

Mathas, S.; Hinz, M.; Anagnostopoulos, I.; Krappmann, D.; Lietz, A.; Jundt, F.; Bommert, K.; Mechta-Grigoriou, F.; Stein, H.; Dorken, B. & Scheidereit, C. (2002). Aberrantly expressed c-Jun and JunB are a hallmark of Hodgkin lymphoma cells, stimulate proliferation and synergize with NF-kappa B. *Embo J*, Vol.21, No.15, pp. 4104-4113, 0261-4189

Mathas, S.; Janz, M.; Hummel, F.; Hummel, M.; Wollert-Wulf, B.; Lusatis, S.; Anagnostopoulos, I.; Lietz, A.; Sigvardsson, M.; Jundt, F.; Johrens, K.; Bommert, K.; Stein, H. & Dorken, B. (2006). Intrinsic inhibition of transcription factor E2A by HLH proteins ABF-1 and Id2 mediates reprogramming of neoplastic B cells in Hodgkin lymphoma. *Nat Immunol*, Vol.7, No.2, pp. 207-215, 1529-2908

Medema, J.P.; de Jong, J.; Peltenburg, L.T.; Verdegaal, E.M.; Gorter, A.; Bres, S.A.; Franken, K.L.; Hahne, M.; Albar, J.P.; Melief, C.J. & Offringa, R. (2001). Blockade of the granzyme B/perforin pathway through overexpression of the serine protease inhibitor PI-9/SPI-6 constitutes a mechanism for immune escape by tumors. *Proc Natl Acad Sci U S A*, Vol.98, No.20, pp. 11515-11520, 0027-8424

Messineo, C.; Jamerson, M.H.; Hunter, E.; Braziel, R.; Bagg, A.; Irving, S.G. & Cossman, J. (1998). Gene expression by single Reed-Sternberg cells: pathways of apoptosis and activation. *Blood*, Vol.91, No.7, pp. 2443-2451, 0006-4971

Metkar, S.S.; Manna, P.P.; Anand, M.; Naresh, K.N.; Advani, S.H. & Nadkarni, J.J. (2001). CD40 Ligand--an anti-apoptotic molecule in Hodgkin's disease. *Cancer Biother Radiopharm*, Vol.16, No.1, pp. 85-92, 1084-9785

Montalban, C.; Abraira, V.; Morente, M.; Acevedo, A.; Aguilera, B.; Bellas, C.; Fraga, M.; Del Moral, R.G.; Menarguez, J.; Oliva, H.; Sanchez-Beato, M. & Piris, M.A. (2000). Epstein-Barr virus-latent membrane protein 1 expression has a favorable influence in the outcome of patients with Hodgkin's Disease treated with chemotherapy. *Leuk Lymphoma*, Vol.39, No.5-6, pp. 563-572, 1042-8194

Montalban, C.; Garcia, J.F.; Abraira, V.; Gonzalez-Camacho, L.; Morente, M.M.; Bello, J.L.; Conde, E.; Cruz, M.A.; Garcia-Sanz, R.; Garcia-Larana, J.; Grande, C.; Llanos, M.; Martinez, R.; Flores, E.; Mendez, M.; Ponderos, C.; Rayon, C.; Sanchez-Godoy, P.; Zamora, J. & Piris, M.A. (2004). Influence of biologic markers on the outcome of Hodgkin's lymphoma: a study by the Spanish Hodgkin's Lymphoma Study Group. *J Clin Oncol*, Vol.22, No.9, pp. 1664-1673, 0732-183X

Montesinos-Rongen, M.; Roers, A.; Kuppers, R.; Rajewsky, K. & Hansmann, M.L. (1999). Mutation of the p53 gene is not a typical feature of Hodgkin and Reed-Sternberg cells in Hodgkin's disease. *Blood,* Vol.94, No.5, pp. 1755-1760, 0006-4971

Morente, M.M.; Piris, M.A.; Abraira, V.; Acevedo, A.; Aguilera, B.; Bellas, C.; Fraga, M.; Garcia-Del-Moral, R.; Gomez-Marcos, F.; Menarguez, J.; Oliva, H.; Sanchez-Beato, M. & Montalban, C. (1997). Adverse clinical outcome in Hodgkin's disease is associated with loss of retinoblastoma protein expression, high Ki67 proliferation index, and absence of Epstein-Barr virus-latent membrane protein 1 expression. *Blood,* Vol.90, No.6, pp. 2429-2436

Muschen, M.; Kuppers, R.; Spieker, T.; Brauninger, A.; Rajewsky, K. & Hansmann, M.L. (2001). Molecular single-cell analysis of Hodgkin- and Reed-Sternberg cells harboring unmutated immunoglobulin variable region genes. *Lab Invest,* Vol.81, No.3, pp. 289-295, 0023-6837

Muschen, M.; Rajewsky, K.; Brauninger, A.; Baur, A.S.; Oudejans, J.J.; Roers, A.; Hansmann, M.L. & Kuppers, R. (2000). Rare occurrence of classical Hodgkin's disease as a T cell lymphoma. *J Exp Med,* Vol.191, No.2, pp. 387-394, 0022-1007

Newcom, S.R.; Kadin, M.E.; Ansari, A.A. & Diehl, V. (1988). L-428 nodular sclerosing Hodgkin's cell secretes a unique transforming growth factor-beta active at physiologic pH. *J Clin Invest,* Vol.82, No.6, pp. 1915-1921, 0021-9738

Ng, A.K.; Bernardo, M.V.; Weller, E.; Backstrand, K.; Silver, B.; Marcus, K.C.; Tarbell, N.J.; Stevenson, M.A.; Friedberg, J.W. & Mauch, P.M. (2002). Second malignancy after Hodgkin disease treated with radiation therapy with or without chemotherapy: long-term risks and risk factors. *Blood,* Vol.100, No.6, pp. 1989-1996, 0006-4971

Nie, L.; Xu, M.; Vladimirova, A. & Sun, X.H. (2003). Notch-induced E2A ubiquitination and degradation are controlled by MAP kinase activities. *Embo J,* Vol.22, No.21, pp. 5780-5792, 0261-4189

Niens, M.; Visser, L.; Nolte, I.M.; van der Steege, G.; Diepstra, A.; Cordano, P.; Jarrett, R.F.; Te Meerman, G.J.; Poppema, S. & van den Berg, A. (2008). Serum chemokine levels in Hodgkin lymphoma patients: highly increased levels of CCL17 and CCL22. *Br J Haematol,* Vol.140, No.5, pp. 527-536, 1365-2141

Nogova, L.; Reineke, T.; Brillant, C.; Sieniawski, M.; Rudiger, T.; Josting, A.; Bredenfeld, H.; Skripnitchenko, R.; Muller, R.P.; Muller-Hermelink, H.K.; Diehl, V. & Engert, A. (2008). Lymphocyte-predominant and classical Hodgkin's lymphoma: a comprehensive analysis from the German Hodgkin Study Group. *J Clin Oncol,* Vol.26, No.3, pp. 434-439, 1527-7755

Obeid, M.; Panaretakis, T.; Joza, N.; Tufi, R.; Tesniere, A.; van Endert, P.; Zitvogel, L. & Kroemer, G. (2007a). Calreticulin exposure is required for the immunogenicity of gamma-irradiation and UVC light-induced apoptosis. *Cell Death Differ,* Vol.14, No.10, pp. 1848-1850, 1350-9047

Obeid, M.; Tesniere, A.; Ghiringhelli, F.; Fimia, G.M.; Apetoh, L.; Perfettini, J.L.; Castedo, M.; Mignot, G.; Panaretakis, T.; Casares, N.; Metivier, D.; Larochette, N.; van Endert, P.; Ciccosanti, F.; Piacentini, M.; Zitvogel, L. & Kroemer, G. (2007b). Calreticulin exposure dictates the immunogenicity of cancer cell death. *Nat Med,* Vol.13, No.1, pp. 54-61, 1078-8956

Ohshima, K.; Haraoka, S.; Fujiki, T.; Yoshioka, S.; Suzumiya, J.; Kanda, M. & Kikuchi, M. (1999). Expressions of cyclin E, A, and B1 in Hodgkin and Reed-Sternberg cells: not suppressed by cyclin-dependent kinase inhibitor p21 expression. *Pathol Int,* Vol.49, No.6, pp. 506-512, 1320-5463

Ohshima, K.; Suzumiya, J.; Akamatu, M.; Takeshita, M. & Kikuchi, M. (1995). Human and viral interleukin-10 in Hodgkin's disease, and its influence on CD4+ and CD8+ T lymphocytes. *Int J Cancer,* Vol.62, No.1, pp. 5-10

Okeley, N.M.; Miyamoto, J.B.; Zhang, X.; Sanderson, R.J.; Benjamin, D.R.; Sievers, E.L.; Senter, P.D. & Alley, S.C. (2010). Intracellular activation of SGN-35, a potent anti-CD30 antibody-drug conjugate. *Clin Cancer Res,* Vol.16, No.3, pp. 888-897, 1078-0432

Oudejans, J.J.; Jiwa, N.M.; Kummer, J.A.; Ossenkoppele, G.J.; van Heerde, P.; Baars, J.W.; Kluin, P.M.; Kluin-Nelemans, J.C.; van Diest, P.J.; Middeldorp, J.M. & Meijer, C.J. (1997). Activated cytotoxic T cells as prognostic marker in Hodgkin's disease. *Blood,* Vol.89, No.4, pp. 1376-1382, 0006-4971

Pages, F.; Galon, J.; Dieu-Nosjean, M.C.; Tartour, E.; Sautes-Fridman, C. & Fridman, W.H. (2010). Immune infiltration in human tumors: a prognostic factor that should not be ignored. *Oncogene,* Vol.29, No.8, pp. 1093-1102, 1476-5594

Parsons, J.T.; Slack-Davis, J.; Tilghman, R. & Roberts, W.G. (2008). Focal adhesion kinase: targeting adhesion signaling pathways for therapeutic intervention. *Clin Cancer Res,* Vol.14, No.3, pp. 627-632, 1078-0432 (

Peh, S.C.; Kim, L.H. & Poppema, S. (2001). TARC, a CC chemokine, is frequently expressed in classic Hodgkin's lymphoma but not in NLP Hodgkin's lymphoma, T-cell-rich B-cell lymphoma, and most cases of anaplastic large cell lymphoma. *Am J Surg Pathol,* Vol.25, No.7, pp. 925-929, 0147-5185

Peipp, M. & Valerius, T. (2002). Bispecific antibodies targeting cancer cells. *Biochem Soc Trans,* Vol.30, No.4, pp. 507-511, 0300-5127

Pham, P.T.; Wilkinson, A.H.; Gritsch, H.A.; Pham, P.C.; Miller, J.M.; Lassman, C.R. & Danovitch, G.M. (2002). Monotherapy with the anti-CD20 monoclonal antibody rituximab in a kidney transplant recipient with posttransplant lymphoproliferative disease. *Transplant Proc,* Vol.34, No.4, pp. 1178-1181, 0041-1345

Piccaluga, P.P.; Agostinelli, C.; Gazzola, A.; Tripodo, C.; Bacci, F.; Sabattini, E.; Sista, M.T.; Mannu, C.; Sapienza, M.R.; Rossi, M.; Laginestra, M.A.; Sagramoso-Sacchetti, C.A.; Righi, S. & Pileri, S.A. (2011). Pathobiology of hodgkin lymphoma. *Adv Hematol,* Vol.2011, pp. 920898, 1687-9112

Pileri, S.; Sabattini, E.; Tazzari, P.L.; Gherlinzoni, F.; Zucchini, L.; Bigerna, B.; Leoncini, L.; Rosso, R.; Stein, H. & Falini, B. (1991). Hodgkin's disease: update of findings. *Haematologica,* Vol.76, No.3, pp. 175-182, 0390-6078

Pileri, S.A.; Poggi, S.; Sabattini, E.; De Vivo, A.; Falini, B. & Stein, H. (1995). Is Hodgkin's disease a unique entity? *Leuk Lymphoma,* Vol.15 Suppl 1, pp. 3-6, 1042-8194

Poppema, S.; Potters, M.; Emmens, R.; Visser, L. & van den Berg, A. (1999). Immune reactions in classical Hodgkin's lymphoma. *Semin Hematol,* Vol.36, No.3, pp. 253-259, 0037-1963

Poppema, S.; Potters, M.; Visser, L. & van den Berg, A.M. (1998). Immune escape mechanisms in Hodgkin's disease. *Ann Oncol,* Vol.9, No.Suppl 5, pp. S21-24, 0923-7534

Poppema, S. & Visser, L. (1994). Absence of HLA class I expression by Reed-Sternberg cells. *Am J Pathol,* Vol.145, No.1, pp. 37-41, 0002-9440

Portis, T.; Dyck, P. & Longnecker, R. (2003). Epstein-Barr Virus (EBV) LMP2A induces alterations in gene transcription similar to those observed in Reed-Sternberg cells of Hodgkin lymphoma. *Blood,* Vol.102, No.12, pp. 4166-4178, 0006-4971

Powles, T. & Bower, M. (2000). HIV-associated Hodgkin's disease. *Int J STD AIDS,* Vol.11, No.8, pp. 492-494.

Powles, T.; Robinson, D.; Stebbing, J.; Shamash, J.; Nelson, M.; Gazzard, B.; Mandelia, S.; Moller, H. & Bower, M. (2009). Highly active antiretroviral therapy and the incidence of non-AIDS-defining cancers in people with HIV infection. *J Clin Oncol,* Vol.27, No.6, pp. 884-890, 1527-7755

Prehn, R.T. (1972). The immune reaction as a stimulator of tumor growth. *Science,* Vol.176, No.31, pp. 170-171, 0036-8075

Puthier, D.; Derenne, S.; Barille, S.; Moreau, P.; Harousseau, J.L.; Bataille, R. & Amiot, M. (1999). Mcl-1 and Bcl-xL are co-regulated by IL-6 in human myeloma cells. *Br J Haematol,* Vol.107, No.2, pp. 392-395, 0007-1048

Quezada, S.A.; Simpson, T.R.; Peggs, K.S.; Merghoub, T.; Vider, J.; Fan, X.; Blasberg, R.; Yagita, H.; Muranski, P.; Antony, P.A.; Restifo, N.P. & Allison, J.P. (2010). Tumor-reactive CD4(+) T cells develop cytotoxic activity and eradicate large established melanoma after transfer into lymphopenic hosts. *J Exp Med,* Vol.207, No.3, pp. 637-650, 1540-9538

Raphael, M.; Said, J.; Borish, B. & al., e. (2008). Lymphomas associated with HIV infection. In: *World Health Organization Classification of Tumours, Pathology and Genetics of Tumours of Haematopoietic and Lymphoid Tissues.* , Swerdlow SH C.E., Harris NL, et al. (eds) (eds), 340-342. IARC Press Lyon

Rassidakis, G.Z.; Medeiros, L.J.; McDonnell, T.J.; Viviani, S.; Bonfante, V.; Nadali, G.; Vassilakopoulos, T.P.; Giardini, R.; Chilosi, M.; Kittas, C.; Gianni, A.M.; Bonadonna, G.; Pizzolo, G.; Pangalis, G.A.; Cabanillas, F. & Sarris, A.H. (2002a). BAX expression in Hodgkin and Reed-Sternberg cells of Hodgkin's disease: correlation with clinical outcome. *Clin Cancer Res,* Vol.8, No.2, pp. 488-493, 1078-0432

Rassidakis, G.Z.; Medeiros, L.J.; Vassilakopoulos, T.P.; Viviani, S.; Bonfante, V.; Nadali, G.; Herling, M.; Angelopoulou, M.K.; Giardini, R.; Chilosi, M.; Kittas, C.; McDonnell, T.J.; Bonadonna, G.; Gianni, A.M.; Pizzolo, G.; Pangalis, G.A.; Cabanillas, F. & Sarris, A.H. (2002b). BCL-2 expression in Hodgkin and Reed-Sternberg cells of classical Hodgkin disease predicts a poorer prognosis in patients treated with ABVD or equivalent regimens. *Blood,* Vol.100, No.12, pp. 3935-3941, 0006-4971

Rathore, B. & Kadin, M.E. (2010). Hodgkin's lymphoma therapy: past, present, and future. *Expert Opin Pharmacother,* Vol.11, No.17, pp. 2891-2906, 1744-7666

Rautert, R.; Schinkothe, T.; Franklin, J.; Weihrauch, M.; Boll, B.; Pogge, E.; Bredenfeld, H.; Engert, A.; Diehl, V. & Re, D. (2008). Elevated pretreatment interleukin-10 serum level is an International Prognostic Score (IPS)-independent risk factor for early treatment failure in advanced stage Hodgkin lymphoma. *Leuk Lymphoma,* Vol.49, No.11, pp. 2091-2098, 1029-2403

Rehwald, U.; Schulz, H.; Reiser, M.; Sieber, M.; Staak, J.O.; Morschlauser, F.; Driessen, C.; Rudiger, T.; Muller-Hermelin, K.; Diehl, V.; Engert, A. (2003). Treatment of relapsed CD20+ Hodgkin lymphoma with the monoclonal antibody rituximab is effective and well tolerated: results of a phase 2 trial of the German Hodgkin lymphoma study group. *Blood* , Vol 101, No 2, pp 420-424, 0006-4971

Ren, F.; Zhan, X.; Martens, G.; Lee, J.; Center, D.; Hanson, S.K. & Kornfeld, H. (2005). Pro-IL-16 regulation in activated murine CD4+ lymphocytes. *J Immunol,* Vol.174, No.5, pp. 2738-2745, 0022-1767

Renne, C.; Martin-Subero, J.I.; Eickernjager, M.; Hansmann, M.L.; Kuppers, R.; Siebert, R. & Brauninger, A. (2006). Aberrant expression of ID2, a suppressor of B-cell-specific gene expression, in Hodgkin's lymphoma. *Am J Pathol,* Vol.169, No.2, pp. 655-664, 0002-9440

Rickinson, A. & Kieff, E. (2001). Epstein-Barr virus. In: *In Fields Virology,* Knipe DM H.P.e. (eds),2575-2627. Lippincott Williams & Wilkins Philadelphia

Rohr, J.C.; Wagner, H.J.; Lauten, M.; Wacker, H.H.; Juttner, E.; Hanke, C.; Pohl, M. & Niemeyer, C.M. (2008). Differentiation of EBV-induced post-transplant Hodgkin lymphoma from Hodgkin-like post-transplant lymphoproliferative disease. *Pediatr Transplant,* Vol.12, No.4, pp. 426-431, 1399-3046

Roskrow, M.A.; Suzuki, N.; Gan, Y.; Sixbey, J.W.; Ng, C.Y.; Kimbrough, S.; Hudson, M.; Brenner, M.K.; Heslop, H.E. & Rooney, C.M. (1998). Epstein-Barr virus (EBV)-specific cytotoxic T lymphocytes for the treatment of patients with EBV-positive relapsed Hodgkin's disease. *Blood,* Vol.91, No.8, pp. 2925-2934, 0006-4971

Rudant, J.; Orsi, L.; Monnereau, A.; Patte, C.; Pacquement, H.; Landman-Parker, J.; Bergeron, C.; Robert, A.; Michel, G.; Lambilliotte, A.; Aladjidi, N.; Gandemer, V.; Lutz, P.; Margueritte, G.; Plantaz, D.; Mechinaud, F.; Hemon, D. & Clavel, J. (2010). Childhood hodgkin's lymphoma, non-Hodgkin's lymphoma and factors related to the immune system: the Escale study (SFCE). *Int J Cancer,* pp. 1097-0215, 0020-7136

Sabattini, E.; Gerdes, J.; Gherlinzoni, F.; Poggi, S.; Zucchini, L.; Melilli, G.; Grigioni, F.; Del Vecchio, M.T.; Leoncini, L. & Falini, B. (1993). Comparison between the monoclonal antibodies Ki-67 and PC10 in 125 malignant lymphomas. *J Pathol,* Vol.169, No.4, pp. 397-403, 0022-3417

Sanchez-Aguilera, A.; Montalban, C.; de la Cueva, P.; Sanchez-Verde, L.; Morente, M.M.; Garcia-Cosio, M.; Garcia-Larana, J.; Bellas, C.; Provencio, M.; Romagosa, V.; de Sevilla, A.F.; Menarguez, J.; Sabin, P.; Mestre, M.J.; Mendez, M.; Fresno, M.F.; Nicolas, C.; Piris, M.A. & Garcia, J.F. (2006). Tumor microenvironment and mitotic checkpoint are key factors in the outcome of classic Hodgkin lymphoma. *Blood,* Vol.108, No.2, pp. 662-668, 0006-4971

Sanchez-Beato, M.; Piris, M.A.; Martinez-Montero, J.C.; Garcia, J.F.; Villuendas, R.; Garcia, F.J.; Orradre, J.L. & Martinez, P. (1996). MDM2 and p21WAF1/CIP1, wild-type p53-induced proteins, are regularly expressed by Sternberg-Reed cells in Hodgkin's disease. *J Pathol,* Vol.180, No.1, pp. 58-64, 0022-3417

Sanchez-Beato, M.; Sanchez-Aguilera, A. & Piris, M.A. (2003). Cell cycle deregulation in B-cell lymphomas. *Blood,* Vol.101, No.4, pp. 1220-1235, 0006-4971

Sarris, A.H.; Kliche, K.O.; Pethambaram, P.; Preti, A.; Tucker, S.; Jackow, C.; Messina, O.; Pugh, W.; Hagemeister, F.B.; McLaughlin, P.; Rodriguez, M.A.; Romaguera, J.; Fritsche, H.; Witzig, T.; Duvic, M.; Andreeff, M. & Cabanillas, F. (1999). Interleukin-10 levels are often elevated in serum of adults with Hodgkin's disease and are associated with inferior failure-free survival. *Ann Oncol,* Vol.10, No.4, pp. 433-440, 0923-7534

Schmitz, R.; Hansmann, M.L.; Bohle, V.; Martin-Subero, J.I.; Hartmann, S.; Mechtersheimer, G.; Klapper, W.; Vater, I.; Giefing, M.; Gesk, S.; Stanelle, J.; Siebert, R. & Kuppers, R. (2009). TNFAIP3 (A20) is a tumor suppressor gene in Hodgkin lymphoma and primary mediastinal B cell lymphoma. *J Exp Med,* Vol.206, No.5, pp. 981-989, 1540-9538

Schnell, R.; Dietlein, M.; Staak, J.O.; Borchmann, P.; Schomaecker, K.; Fischer, T.; Eschner, W.; Hansen, H.; Morschhauser, F.; Schicha, H.; Diehl, V.; Raubitschek, A. & Engert, A. (2005). Treatment of refractory Hodgkin's lymphoma patients with an iodine-131-labeled murine anti-CD30 monoclonal antibody. *J Clin Oncol,* Vol.23, No.21, pp. 4669-4678, 0732-183X

Schulz, H.; Rehwald, U.; Morschhauser, F.; Elter, T.; Driessen, C.; Rudiger, T.; Borchmann, P.; Schnell, R.; Diehl, V.; Engert, A. & Reiser, M. (2008). Rituximab in relapsed lymphocyte-predominant Hodgkin lymphoma: long-term results of a phase 2 trial by the German Hodgkin Lymphoma Study Group (GHSG). *Blood,* Vol.111, No.1, pp. 109-111, 0006-4971

Schwering, I.; Brauninger, A.; Klein, U.; Jungnickel, B.; Tinguely, M.; Diehl, V.; Hansmann, M.L.; Dalla-Favera, R.; Rajewsky, K. & Kuppers, R. (2003). Loss of the B-lineage-specific gene expression program in Hodgkin and Reed-Sternberg cells of Hodgkin lymphoma. *Blood,* Vol.101, No.4, pp. 1505-1512, 0006-4971

Seitz, V.; Hummel, M.; Marafioti, T.; Anagnostopoulos, I.; Assaf, C. & Stein, H. (2000). Detection of clonal T-cell receptor gamma-chain gene rearrangements in Reed-Sternberg cells of classic Hodgkin disease. *Blood,* Vol.95, No.10, pp. 3020-3024, 0006-4971

Shaffer, A.L.; Yu, X.; He, Y.; Boldrick, J.; Chan, E.P. & Staudt, L.M. (2000). BCL-6 represses genes that function in lymphocyte differentiation, inflammation, and cell cycle control. *Immunity,* Vol.13, No.2, pp. 199-212, 1074-7613

Shimizu, J.; Yamazaki, S.; Takahashi, T.; Ishida, Y. & Sakaguchi, S. (2002). Stimulation of CD25(+)CD4(+) regulatory T cells through GITR breaks immunological self-tolerance. *Nat Immunol,* Vol.3, No.2, pp. 135-142, 1529-2908

Skinnider, B.F.; Elia, A.J.; Gascoyne, R.D.; Patterson, B.; Trumper, L.; Kapp, U. & Mak, T.W. (2002). Signal transducer and activator of transcription 6 is frequently activated in Hodgkin and Reed-Sternberg cells of Hodgkin lymphoma. *Blood,* Vol.99, No.2, pp. 618-626, 0006-4971

Skinnider, B.F. & Mak, T.W. (2002). The role of cytokines in classical Hodgkin lymphoma. *Blood,* Vol.99, No.12, pp. 4283-4297, 0006-4971

Slovak, M.L.; Bedell, V.; Hsu, Y.H.; Estrine, D.B.; Nowak, N.J.; Delioukina, M.L.; Weiss, L.M.; Smith, D.D. & Forman, S.J. (2011). Molecular karyotypes of Hodgkin and Reed-Sternberg cells at disease onset reveal distinct copy number alterations in chemosensitive versus refractory Hodgkin lymphoma. *Clin Cancer Res,* Vol.17, No.10, pp. 3443-3454, 1078-0432

Smith, E.M.; Akerblad, P.; Kadesch, T.; Axelson, H. & Sigvardsson, M. (2005). Inhibition of EBF function by active Notch signaling reveals a novel regulatory pathway in early B-cell development. *Blood,* Vol.106, No.6, pp. 1995-2001, 0006-4971

Smolewski, P.; Robak, T.; Krykowski, E.; Blasinska-Morawiec, M.; Niewiadomska, H.; Pluzanska, A.; Chmielowska, E. & Zambrano, O. (2000). Prognostic factors in

Hodgkin's disease: multivariate analysis of 327 patients from a single institution. *Clin Cancer Res,* Vol.6, No.3, pp. 1150-1160, 1078-0432

Smyth, M.J.; Hayakawa, Y.; Takeda, K. & Yagita, H. (2002). New aspects of natural-killer-cell surveillance and therapy of cancer. *Nat Rev Cancer,* Vol.2, No.11, pp. 850-861, 1474-175X

Song, L.; Li, Y.; Sun, Y. & Shen, B. (2002). Mcl-1 mediates cytokine deprivation induced apoptosis of human myeloma cell line XG-7. *Chin Med J (Engl),* Vol.115, No.8, pp. 1241-1243, 0366-6999

Specht, L. & Hasenclever, D. (1999). Prognostic factors of Hodgkin´s disease. In: *Hodgkin´s disease.* , Mauch PM A.J., Diehl V, Hoppe RT, Weiss LM (eds). (eds),295-325. Lippincott Williams & Wilkins Philadelphia:295-325

Staudt, L.M. (2000). The molecular and cellular origins of Hodgkin's disease. *J Exp Med,* Vol.191, No.2, pp. 207-212, 0022-1007

Steidl, C.; Connors, J.M. & Gascoyne, R.D. (2011a). Molecular pathogenesis of Hodgkin's lymphoma: increasing evidence of the importance of the microenvironment. *J Clin Oncol,* Vol.29, No.14, pp. 1812-1826, 1527-7755

Steidl, C.; Lee, T.; Shah, S.P.; Farinha, P.; Han, G.; Nayar, T.; Delaney, A.; Jones, S.J.; Iqbal, J.; Weisenburger, D.D.; Bast, M.A.; Rosenwald, A.; Muller-Hermelink, H.K.; Rimsza, L.M.; Campo, E.; Delabie, J.; Braziel, R.M.; Cook, J.R.; Tubbs, R.R.; Jaffe, E.S.; Lenz, G.; Connors, J.M.; Staudt, L.M.; Chan, W.C. & Gascoyne, R.D. (2010). Tumor-associated macrophages and survival in classic Hodgkin's lymphoma. *N Engl J Med,* Vol.362, No.10, pp. 875-885, 1533-4406

Steidl, C.; Shah, S.P.; Woolcock, B.W.; Rui, L.; Kawahara, M.; Farinha, P.; Johnson, N.A.; Zhao, Y.; Telenius, A.; Neriah, S.B.; McPherson, A.; Meissner, B.; Okoye, U.C.; Diepstra, A.; van den Berg, A.; Sun, M.; Leung, G.; Jones, S.J.; Connors, J.M.; Huntsman, D.G.; Savage, K.J.; Rimsza, L.M.; Horsman, D.E.; Staudt, L.M.; Steidl, U.; Marra, M.A. & Gascoyne, R.D. (2011b). MHC class II transactivator CIITA is a recurrent gene fusion partner in lymphoid cancers. *Nature,* Vol.471, No.7338, pp. 377-381, 1476-4687

Stein, H.; Delsol, G. & Pileri, S. (2008a). Classical Hodgkin lymphoma, introduction. In: *WHO Classification of Tumours of Haematopoietic and Lymphoid Tissues.* , Swerdlow SH C.E., Harris NL, et al. (eds) (eds),326-329. IARC Lyon

Stein, H.; Marafioti, T.; Foss, H.D.; Laumen, H.; Hummel, M.; Anagnostopoulos, I.; Wirth, T.; Demel, G. & Falini, B. (2001). Down-regulation of BOB.1/OBF.1 and Oct2 in classical Hodgkin disease but not in lymphocyte predominant Hodgkin disease correlates with immunoglobulin transcription. *Blood,* Vol.97, No.2, pp. 496-501, 0006-4971

Stein, R.; Von Wasielewski; Poppema, S.; MacLennan, K. & Guenova, M. (2008b). Nodular sclerosis classical Hodgkin lymphoma. In: *WHO Classification of Tumors of Haematopoietic and Lymphoid Tissues* Swerdlow S., Campo E., Harris N., Jaffe E., Pileri S., Stein H., al. e. (eds),330, IARC, Lyon, France

Stupp, R. & Ruegg, C. (2007). Integrin inhibitors reaching the clinic. *J Clin Oncol,* Vol.25, No.13, pp. 1637-1638, 1527-7755

Sup, S.J.; Alemany, C.A.; Pohlman, B.; Elson, P.; Malhi, S.; Thakkar, S.; Steinle, R. & Hsi, E.D. (2005). Expression of bcl-2 in classical Hodgkin's lymphoma: an independent predictor of poor outcome. *J Clin Oncol,* Vol.23, No.16, pp. 3773-3779, 0732-183X

Suri-Payer, E.; Amar, A.Z.; Thornton, A.M. & Shevach, E.M. (1998). CD4+CD25+ T cells inhibit both the induction and effector function of autoreactive T cells and represent a unique lineage of immunoregulatory cells. *J Immunol,* Vol.160, No.3, pp. 1212-1218,

Sutmuller, R.P.; van Duivenvoorde, L.M.; van Elsas, A.; Schumacher, T.N.; Wildenberg, M.E.; Allison, J.P.; Toes, R.E.; Offringa, R. & Melief, C.J. (2001). Synergism of cytotoxic T lymphocyte-associated antigen 4 blockade and depletion of CD25(+) regulatory T cells in antitumor therapy reveals alternative pathways for suppression of autoreactive cytotoxic T lymphocyte responses. *J Exp Med,* Vol.194, No.6, pp. 823-832

Swerdlow, S.; Campo, E. & Harris, N. (2008a). Pathology and Genetics of Tumours of Haematopoietic and Lymphoid Tissues. In: *World Health Organization Classification of Tumours,* Swerdlow SH C.E., Harris NL (eds). IARC Press Lyon

Swerdlow, S.; Campo, E.; Harris. NL; Jaffe, E.; Pileri, S.; Stein, H.; Thiele, J. & Vardiman, J. (2008b). *WHO classification of tumours of haematopoietic and lymphoid tissues.* IARC Press Lyon, France

Swerdlow, S.; Webber, S.; A., C. & Ferry, J. (2008c). Post-transplant lymphoproliferative disorders. In: *World Health Organization Classification of Tumours, Pathology and Genetics of Tumours of Haematopoietic and Lymphoid Tissues.* , Swerdlow SH C.E., Harris NL, et al. (eds) (eds),343-349. IARC Press Lyon

Takahashi, T.; Tagami, T.; Yamazaki, S.; Uede, T.; Shimizu, J.; Sakaguchi, N.; Mak, T.W. & Sakaguchi, S. (2000). Immunologic self-tolerance maintained by CD25(+)CD4(+) regulatory T cells constitutively expressing cytotoxic T lymphocyte-associated antigen 4. *J Exp Med,* Vol.192, No.2, pp. 303-310, 0022-1007

Tang, T.T.; Dowbenko, D.; Jackson, A.; Toney, L.; Lewin, D.A.; Dent, A.L. & Lasky, L.A. (2002). The forkhead transcription factor AFX activates apoptosis by induction of the BCL-6 transcriptional repressor. *J Biol Chem,* Vol.277, No.16, pp. 14255-14265, 0021-9258

Tazzari, P.L.; Bolognesi, A.; de Totero, D.; Falini, B.; Lemoli, R.M.; Soria, M.R.; Pileri, S.; Gobbi, M.; Stein, H.; Flenghi, L. & et al. (1992). Ber-H2 (anti-CD30)-saporin immunotoxin: a new tool for the treatment of Hodgkin's disease and CD30+ lymphoma: in vitro evaluation. *Br J Haematol,* Vol.81, No.2, pp. 203-211, 0007-1048

Tedoldi, S.; Mottok, A.; Ying, J.; Paterson, J.C.; Cui, Y.; Facchetti, F.; van Krieken, J.H.; Ponzoni, M.; Ozkal, S.; Masir, N.; Natkunam, Y.; Pileri, S.; Hansmann, M.L.; Mason, D.; Tao, Q. & Marafioti, T. (2007). Selective loss of B-cell phenotype in lymphocyte predominant Hodgkin lymphoma. *J Pathol,* Vol.213, No.4, pp. 429-440, 0022-3417

Teichmann, M.; Meyer, B.; Beck, A. & Niedobitek, G. (2005). Expression of the interferon-inducible chemokine IP-10 (CXCL10), a chemokine with proposed anti-neoplastic functions, in Hodgkin lymphoma and nasopharyngeal carcinoma. *J Pathol,* Vol.206, No.1, pp. 68-75, 0022-3417

ten Berge, R.L.; Oudejans, J.J.; Dukers, D.F.; Meijer, J.W.; Ossenkoppele, G.J. & Meijer, C.J. (2001). Percentage of activated cytotoxic T-lymphocytes in anaplastic large cell lymphoma and Hodgkin's disease: an independent biological prognostic marker. *Leukemia,* Vol.15, No.3, pp. 458-464

Teramoto, N.; Pokrovskaja, K.; Szekely, L.; Polack, A.; Yoshino, T.; Akagi, T. & Klein, G. (1999). Expression of cyclin D2 and D3 in lymphoid lesions. *Int J Cancer,* Vol.81, No.4, pp. 543-550, 0020-7136

Tesniere, A.; Apetoh, L.; Ghiringhelli, F.; Joza, N.; Panaretakis, T.; Kepp, O.; Schlemmer, F.; Zitvogel, L. & Kroemer, G. (2008). Immunogenic cancer cell death: a key-lock paradigm. *Curr Opin Immunol,* Vol.20, No.5, pp. 504-511, 0952-7915

Thomas, R.K.; Re, D.; Wolf, J. & Diehl, V. (2004). Part I: Hodgkin's lymphoma--molecular biology of Hodgkin and Reed-Sternberg cells. *Lancet Oncol,* Vol.5, No.1, pp. 11-18, 1470-2045

Thome, M. & Tschopp, J. (2001). Regulation of lymphocyte proliferation and death by FLIP. *Nat Rev Immunol,* Vol.1, No.1, pp. 50-58, 1474-1733

Tirelli, U.; Errante, D.; Dolcetti, R.; Gloghini, A.; Serraino, D.; Vaccher, E.; Franceschi, S.; Boiocchi, M. & Carbone, A. (1995). Hodgkin's disease and human immunodeficiency virus infection: clinicopathologic and virologic features of 114 patients from the Italian Cooperative Group on AIDS and Tumors. *J Clin Oncol,* Vol.13, No.7, pp. 1758-1767, 0732-183X

Tlsty, T.D. & Coussens, L.M. (2006). Tumor stroma and regulation of cancer development. *Annu Rev Pathol,* Vol.1, pp. 119-150, 1553-4006

Tsavaris, N.; Kosmas, C.; Vadiaka, M.; Kanelopoulos, P. & Boulamatsis, D. (2002). Immune changes in patients with advanced breast cancer undergoing chemotherapy with taxanes. *Br J Cancer,* Vol.87, No.1, pp. 21-27, 0007-0920

Tzankov, A.; Krugmann, J.; Fend, F.; Fischhofer, M.; Greil, R. & Dirnhofer, S. (2003a). Prognostic significance of CD20 expression in classical Hodgkin lymphoma: a clinicopathological study of 119 cases. *Clin Cancer Res,* Vol.9, No.4, pp. 1381-1386, 1078-0432

Tzankov, A.; Zimpfer, A.; Lugli, A.; Krugmann, J.; Went, P.; Schraml, P.; Maurer, R.; Ascani, S.; Pileri, S.; Geley, S. & Dirnhofer, S. (2003b). High-throughput tissue microarray analysis of G1-cyclin alterations in classical Hodgkin's lymphoma indicates overexpression of cyclin E1. *J Pathol,* Vol.199, No.2, pp. 201-207

Tzankov, A.; Zimpfer, A.; Pehrs, A.C.; Lugli, A.; Went, P.; Maurer, R.; Pileri, S. & Dirnhofer, S. (2003c). Expression of B-cell markers in classical hodgkin lymphoma: a tissue microarray analysis of 330 cases. *Mod Pathol,* Vol.16, No.11, pp. 1141-1147, 0893-3952

Tzardi, M.; Kouvidou, C.; Panayiotides, I.; Koutsoubi, K.; Stefanaki, K.; Giannikaki, E.; Darivianaki, K.; Zois, M.; Eliopoulos, G.; Kakolyris, S.; Delides, G.; Rontogianni, D. & Kanavaros, P. (1996). Expression of p53 and mdm-2 proteins in Hodgkin's Disease. Absence of correlation with the presence of Epstein-Barr virus. *Anticancer Res,* Vol.16, No.5A, pp. 2813-2819, 0250-7005

Ushmorov, A.; Leithauser, F.; Sakk, O.; Weinhausel, A.; Popov, S.W.; Moller, P. & Wirth, T. (2006). Epigenetic processes play a major role in B-cell-specific gene silencing in classical Hodgkin lymphoma. *Blood,* Vol.107, No.6, pp. 2493-2500, 0006-4971

Ushmorov, A.; Ritz, O.; Hummel, M.; Leithauser, F.; Moller, P.; Stein, H. & Wirth, T. (2004). Epigenetic silencing of the immunoglobulin heavy-chain gene in classical Hodgkin lymphoma-derived cell lines contributes to the loss of immunoglobulin expression. *Blood,* Vol.104, No.10, pp. 3326-3334, 0006-4971

Vaccher, E.; Spina, M.; Talamini, R.; Zanetti, M.; di Gennaro, G.; Nasti, G.; Tavio, M.; Bernardi, D.; Simonelli, C. & Tirelli, U. (2003). Improvement of systemic human immunodeficiency virus-related non-Hodgkin lymphoma outcome in the era of highly active antiretroviral therapy. *Clin Infect Dis,* Vol.37, No.11, pp. 1556-1564, 1537-6591

van den Berg, A.; Visser, L. & Poppema, S. (1999). High expression of the CC chemokine TARC in Reed-Sternberg cells. A possible explanation for the characteristic T-cell infiltratein Hodgkin's lymphoma. *Am J Pathol,* Vol.154, No.6, pp. 1685-1691, 0002-9440

Vassilakopoulos, T.P.; Nadali, G.; Angelopoulou, M.K.; Siakantaris, M.P.; Dimopoulou, M.N.; Kontopidou, F.N.; Rassidakis, G.Z.; Doussis-Anagnostopoulou, I.A.; Hatzioannou, M.; Vaiopoulos, G.; Kittas, C.; Sarris, A.H.; Pizzolo, G. & Pangalis, G.A. (2001). Serum interleukin-10 levels are an independent prognostic factor for patients with Hodgkin's lymphoma. *Haematologica,* Vol.86, No.3, pp. 274-281, 0390-6078

Viviani, S.; Notti, P.; Bonfante, V.; Verderio, P.; Valagussa, P. & Bonadonna, G. (2000). Elevated pretreatment serum levels of Il-10 are associated with a poor prognosis in Hodgkin's disease, the milan cancer institute experience. *Med Oncol,* Vol.17, No.1, pp. 59-63, 1357-0560

Wagner, E.F.; Hleb, M.; Hanna, N. & Sharma, S. (1998). A pivotal role of cyclin D3 and cyclin-dependent kinase inhibitor p27 in the regulation of IL-2-, IL-4-, or IL-10-mediated human B cell proliferation. *J Immunol,* Vol.161, No.3, pp. 1123-1131, 0022-1767

Watanabe, K.; Yamashita, Y.; Nakayama, A.; Hasegawa, Y.; Kojima, H.; Nagasawa, T. & Mori, N. (2000). Varied B-cell immunophenotypes of Hodgkin/Reed-Sternberg cells in classic Hodgkin's disease. *Histopathology,* Vol.36, No.4, pp. 353-361, 0309-0167

Wei, W.Z.; Morris, G.P. & Kong, Y.C. (2004). Anti-tumor immunity and autoimmunity: a balancing act of regulatory T cells. *Cancer Immunol Immunother,* Vol.53, No.2, pp. 73-78

Weihrauch, M.R.; Manzke, O.; Beyer, M.; Haverkamp, H.; Diehl, V.; Bohlen, H.; Wolf, J. & Schultze, J.L. (2005). Elevated serum levels of CC thymus and activation-related chemokine (TARC) in primary Hodgkin's disease: potential for a prognostic factor. *Cancer Res,* Vol.65, No.13, pp. 5516-5519, 0008-5472

Weniger, M.A.; Melzner, I.; Menz, C.K.; Wegener, S.; Bucur, A.J.; Dorsch, K.; Mattfeldt, T.; Barth, T.F. & Moller, P. (2006). Mutations of the tumor suppressor gene SOCS-1 in classical Hodgkin lymphoma are frequent and associated with nuclear phospho-STAT5 accumulation. *Oncogene,* Vol.25, No.18, pp. 2679-2684, 0950-9232

Willenbrock, K.; Roers, A.; Blohbaum, B.; Rajewsky, K. & Hansmann, M.L. (2000). CD8(+) T cells in Hodgkin's disease tumor tissue are a polyclonal population with limited clonal expansion but little evidence of selection by antigen. *Am J Pathol,* Vol.157, No.1, pp. 171-175

Wolf, A.M.; Wolf, D.; Steurer, M.; Gastl, G.; Gunsilius, E. & Grubeck-Loebenstein, B. (2003). Increase of regulatory T cells in the peripheral blood of cancer patients. *Clin Cancer Res,* Vol.9, No.2, pp. 606-612, 1078-0432

Wood, K.M.; Roff, M. & Hay, R.T. (1998). Defective IkappaBalpha in Hodgkin cell lines with constitutively active NF-kappaB. *Oncogene,* Vol.16, No.16, pp. 2131-2139, 0950-9232

Xicoy, B.; Ribera, J.M.; Miralles, P.; Berenguer, J.; Rubio, R.; Mahillo, B.; Valencia, M.E.; Abella, E.; Lopez-Guillermo, A.; Sureda, A.; Morgades, M.; Navarro, J.T. & Esteban, H. (2007). Results of treatment with doxorubicin, bleomycin, vinblastine and dacarbazine and highly active antiretroviral therapy in advanced stage, human immunodeficiency virus-related Hodgkin's lymphoma. *Haematologica,* Vol.92, No.2, pp. 191-198, 1592-8721

Yamamoto, R.; Nishikori, M.; Kitawaki, T.; Sakai, T.; Hishizawa, M.; Tashima, M.; Kondo, T.; Ohmori, K.; Kurata, M.; Hayashi, T. & Uchiyama, T. (2008). PD-1-PD-1 ligand interaction contributes to immunosuppressive microenvironment of Hodgkin lymphoma. *Blood,* Vol.111, No.6, pp. 3220-3224, 0006-4971

Younes, A. (2009). Novel treatment strategies for patients with relapsed classical Hodgkin lymphoma. *Hematology Am Soc Hematol Educ Program,* pp. 507-519, 1520-4383

Younes, A.; Bartlett, N.L.; Leonard, J.P.; Kennedy, D.A.; Lynch, C.M.; Sievers, E.L. & Forero-Torres, A. (2010). Brentuximab vedotin (SGN-35) for relapsed CD30-positive lymphomas. *N Engl J Med,* Vol.363, No.19, pp. 1812-1821, 1533-4406

Young, L.S. & Rickinson, A.B. (2004). Epstein-Barr virus: 40 years on. *Nat Rev Cancer,* Vol.4, No.10, pp. 757-768, 1474-175X

Zheng, B.; Fiumara, P.; Li, Y.V.; Georgakis, G.; Snell, V.; Younes, M.; Vauthey, J.N.; Carbone, A. & Younes, A. (2003). MEK/ERK pathway is aberrantly active in Hodgkin disease: a signaling pathway shared by CD30, CD40, and RANK that regulates cell proliferation and survival. *Blood,* Vol.102, No.3, pp. 1019-1027, 0006-4971

Zhu, J. & Paul, W.E. (2008). CD4 T cells: fates, functions, and faults. *Blood,* Vol.112, No.5, pp. 1557-1569, 1528-0020

Part 5

Treatment of Early Stage Hodgkin's Lymphoma

5

Treatment of Early Stage Hodgkin Lymphoma

Samer A. Srour and Luis E. Fayad
The University of Oklahoma Health Sciences Center
University of Texas MD Anderson Cancer Center,
USA

1. Introduction

Hodgkin lymphoma (HL) is an uncommon lymphoid malignancy which accounts for about 0.5% to 1% of all cancers. In 2010, an estimated 8,490 new cases and 1,320 deaths will occur in the United States (Jemal, Siegel, Xu, *et al*, 2010). HL incidence appears to be stable over the past few decades, in contrast to the incompletely understood continued increase in frequency of non-Hodgkin lymphomas. HL has a bimodal incidence with most patients diagnosed in the third decade, followed by another peak in adults aged 55 years or older. There has been correlation between incidence of certain histologic sybtypes of HL and age and sex; for example, nodular-sclerosis HL is more common in women and young adults in contrast to mixed cellularity HL which is more common in men and lymphocyte-rich HL which is more common in older males (Correa, O'Conor, Berard, *et al*, 1973).

The cause of HL remains unknown, but there has been some progress in identifying risk factors in development of HL. Factors associated with HL include genetic predisposition (increased incidence in certain ethnic populations such as Jews and in first degree relatives such as siblings, twins and children), viral exposures, and immune suppression (Bernard, Cartwright, Darwin, *et al*, 1987; Glaser & Jarrett, 1996; Lynch, Marcus & Lynch, 1992; Mack, Cozen, Shibata, *et al*, 1995). Epstein-Bar virus (EBV) has been implicated in the etiology of HL based on epidemiological and serologic studies (Weiss, Strickler, Warnke, *et al*, 1987), as well as by the detection of the EBV genome in tumor specimens of about half of HL nodes. Moreover, HIV-infected patients have been noted in many studies to have a significantly increased risk of HL with the majority of patients presenting with advanced stages, having extranodal involvement and unfavorable histological subtypes, and associated with a poorer outcome after initial therapy (Levy, Colonna, Tourani, *et al*, 1995; Tirelli, Errante, Dolcetti, *et al*, 1995).

The past few decades have seen major advances in treatment of HL using both, radiation therapy (RT) and chemotherapy. With advances in combination chemotherapy regimens and RT techniques over the past four-five decades, HL has changed from an incurable disease to one with the best survival rates to date among other cancers. HL is currently curable in 85% to 95% of cases, depending on disease stage at time of diagnosis and other risk factors (Diehl, 2007). In the H8-F trial, Ferme' et al. reported a 10-year overall survival (OS) estimates of 97% in early-stage disease (Ferme, Eghbali, Meerwaldt, *et al*, 2007). In fact, cure rates for HL have increased so extensively that the overriding treatment considerations often relate to long-term toxicity, especially for patients with early- or intermediate-stage disease (Hoppe, Advani, Ai, *et al*, 2011). For advanced disease, clinical trials still emphasize improvement in cure rates, but the potential long-term effect of treatments remain an important consideration as well. New innovative treatment strategies are clearly needed for the refractory and recurrent disease, as the cure rates in these patients are still low, especially for those who relapse after autologous stem cell transplantation (ASCT).

In this chapter, we will discuss briefly the initial workup and staging at the time of diagnosis with brief review of the role of positron emission tomography (PET) scan in HL. We will then go through the revised response criteria, followed by a thorough review for the management of early stage HL including the various definitions of the favorable and unfavorable risk groups as determined by major study groups. Management of HL in specific populations such as the NLPHL, elderly, and pregnant patients will be reviewed in this chapter as well.

2. Diagnosis/staging

Hodgkin lymphomas are defined as lymphomas containing one of the characteristic types of Reed-Stenberg (RS) cells in a background of nonneoplastic cells. Based on the morphology and immunophenotype of the RS cells and the composition of the cellular background, the WHO classification system published in 2001 divided HL into two disease entities: classical HL (cHL) which accounts for 95% and nodular lymphocyte-predominant HL (NLPHL) which accounts for 5% of all HL cases. cHL is further divided into 4 subtypes: nodular sclerosis (grades I or II), mixed cellularity, lymphocyte depleted, and lymphocyte-rich cHL (Diehl V, 2005b; Harris, Jaffe, Diebold, *et al*, 1999; Jaffe ES, 2001). cHL and NLPHL share the same diagnostic workup, though they have different natural history and distinctive morphologic and immunophenotypic features (**Table 1**), and ultimately different approach of therapy.

	Classic HL	NLPHL
Pattern	Diffuse, interfollicular, nodular	Nodular, at least in part
Tumor cells	Diagnostic RS cells; mononuclear or lacunar cells	L&H or popcorn cells
Background	Lymphocytes (T cells > B cells), histiocytes, eosinophils, plasma cells	Lymphocytes (B cells > T cells), histiocytes
Fibrosis	Common	Rare
CD15, CD30	+	–
CD45 & CD57 + T cells	–	+
EMA	–	+
CD20	±	+
EBV (in RS cells)	+ (~50%)	–
Nuclear bcl-6 protein	–	+
Ig genes (single-cell PCR)	Rearranged, clonal, mutated, "crippled"	Rearranged, clonal, mutated, ongoing

EBV, Epstein-Barr virus; EMA, epithelial membrane antigen; Ig, immunoglobulin; L&H, lymphocytes and histiocytes; PCR, polymerase chain reaction; RS, Reed-Sternberg.
Adapted from De Vita et al. Cancer. Principles & practice of oncology. Philadelphia: Lippincott Williams and Wilkins; 2005.

Table 1. Morphologic and Immunophenotypic Features of cHL Compared to NLPHL.

Diagnosis of HL should always be established by a tissue biopsy; though a core needle biopsy may be adequate, an excisional lymph node biopsy is preferred and highly recommended. FNA alone is generally insufficient for the evaluation of architecture and for immunophenotyping, and should be avoided (Caraway, 2005; Hehn, Grogan & Miller, 2004; Meda, Buss, Woodruff, *et al*, 2000). Rarely, multiple LN biopsies may be necessary for the diagnosis, as the cytokines associated with HL can produce reactive hyperplastic changes in adjacent lymph nodes (Ansell & Armitage, 2006).

Though it might not be necessary for typical cases of cHL, immunohistochemistry staining is recommended for accurate diagnosis of any case of HL with atypical features and many cases of NLPHL. cHL is usually positive for CD15 and CD30, but negative for CD3 and CD45. NLPHL usually stains positive for CD45 and CD20, but negative for CD15, and rarely expresses CD30 (Hoppe, Advani, Ai, *et al*, 2011)(**Table 1**). Also, in contrast to NLPHL, the RS cells of cHL lack the nuclear bcl-6 protein associated with follicle center B cells (Falini B, 1995).

Staging of HL is based on the Ann Arbor staging system that was developed in 1971 (Carbone, Kaplan, Musshoff, *et al*, 1971) and further modified in 1989 through a consensus meeting held in Cotswolds, England (Lister, Crowther, Sutcliffe, *et al*, 1989) (**Table 2**).

Stage	Definition/Disease Involvement
I	Involvement of a single lymph node region (I) or a single extralymphatic site (IE).
II	Involvement of two or more lymph node regions on the same side of the diaphragm (II) or localized involvement of only one extranodal organ or site and of ≥1 lymph node regions on the same side of the diaphragm (IIE).
III	Involvement of lymph node regions on both sides of the diaphragm (III), which may also be accompanied by involvement of the spleen (III_S) or by localized involvement of an extranodal organ or site (IIIE) or both (III_{S+E}).
IV	Diffuse involvement of one or more extranodal organs or sites, with or without associated lymph node involvement.
Each Stage may be subdivided into:	
A	No symptoms.
B	General symptoms include any of the following: fever (unexplained temperatures >38°C over the preceding one month), drenching night sweats, unexplained loss of >10% body weight within the preceding 6 months.
X	Bulky disease which is defined by any nodal mass with a maximal dimension ≥10 cm or a mediastinal mass exceeding one third of the widest transverse transthoracic diameter measured on a standard PA chest radiography.
E	Involvement of a single extranodal site that is contiguous or proximal to the known nodal site.

Table 2. Modified Ann Arbor Staging System for HL.

Initial staging evaluation starts with a detailed history and physical examination. History should focus on the presence or absence of systemic B symptoms (unexplained fevers >38 °C within the preceding month, drenching night sweats, and unexplained weight loss of >10%

body weight within the preceding 6 months), performance status, pruritus, alcohol intolerance, and any history of prior cancers and treatments received (chemotherapy and/or RT). Of notice, cHL compared to NLPHL, presents more commonly with B symptoms (about one third of patients with HL), pruritus, alcohol-induced pain, and extra nodal disease involvement. Physical examination should be focused on all lymphoid regions in addition to the liver and spleen.

The National Comprehensive Cancer Network (NCCN) established certain laboratory and radiographic studies which are recommended at the initial evaluation of patients with HL. These include (NCCN, v.2.2011) CBC with differential and platelets, ESR, LDH, albumin, liver and kidney function tests, and a pregnancy test for women of childbearing age. An adequate bone marrow (BM) biopsy should be performed for stages IB-IIB and stages III-IV disease. More invasive procedures such as liver biopsy, diagnostic laparotomy, or splenectomy are restricted to a very small subgroup of patients where initial staging is inconclusive. Radiographic studies should include at least chest x-ray and diagnostic computed tomography (CT) of the chest, abdomen and pelvis. CT-PET scan has become an integral part of initial staging as well. Neck CT is recommended if RT is planned.

2.1 Role of PET in HL

The role of PET in HL has been markedly evolving over the past few years. It has been used and shown to have high positivity and specificity for initial staging and restaging in patients with lymphoma (Isasi, Lu & Blaufox, 2005; Seam, Juweid & Cheson, 2007). In a review done by Juweid ME (Juweid, 2006a), the use of PET scan in HL results in a modification of disease stage (usually upstaging) in about 15-20% of patients with an impact on management in about 5-15%. However, it remains unclear whether patients would benefit from a subsequent change in the treatment plan, and therefore, the value of PET for initial staging of HL patients outside a clinical trial is still debatable. On the other hand, as reviewed by Juweid, response assessment after completion of therapy is currently the most widely utilized application of restaging PET in HL and can be considered the standard of care for post treatment assessment of patients with HL. In this setting, PET shows an excellent negative predictive value between 91 and 95% in several studies, but the positive predictive value is substantially lower and considerably more variable averaging approximately 65% (de Wit, Bohuslavizki, Buchert, *et al*, 2001; Juweid, 2006a; Weihrauch, Re, Scheidhauer, *et al*, 2001). To decrease the false positive results, the International Harmonization Project (IHP), recommends that PET not be performed for at least 3 weeks following chemotherapy and preferably 8-12 weeks after completion of radiotherapy (Juweid, 2006b). The role of PET scan for routine post therapy surveillance remains controversial, primarily because of the potential for a disproportionate fraction of false-positive findings, potentially resulting in increasing cost without proven benefit from earlier PET detection of disease compared to standard surveillance methods (Cheson, Pfistner, Juweid, *et al*, 2007; Jerusalem, Beguin, Fassotte, *et al*, 2003).

Another evolving and interesting use of PET scan is in the assessment of early response; interim PET scan findings has been significantly correlated with treatment outcomes in terms of progression-free survival (PFS) and OS. Recently, PET scanning was proposed to assist in determining the choice of therapy. Patients with negative PET scans after 2-3 cycles of treatment are being considered for an abbreviated course of chemotherapy alone, whereas those with positive PET scan are treated in a more standard fashion with the combined modality. The ongoing United Kingdom (RAPID trial) is testing whether PET scanning can guide therapy in early HL after 3 cycles of chemotherapy; PET-negative patients are randomized to involved field RT (IF-RT) versus observation while PET-positive are treated with 4th cycle ABVD (doxorubicin, bleomycin, vinblastine, dacarbazine) followed by IFRT. The recently initiated EORTC/GELA H10 Intergroup trial is comparing 'standard therapy' to PET-based response-adapted therapy (i.e. PET after 2 cycles ABVD) for favorable and intermediate group patients with early-stage HL.

3. Response criteria

Uniform and standardized criteria for assessment of initial treatment response are essential since they guide for additional treatment and are required for interpreting and comparing clinical trials. Hence, the International Working Group (IWG) published guidelines for non-Hodgkin's lymphoma response criteria first time in 1999 (Cheson, Horning, Coiffier, *et al*, 1999; Cheson, Pfistner, Juweid, *et al*, 2007). The HL study groups have adopted these IWG criteria which were based on the size reduction of the enlarged lymph nodes (as measured with CT scan) and the extent of BM involvement; bone marrow aspirate and biopsy should only be performed to confirm a CR if they were initially positive or if it is clinically indicated by new abnormalities in the peripheral blood counts or blood smear.

The IWG guidelines were revised in 2007, by the IHP, after incorporating the PET scans, immunohistochemistry, and flow cytometry in the definitions of response for both NHL and HL (**Table 3**). Using the revised system, response is simplified to complete response (CR), partial response (PR), stable disease (SD), relapsed disease, or progressive disease (PD) (see table 3). CRU (complete response uncertain) category was eliminated from the new guidelines, based on the improved ability of PET scans to distinguish between viable tumor and necrosis or fibrosis in residual masses present after treatment (Buchmann, Reinhardt, Elsner, *et al*, 2001; Jerusalem, Beguin, Fassotte, *et al*, 1999; Jerusalem, Warland, Najjar, *et al*, 1999; Wirth, Seymour, Hicks, *et al*, 2002).

More recently integrated PET/CT scan, which combines a PET and a CT scan in a single study, has been shown to provide at least equal information to that obtained separately by PET and CT scans. This is supported mostly by retrospective and small trials (Juweid, 2006a). The recent increase in use of combined PET/CT scans may further help in distinction between viable and nonviable tumors.

4. Treatment

4.1 Background

Traditionally, treatment modality for HL had been chosen based on clinical stage. Early-stage HL includes the limited stages I, II, and IIIA whereas advanced HL includes stage IIIB and stage IV, according to the Cotswolds modification of the Ann Arbor classification (Josting, Wolf & Diehl, 2000). Major advances in treatment modalities over past 3 decades made early stage HL highly curable with rates achieving up 97% after 10-year follow up as reported by Ferme et al (Ferme, Eghbali, Meerwaldt, *et al*, 2007). Such high cure rates for

Table 3. Revised Response Criteria/Definitions for Lymphoma.

Response	Definition	Nodal Masses	Spleen, Liver	Bone Marrow
CR	Disappearance of all evidence of disease	(a) FDG-avid or PET positive prior to therapy; mass of any size permitted if PET negative (b) Variably FDG-avid or PET negative; regression to normal size on CT	Not palpable, nodules disappeared	Infiltrate cleared on repeat biopsy; if indeterminate by morphology, immunohistochemistry should be negative
PR	Regression of measuable disease and no new sites	≥50% decrease in SPD of up to 6 largest dominant masses; no increase in size of other nodes (a) FDG-avid or PET positive prior to therapy; one or more PET positive at previously involved site (b) Variably FDG-avid or PET negative; regression on CT	≥50% decrease in SPD of nodules (for single nodule in greatest transverse diameter); no increase in size of liver or spleen	Irrelevant if positive prior to therapy; cell type should be specified
SD	Failure to attain CR/PR or PD	(a) FDG-avid or PET positive prior to therapy; PET positive at prior sites of disease and no new sites on CT or PET (b) Variably FDG-avid or PET negative; no change in size of previous lesions on CT		
Relapsed disease or PD	Any new lesion or increase by ≥50% of previously involved sites from nadir	Appearance of a new lesion(s) > 1.5 cm in any axis, ≥50% increase in SPD of more than one node, or ≥50% increase in longest diameter of a previously identifed node > 1 cm in short axis Lesions PET positive if FDG-avid lymphoma or PET positive prior to therapy	> 50% increase from nadir in the SPD of any previous lesions	New or recurrent involvement

Abbreviations: CR, complete remission; FDG, [18F]fluorodeoxyglucose; PET, positron emission tomography; CT, computed tomography; PR, partial remission; SPD, sum of the product of the diameters; SD, stable disease; PD, progressive disease. Source: Table 3 from Cheson BD, Pfistner B, Juweid ME, et al. Revised response criteria for malignant lymphoma. J of Clin Oncol 2007;25(5):579-586.

early stage HL made the focus of recent studies on minimizing acute and late therapy related toxicities without decreasing the excellent treatment outcomes. Hence, there have been various attempts to modify different treatment modalities such as omitting RT, decreasing the dose and/or field of RT, and modifying the chemotherapy. In order to maintain efficacy and decrease toxicity, clinical investigators, through major randomized studies, were able to identify adverse prognostic factors that may predict treatment outcomes in different groups of patients. We will discuss and define below these risk groups according to published data from major study groups in Europe and North America. Subsequently, we will discuss the management of early stage HL according to different risk groups.

4.2 Definitions of favorable and unfavorable early-stage HL

In addition to the clinical stage and B symptoms which have traditionally known to be of prognostic value, various other adverse factors have been identified based on large cohorts over several years. As there have been different approaches to treat HL among major study groups which ultimately lead to different prognostic variables, various definitions for different risk groups do exist among these cooperative research groups.

In Europe, three different risk groups are defined: early-stage favorable, early-stage unfavorable (intermediate) and advanced-stage HL (**Table 4**). The NCCN divides HL into 3 groups: early-stage favorable (stage I-II with no B symptoms or large mediastinal adenopathy), early-stage unfavorable (stage I-II with large mediastinal mass, with or without B symptoms; stage I-II with B symptoms; numerous sites of disease; or significantly elevated ESR), and advanced-stage disease (stage III-IV). However, some centers in Northern America define only two risk groups, namely limited-stage (IA and IIA without bulky disease) and advanced-stage HL [III and IV; B symptoms; bulky disease (≥10 cm)] (Fuchs, Diehl & Re, 2006).

NCCN unfavorable risk factors for stage I-II disease include bulky mediastinal disease (mediastinal mass ratio >0.33) or bulky disease >10 cm, B symptoms, ESR >50 and more than 3 nodal sites of disease. NCCN further classifies unfavorable stage I-II disease into stage I-II (unfavorable with bulky disease) and unfvaorable stage I-II with bulky disease and unfvaorable stage I-II with non-bulky disease. The European Organization for Research and Treatment of Cancers (EORTC) definitions of favorable and unfavorable early stage HL are very similar to those for early stage HL in the German HL Study Group (GHSG) (**Table 4**) (Carde, Burgers, Henry-Amar, *et al*, 1988; Loeffler, Pfreundschuh, Ruhl, *et al*, 1989; Mauch, Tarbell, Weinstein, *et al*, 1988; Tubiana, Henry-Amar, Carde, *et al*, 1989). The EORTC criteria differs by substituting age ≥50 years in place of the extra nodal disease criterion and specifying ≥4 involved regions rather than ≥3, as in GHSG (Noordijk, Carde, Dupouy, *et al*, 2006). Moreover, the National Cancer Institute of Canada (NCIC) and the Eastern Cooperative Oncology Group (ECOG) subdivided early-stage HL into risk categories, with 'low risk' being NLPHL and nodular sclerosis histology, age <40 years, erythrocyte sedimentation rate (ESR) <50, and ≤3 disease regions. 'High risk' group patients were all other cases with stage I-II disease, except those with bulky disease > 10 cm, which are assigned to advanced-stage disease (**Table 4**) (Evens, Hutchings & Diehl, 2008; Meyer, Gospodarowicz, Connors, *et al*, 2005).

	GHSG		EORTC/GELA		NCIC/ECOG		NCCN	
Risk Factors (RF)	A	Large mediastinal mass	A	Large mediastinal mass	A	Bulky disease >10 cm	A	Large mediastinal mass (MMR >0.33) or bulky disease (>10 cm)
	B	Extranodal disease	B	Age ≥50 y	B	Age ≥40	B	ESR ≥50, if asymptomatic
	C	ESR ≥50 or B symptoms[a] with ESR ≥30	C	Same as for GHSG[1]	C	ESR ≥50 or any B symptom[a]	C	B symptoms[a]
	D	≥3 involved nodal regions	D	≥4 involved nodal regions	D	>3 involved nodal regions	D	>3 involved nodal regions
					E	MCHL or LDHL		
Treatment groups								
Lymphocyte predominant	NLPHL histology in CS I–II with no RF		NLPHL histology in supradiaphragmatic CS I–II		Low risk early stage	CS I–II with no RF		
Early stage favorable	CS I–II with no RF		CS I–II supradiaphragmatic with no RF		Low risk early stage	CS I–II with no RF	CS I–II with none of the RFs	
Early stage unfavorable	CS I, CS IIA with any RF; CS IIB with C/D but without A/B		CS I–II supradiaphragmatic with any RF		High risk early stage	CS I–II with any RF except A	CS I–II with any of the RFs	
Advanced stage	CS IIB with A/B; CS III–IV		CS III–IV		CS I–II with A; CS III–IV		CS III–IV	

Abbreviations: CS, clinical stage; EORTC, European Organization for Research and Treatment of Cancer; ESR, erythrocyte sedimentation rate; GELA, Groupe d'Etude des Lymphomes de l'Adulte; GHSG, German Hodgkin Study Group; LDHL, lymphocyte depleted HL; MCHL, mixed cellularity HL; MMR, mediastinal mass ratio, maximum width of mass/maximum intrathoracic diameter; NCIC/ECOG, National Cancer Institute of Canada/ Eastern Cooperative Oncology Group; NCCN, National Comprehensive Cancer Network; NLPHL, nodular lymphocyte-predominant Hodgkin's lymphoma; RF, risk factor

[a]B symptoms include fever with temperature >38°C, drenching night sweats, and unexplained weight loss of >10% body weight within 6 months.

[b]Source: Derived from Table 21.2 by Srour S.A. and Fayad L.E. (Srour & Fayad, 2010).

Table 4. Unfavorable Factors and Treatment Groups According to Major Study Groups and NCCN.

4.3 Treatment of early stage cHL

Treatment of HL is becoming more standardized in the current era of rapidly evolving medical literature and with the marked advances in high technique imaging studies. The most accepted standard of care to date is the combined modality treatment (CMT) with chemotherapy and radiotherapy (**Table 5**). However, there has been some controversy about the best RT field/dose and/or the best chemotherapy regimens. We will discuss below some of these issues.

Histology	Prognostic Group	Recommended Treatment
Early Stage cHL	Favorable[a]	Chemotherapy[b, d] + 20 Gy to 30 Gy IF-RT (most commonly accepted protocol) or Chemotherapy alone with 4-6 cycles of ABVD (category 2B[e] per NCCN Guidelines)
	Unfavorable[a]	Chemotherapy[c, d] + 30 Gy to 36 Gy IF-RT
Early Stage NLPHL	CS IA	Local LN excision (limited data) or IF-RT alone (preferred option)
	CS IIA	Regional RT or IF-RT alone[f] (preferred option by most investigators)
	CS IB–IIB	Chemotherapy[g] followed by IF-RT

[a]See Table 4 for the definitions of favorable and unfavorable prognostic groups
[b]For favorable early stage cHL, the most commonly used regimens are the ABVD (2 to 4 cycles) and the Stanford V regimen (2 cycles)
[c]For unfavorable early stage cHL, either ABVD is given for 4 to 6 cycles or Stanford V for 3 cycles
[d]See Table x for the chemotherapy regimen abbreviations and dosages
[e]Category 2B, per NCCN, is defined as follows: the recommendation is based on lower-level evidence and there is nonuniform NCCN consensus (but no major disagreement)
[f]In the setting of non-bulky CS IIA NLPHL
[g]Given the rarity of NLPHL, no large randomized trials regarding the best chemotherapeutic regimen are done. ABVD is widely used based on data for cHL. Immunotherapy with rituximab has been shown recently to have excellent response rates in NLPHL. See text for further details.
CS, clinical stage; IF-RT, involved field radiation therapy; NCCN, National Comprehensive Cancer network; RT, radiation therapy

Table 5. Recommended Treatments for Early Stage HL Commonly Adopted in Europe and USA.

4.3.1 Radiotherapy alone

It was first noticed in 1950, by Peters (Peters, 1950), that aggressive RT might cure patients with limited stage HL. It was not then until early 1960's when extended field RT (EF-RT) was adopted as standard of care for early stage HL. However, EF-RT was complicated by high relapse rates (Horwich, Specht & Ashley, 1997) and serious long-term side effects including pulmonary dysfunction, heart disease and secondary cancers (Gustavsson, Osterman & Cavallin-Stahl, 2003). Hence, in an attempt to lessen toxicity and improve treatment outcomes, several studies over the past 3 decades addressed those concerns through modifying the radiation field/dose and/or incorporating chemotherapy to RT. Multiple randomized studies revealed that combined modality treatment (RT plus chemotherapy) has superior outcomes and less toxicity to RT alone. Of importance are the two randomized studies by Press et al (Press, LeBlanc, Lichter, *et al*, 2001) and Engert et al (Engert, Franklin, Eich, *et al*, 2007) which compared RT alone in early stage favorable HL to combined modality with chemotherapy followed by RT. Press el al compared 3 cycles of chemotherapy (doxorubicin + vinblastine) followed by subtotal lymphoid irradiation (STLI) to STLI alone with freedom from treatment failure (FFTF) of 94% vs. 81% after 3 years of follow up in favor to combined modality arm. Engert et al compared EF-RT alone to combined modality with 2 cycles of ABVD followed by EF-RT. Superior outcomes were in favor to the combined therapy after 7 years of follow up with FFTF of 88% vs. 67%.

Therefore, treatment with large radiation fields alone has been abandoned and the availability of less toxic and more effective chemotherapy made the combined modality therapy the standard of care in treating early HL over the past 10-15 years. The only exception is those patients with stage IA NLPHL who might benefit from RT alone as will be discussed below.

4.3.2 Early stage favorable cHL

Almost all investigators in Europe and US now agree that patients with favorable early stages HL should receive combined modality therapy. However, there is still no consensus as to what chemotherapy should be used, how many cycles should be delivered, and how much RT should be administered, if at all. The application of chemotherapy prior to irradiation not only led to better treatment results but also enabled the reduction of EF-RT to IF-RT in this group of patients (Bonadonna, Bonfante, Viviani, *et al*, 2004; Diehl V, 2005a, Hagenbeek A, 2000; Noordijk EM, 2005) and also lead to a meaningful reduction (up to 50%) in the effective prescribed radiation dose (Yahalom, 2006).

Among other regimens (chemotherapy regimens abbreviations are listed in Tables 6-8), ABVD and Stanford V have been favored as frontline regimens in the combined modality with RT in the early stage HL (see **Table 6** for regimen details and dosages). ABVD was first introduced by Bonadonna et al in 1975 for patients who failed MOPP with very promising results. Hence, Santoro and colleagues (Santoro, Bonadonna, Valagussa, *et al*, 1987) compared then three cycles of MOPP vs. ABVD as frontline therapy followed by EF-RT and three additional chemotherapy cycles in an attempt to improve outcomes and decrease toxicities associated with MOPP. ABVD arm had superior outcomes with better freedom from progression (FFP) rates (81% vs. 63%) and lower rates of sterility and leukemia. Since then, many studies were conducted by major study groups in Europe and USA and compared the combination of either EF-RT or IF-RT with different chemotherapy regimens like ABVD, MOPP, MOPP/ABV, EBVP, COPP and BEACOPP, among others. **Table 7** summarizes some of the major studies addressed the combined modality treatment with the treatment outcomes.

The Stanford V regimen, which incorporated the active agents from ABVD and MOPP into a brief dose-intense regimen, is one of the relatively new regimens that also has been proven, combined with radiotherapy, to be highly effective in early stage favorable and unfavorable or locally extensive HL with low toxicity profile.

The number of chemotherapy cycles (2 to 4 ABVD versus 2 to 3 Stanford V), and the intensity of radiation, have been addressed by multiple randomized studies to date with major impact on current therapy guidelines. Bonadonna et al (Bonadonna, Bonfante, Viviani, *et al*, 2004) revealed a noninferiority outcomes with 4 cycles of ABVD followed by IF-RT compared to same chemotherapy followed by EF-RT after 12 years of follow up (FFP rates of 93% for ABVD followed by EF-RT vs. 94% for ABVD followed by IF-RT). Horning S (Horning SJ, 2004), in a single arm study, showed as well that the 8-week modified Stanford V chemotherapy (rather than the standard 12 -week cycle) followed by IF-RT has

Regimen	Dosage and schedule	Frequency[a]
ABVD[b]		
Doxorubicin	25 mg/m^2 IV on days 1 and 15	
Bleomycin	10 units/m^2 IV on days 1 and 15	Repeat cycle every 28 days
Vinblastine	6 mg/m^2 IV on days 1 and 15	
Dacarbazine[b]	375 mg/m^2 IV on days 1-5	
Standard BEACOPP[c]		
Bleomycin	10 units/m^2 IV on day 8	
Etoposide	100 mg/m^2 IV on days 1, 2, and 3	
Doxorubicin	25 mg/m^2 IV on day 1	Repeat cycle every 21 days
Cyclophosphamide	650 mg/m^2 IV on day 1	
Vincristine[d]	1.4 mg/m^2 IV on day 8	
Procarbazine	100 mg/m^2 PO on days 1-7	
Prednisone	40 mg/m^2 PO on days 1-14	
Esc-BEACOPP[c]		
Bleomycin	10 mg/m^2 IV on day 8	Repeat cycle every 21 days
Etoposide	200 mg/m^2 IV on days 1, 2, and 3	
Doxorubicin	35 mg/m^2 IV on day 1	
Cyclophosphamide	1200 mg/m^2 IV on day 1	
Vincristine[d]	1.4 mg/m^2 IV on day 8	
Procarbazine	100 mg/m^2 PO on days 1-7	
Prednisone	40 mg/m^2 PO on days 1-14	
Filgrastim[e]	300 mcg/day starting on day 8	
STANFORD V[f]		
Doxorubicin	25 mg/m^2 IV on days 1 and 15	
Vinblastine[g]	6 mg/m^2 IV on days 1 and 15	
Mechlorethamine	6 mg/m^2 IV on day 1	
Vincristine[g]	1.4 mg/m^2 IV on days 8 and 22	Repeat cycle every 28 days
Bleomycin	5 units/m^2 IV on days 8 and 22	
Etoposide	60 mg/m^2 IV on days 15 and 16	
Prednisone[h]	40 mg/m^2 PO every other day	

[a]The duration of chemotherapy and number of cycles are determined by the stage of the disease and the prognostic stratification (see text for details)
[b]ABVD regimen was used first as described in the table by Bonadonna G et al (Bonadonna G et al., 1975). On subsequent studies, dacarbazine was administered on days 1 and 15 rather than on days 1-5 (Canellos GP et al., 1992)
[c]Derived from Diehl V et al. 2003
[d]Maximum dose 2 mg.
[e]Filgrastrim is given subcutaneously starting on day 8 and continuing until WBC ≥13,000/mm^{3}on 3 consecutive days. The dose is 300 mcg/day for patients with body weight <75 kg and 400 mcg/day for those ≥75 kg
[f]Derived from Bartlett NL et al. 1995
[g]Vinblastine dose reduced to 4mg/m^2 and vincristine dose to 1mg/m^2 during cycle 3 for patients 50 years of age or older
[h]Prednisone is started on day 1 and continued every other day. It is tapered by 10 mg/dose every other day starting on day 14 of the third cycle

Table 6. Common Chemotherapy Regimens Used for the Treatment of HL in Europe and USA.

Trial/Study Group	Treatment Protocols	No. of Patients	Median Follow-up	Treatment Outcomes
Engert A et al. (2007) GHSG HD7	A: RT alone (30 Gy EF-RT or 40 Gy IF-RT)	311	87 months	7-yr FFTF, 67%; 7-yr OS: 92%
	B: 2 ABVD + RT (30 Gy EF-RT or 40 Gy IF-RT)	316		7-yr FFTF: 88%; 7-yr OS: 94%
Engert A et al. (2010) GHSG HD10, 1998–2003	A: 2 ABVD + IF-RT (30 Gy)	295	91 months for OS and 79 months for FFTF	8-yr FFTF: 85.5 8-yr OS: 93.6
	B: 2 ABVD + IF-RT (20 Gy)	299		8-yr FFTF: 85.9 8-yr OS: 95.1
	C: 4 ABVD + IF-RT (30 Gy)	298		8-yr FFTF: 87.2 8-yr OS: 94.4
	D: 4 ABVD + IF-RT (20 Gy)	298		8-yr FFTF: 89.9 8-yr OS: 94.7
Advani RH et al. (2010) Stanford[a]	A: Stanford V for 8 wk + IF-RT (mostly 30 Gy, but some with 20 Gy)	46 (favorable factors GHSG)	8.5 years	10-yr FFP: 100% 10-yr OS: 97%
Press OW et al. (2001) SWOG 9133/CALGB 9391	A: 3 (doxorubicin + vinblastine) + STLI (S) (36–40 Gy)	165	3.3 years	3-yr FFS: 94% 3-yr OS: 98%
	B: STLI (S) (36–40 Gy)	161		3-yr FFS: 81% 3-yr OS: 96%
Ferme C et al. (2007) EORTC/GELA H8F	A: 3 MOPP/ABV + IF-RT (36 Gy)	270	92 months	10-yr EFS: 93% 10-yr OS 97%
	B: STLI (S)	272		10-yr EFS 68%; 10-yr OS 92%
Horning SJ et al. (1999) Stanford[a]	Stanford V for 8 wk + modified IF-RT (30 Gy)	65	16 months	3-yr FFP: 94.6% 3-yr OS: 96.6%
Noordijik EM et al. (2006) EORTC/GELA H7F	A: 6 EBVP + IF-RT (36 GY)	164	9 years	10-yr EFS: 88%; 10-yr OS: 92%
	B: EF-RT	165		10 yr FFTF: 78%; 10 yr OS: 92%
Meyer RM et al. (2005) NCIC-CTG/ECOG	A: EF-RT alone	64	4.2 years	5-yr EFS: 88% 5-yr OS: 100%
	B: 4-6 cycles of ABVD alone	59		5-yr EFS: 87% 5-yr OS: 97%
Eghbali H et al. (2005) EORTC-GELA H9-F	A: 6 EBVP + IF-RT (36 Gy)	239	51 months	4-yr EFS: 88% 4-yr OS: 99%
	B: 6 EBVP + IF-RT (20 Gy)	209		4-yr EFS: 85% 4-yr OS: 100%
	C: 6 EBVP alone	130		4-yr EFS: 69% 4-yr OS: 98%
Wirth A et al. (2011) ALLG/TTROG[a]	3 ABVD followed by 30 Gy IF-RT	?75	5.9 years	5-yr FFP: 97%

ABV, doxorubicin (Adriamycin), bleomycin, vinblastine; ABVD, doxorubicin, bleomycin, vinblastine, dacarbazine; ALLG/TTROG, Australasian Leukaemia and Lymphoma Group/Trans-Tasman Radiation

Oncology Group; AV, doxorubicin and vinblastine; AVD, doxorubicin, vinblastine, dacarbazine; CALGB, Cancer and Leukemia Group B; EF-RT, extended-field radiotherapy; EBVP regimen, epirubicin, bleomycin, vinblastine, and prednisone; ECOG, Eastern Cooperative Oncology Group; EFS, event-free survival; EORTC, European Organization for Research and Treatment of Cancer; FFP, freedom from progression; FFS, failure-free survival; FFTF, freedom from treatment failure; GELA, Groupe d'Etude des Lymphomes de l'Adulte; GHSG, German Hodgkin Study Group; IF-RT, involved-field radiation therapy; MOPP, mechlorethamine, vincristine, procarbazine, prednisone; OS, overall survival; NCIC-CTG, National Cancer Institute of Canada Clinical Trials Group; RFS, relapse-free survival; RT, radiotherapy; Stanford V, mechlorethamine, doxorubicin, vinblastine, prednisone, vincristine, bleomycin, VP-16; STLI (S), subtotal nodal irradiation (splenic irradiation); SWOG, Southwest Oncology Group; VAPEC-B, doxorubicin, cyclophosphamide, etoposide, vincristine, bleomycin, prednisone; yr, year.
[a]Used GHSG definition for early stage favorable HL

Table 7. Selected Trials in Favorable Early Stage HL Derived from Major Study Groups.

comparable outcomes to more intense regimens with FFP of 96% and OS of 98% after a median follow-up of 5.7 years.

Furthermore, one of the recent "practice changing" important studies, the GHSG HD 10 trial by Engert A et al (Engert, Plutschow, Eich, *et al*, 2010), randomized 1370 patients (age range, 16 to 75) with early stage favorable HL in a 4 arm study into 2 or 4 cycles of ABVD followed by 20 or 30 Gy IF-RT. Favorable disease included patients with no bulky disease, no extranodal extension, and without elevated ESR (see Table 4 for definitions of risk groups). With a median follow-up of 79-91 months, there were no significant differences in FFTF and OS in the 4 arms with FFTF rates in the range of 85.5% to 89.9% and OS rates in the range of 93.6% to 95.1% (**Table 7**). Furthermore, patients who received only two cycles of ABVD and low dose of radiation have less adverse events and acute toxic effects.

The HD 13 randomized trial is trying to address the question, in order to decrease toxicity from ABVD, whether the number of drugs can be reduced. Patients in this study are randomly assigned to one of the 4 arms: ABVD, ABV, AVD, or AV chemotherapy followed by 30 Gy of IF-RT. An interim safety analysis in 2006 showed increased failure rates in the ABV and AV arms, hence those arms were closed. Until further evidence, dacarbazine should be considered an integral part of the ABVD regimen in early stage favorable HL. Future analyses of the HD 13 study would hopefully answer the question whether ABVD and AVD are equivalent or not (Borchmann & Engert, 2010).

4.3.3 Early stage unfavorable cHL

The standard of care based on multiple randomized studies remains the combined modality treatment with chemotherapy and RT, as for the early stage favorable HL. However, there has been a trend towards more intense therapy than early favorable stage HL with some investigators suggesting therapy approaches similar to those adopted for advanced HL. However, giving the high cure rates and prolonged CR rates, there have been many randomized studies trying to address the need for less intense chemotherapy and/or RT in order to decrease long term toxicity from RT and maintain the best response rates. **Table 8** summarizes some of the major studies addressing the therapeutic approaches for early stage unfavorable HL with the associated response rates.

4.3.3.1 Brief historical background for chemotherapy use in early stage unfavorable cHL

Various chemotherapeutic regimens have been investigated in the combined modality treatment for early stage unfavorable HL since early 1980's. However, studies didn't identify significant survival advantages among different modalities. Based on data derived from major studies in advanced HL, ABVD has been favored in most recent studies as first line therapy combined with RT in this population. ABVD has been favored for its superior outcomes and low late toxicity profile compared to other more intense regimens. Stanford V has been studied as well with some promising data and more recently ABVD has been compared to more intense regimens such as BEACOPP in early stage unfavorable HL.

Earlier studies in unfavorable HL patients compared CMT with MOPP to ABVD and MOPP-like combinations. One of the earlier studies is the Milan study (Santoro, Viviani & Zucali, 1983) which randomized patients in a split fashion for 3 cycles of MOPP followed by subtotal nodal irradiation followed by another 3 cycles of MOPP versus same course but with ABVD rather than MOPP. No significant differences in FFP were noticed initially. However, the EORTC H6U trial (Cosset, Ferme, Noordijk, *et al*, 1996) showed a better 10-year FFTF with ABVD compared to MOPP, though there was no significant survival advantage as in many other subsequent studies.

In an attempt to improve efficacy and reduce toxicity, few studies were conducted with modified combinations such as reducing alkylating agents or total cumulative dosage of chemotherapy. However, inferior outcomes were noticed in the unfavorable early stage HL with these approaches (**Table 8**).

One of such experiences was the Cancer and Leukemia Group B 9051 phase II study (Wasserman, Petroni, Millard, *et al*, 1999) which tested three cycles of etoposide, vinblastine, and doxorubicin (EVA) followed by subtotal lymphoid irradiation in 59 patients with CS I-III disease and unfavorable features (bleomycin was eliminated). CR rate was about 66% with high relapse rate of 20%.

In a more recent study (the EORTC H7U trial) conducted by the EORTC group (Noordijk, Carde, Dupouy, *et al*, 2006), 389 patients with unfavorable prognosis early stage HL were randomized to receive CMT with six cycles of epirubicin, bleomycin, vinblastine, and prednisone (EBVP) and IF-RT versus 6 cycles of mechlorethamine, vincristine, procarbazine, prednisone, doxorubicin, bleomycin, and vinblastine (MOPP/ABV hybrid) and IF-RT. The EBVP regimen, given one time per month (compared with two times per month for ABVD), was anticipated to be a less toxic regimen. However, the 10-year EFS rate was 88% in the MOPP/ABV arm compared with 68% in the EBVP arm ($P < .001$), leading to 10-year OS rates of 87% and 79%, respectively ($P = .0175$). Also, the failure-free survival rate at three years was significantly lower with EBVP (72 versus 88 percent) and further entry into the trial was discontinued.

4.3.3.2 Popular chemotherapy regimens, number of cycles, and dose/field of radiation

Recent studies, focused on the more popular regimens such as the ABVD, Stanford V, and BEACOPP, and as well on the number of cycles and dose/field of RT in order to enhance the outcomes and decrease toxicities (**Table 8**).

Trial/Study Group	Treatment Protocols	No. of Patients	Median Follow-up	Treatment Outcomes
Cosset J et al. (1996) EORTC H6U	A: 3 MOPP + mantle RT + 3 MOPP	165		10-yr FFP: 68% 10-yr OS: 87%
	B: 3 ABVD + mantle RT + 3 ABVD	151		10-yr FFP: 90% 10-yr OS: 87%
Santoro A et al. (1983) Istituto Nazionale Tumori, Milan	A: 3 MOPP + STLI/TLI + 3 MOPP	33		5-yr FFP: 66%
	B: 3 ABVD + STLI/TLI + 3 ABVD	36		5-yr FFP: 72%
Pavlovsky S et al. (1997) GATLA	A: 3 CVPP + IF-RT (30 Gy) + 3 CVPP	92		5-yr EFS: 85% 5-yr OS: 95%
	B. 3 AOPE + IF-RT (30 Gy) + 3 AOPE	84		5-yr EFS: 66% 5-yr OS: 87%
Noordijik EM et al. (2006) EORTC H7U	A: 6 EBVP II + IF-RT (36 GY)	194	9 years	10-yr EFS: 68%; 10-yr OS: 79%
	B: 6 MOPP/ABV + IF-RT	195		5-yr EFS, 88%; 5-yr OS 87%
Meyer RM et al. (2005) NCIC-CTG/ECOG	A: 2 ABVD followed by EF-RT	139	4.2 years	5-yr EFS: 88% 5-yr OS: 92%
	B: 4-6 ABVD alone	137		5-yr EFS: 85% 5-yr OS: 95%
Eich HT et al. (2010) GHSG HD11	A: 4 ABVD + IF-RT (30 Gy)	356	6.8 years	5-yr FFTF: 85.3% 5-yr OS: 94.3%
	B: 4 ABVD + IF-RT (20 Gy)	347		5-yr FFTF: 81.1% 5-yr OS: 93.8%
	C: 4 baseline BEACOPP + IF-RT (30 Gy)	341		5-yr FFTF: 87% 5-yr OS: 94.6%
	D: 4 baseline BEACOPP + IF-RT (20 Gy)	351		5-yr FFTF: 86.8% 5-yr OS: 95.1%
Advani RH et al. (2010) Stanford[a]	A: Stanford V for 8 wk + IF-RT (20 or mostly 30 Gy)	55	8.5 years	10-yr FFP: 89% 10-yr OS: 96%
Wirth A et al. (2011) ALLG/TTROG[a]	4 ABVD followed by 30 Gy IF-RT for: A. Stage IA-IIA with any risk factor B. Stage IB-IIB:	A. 47 B. ?26	5.9 years	A. 5-yr FFP: 89% B. 5-yr FFP: 73%
Zittoun R et al. (1985)	A: 3 MOPP + IF-RT (40 Gy) + 3 MOPP	82		6-yr DFS: 87% 6-yr OS: 92%

Trial/Study Group	Treatment Protocols	No. of Patients	Median Follow-up	Treatment Outcomes
French Cooperation				
	B: 3 MOPP + EF-RT (40 Gy) + 3 MOPP	91		6-yr DFS: 93% 6-yr OS: 91%
Bonadonna G e al. (2004) Istituto Nazionale Tumori, Milan[b]	A: 4 ABVD + STLI	66	116 months	12 yr FFP: 93% 12-yr OS: 96%
	B: 4 ABVD + IF-RT	70		12-yr FFP: 94% 12-yr OS: 94%
Ferme C et al. (2007) EORTC/GELA H8U	A: 6 MOPP/ABV + IF-RT (36 Gy)	336	92 months	10-yr EFS: 82% 10-OS: 88%
	B: 4 MOPP/ABV + IF-RT (36 Gy)	333		10-yr EFS: 80% 10-yr OS: 85%
	C: 4 MOPP/ABV + STLI	327		10-yr EFS: 80% 10-yr OS: 84%
Engert A et al. (2003) GHSG HD8	A: 4 COPP/ABVD + 30 Gy EF-RT (+ 10 Gy to bulky disease)	532	54 months	5-yr FFTF: 85.8% 5-yr OS: 90.8%
	A: 4 COPP/ABVD + 30 Gy IF-RT (+ 10 Gy to bulky disease)	532		5-yr FFTF: 84.2% 5-yr OS: 92.4%

ABV, doxorubicin (Adriamycin), bleomycin, vinblastine; ABVD, doxorubicin, bleomycin, vinblastine, dacarbazine; ALLG/TTROG, Australasian Leukaemia and Lymphoma Group/Trans-Tasman Radiation Oncology Group; AOPE, doxorubicin, vincristine, prednisone, etoposide; BEACOPP, bleomycin, etoposide, doxorubicin, cyclophosphamide, vincristine, procarbazine, prednisone; COPP, cyclophosphamide, vincristine, procarbazine, prednisone; CVPP, cyclophosphamide, vinblastine, procarbazine, prednisone; DFS, disease-free survival; EBVP, epirubicin, bleomycin, vinblastine, prednisone; ECOG, Eastern Cooperative Oncology Group; EF-RT, extended-field radiotherapy; EFS, event-free survival; EORTC, European Organization for Research and Treatment of Cancer; FFP, freedom from progression; FFTF, freedom from treatment failure; GATLA, Grupo Argentino de Tratamiento de la Leucemia Aguda; GELA, Groupe d'Etude des Lymphomes de l'Adulte; GHSG, German Hodgkin Study Group; IF-RT, involved-field irradiation; MOPP, mechlorethamine, vincristine, procarbazine, prednisone; NCIC-CTG, National Cancer Institute of Canada Clinical Trials Group; OS, overall survival; Stanford V, mechlorethamine, doxorubicin, vinblastine, prednisone, vincristine, bleomycin, VP-16; RT, radiation therapy; STLI, subtotal nodal irradiation; TLI, total lymphoid irradiation.

[a]Used GHSG definitions for favorable and unfavorable early stage HL

[b]Included unfavorable stage I and all clinical stage II patients

Table 8. Selected Trials in Unfavorable Early Stage HL Derived from Major Study Groups.

Trying to address the number of cycles and/or radiation field, Ferme C, et al. randomized 996 patients with early unfavorable HL in the GELA H8U trial into one of the following three arms: six cycles of the hybrid MOPP/ABV regimen plus IF-RT versus four cycles plus IF-RT versus 4 cycles plus subtotal nodal irradiation (STNI). All arms had similar 5-year EFS and 10-year OS rates (Ferme, Eghbali, Meerwaldt, *et al*, 2007). Hence, 4 cycles of chemotherapy followed by IF-RT was proposed as standard treatment for early stage unfavorable HL. EF-RT versus IF-RT has been addressed as well by the large HD8 randomized trial from the German Hodgkin's Lymphoma Study Group (Engert, Schiller,

Josting, *et al*, 2003), where 1204 patients were randomly assigned to receive four cycles of COPP/ABVD followed by either IF-RT or EF-RT. At 5-years of follow-up, there was no significant difference in FFTF and OS between the 2 groups, but increased acute toxicity with the EF-RT group (leukopenia, thrombocytopenia, and GI toxicities).

ABVD and BEACOPP have been compared head to head in early stage unfavorable HL. In the EORTC/GELA H9U study (Noordijk EM, 2005) patients were randomly assigned to 6 cycles of ABVD or 4 cycles of ABVD or 4 cycles of baseline BEACOPP, all followed by 30 Gy IF-RT. At an interim analysis with a median follow-up of 4 years, no EFS and OS differences were noted, but increased toxicity with baseline BEACOPP. More recently, the final analysis of the GHSG HD11 trial (Eich, Diehl, Gorgen, *et al*, 2010) has been published with similar results to the H9U study, but with more information about the RT dosage. In this 4-arm study, 1395 patients with early stage unfavorable HL were randomized to either 4 cycles of ABVD or 4 cycles of baseline BEACOPP. Patients in each group of chemotherapy were then randomized to either 20 or 30 Gy IF-RT. At a median follow-up of 7.5 years, the OS was similar in all 4 arms. FFTF and PFS were similar as well between the 2 chemotherapy arms with the 30 Gy IF-RT. Baseline BEACOPP arm with 20 Gy IF-RT showed superior FFTF compared to ABVD followed by same RT. However, treatment-related toxicity was more frequently observed in the baseline BEACOPP arm and hence the BEACOPP is not adopted as new standard of care.

More recently, Wirth and colleagues (Wirth, Grigg, Wolf, *et al*, 2011) reported the results of the Australian Leukemia and Lymphoma Group/Trans-Tasman Radiation Oncology Group which tested combined modality treatment in stages I-II HL with IF-RT, with the number of cycles of ABVD determined by risk group (according to GHSG). 150 patients were classified into three groups as follows: group 1 with no risk factors who received 3 cycles of ABVD and IF-RT, group 2 with stages IA-IIA disease and any of the risk factors and group 3 included patients with stage IB-IIB; groups 2 and 3 received the same therapy with 4 cycles of ABVD and IF-RT. With a median follow-up of 5.9 years, the 5-year FFP and OS were comparable to those in the HD10 and HD11 trials for groups 1 and 2, but not group 3 which showed lower 5-year FFP and OS of 73% and 85%, respectively. The lower rates in group 3 may be explained by the inclusion of stage IIBX disease (44% of patients) in this study (those were excluded from HD10 and HD11 studies).

As with ABVD and BEACOPP, clinical studies has shown promising response rates with the Stanford V regimen. Advani RH, et al (Advani, Hoppe, Baer, *et al*, 2009) updated recently the initial results of the G4 study published by Horning SJ et al (Horning SJ, 2004). Among the 87 patients with non-bulky stage IA-IIA HL, 47 patients had unfavorable risk factors (according to GHSG criteria). At a median follow-up of 9 years, the FFP and OS rates for the whole group were 94% and 96%, respectively. However, FFP was 100% for favorable disease patients compared to 89% of those with unfavorable factors, but with no significant OS differences. Hence, Stanford V (8 weeks; 2 cycles) and 30 Gy IF-RT is considered safe and highly effective in this group of patients.

Few other studies confirmed as well that combined modality with Stanford V regimen is highly effective for locally extensive and advanced HL with low toxicity profile. More recently, the MSKCC study (Edwards-Bennett, Jacks, Moskowitz, *et al*, 2010) tested 126 patients with either locally extensive or advanced disease with 12-week Stanford V chemotherapy regimen followed by 36 Gy IF-RT to bulky sites and/or macroscopic splenic disease. The 5-and 7-year OS rates were 90% and 88%, respectively. On the other hand, at least 3 randomized trials were conducted comparing combined modality treatment with Stanford V versus ABVD. The final results confirm that ABVD should stay the standard therapy, but offers Stanford V as an acceptable and effective alternative (NCCN, v2.2011).

4.3.4 Chemotherapy alone

Giving the high cure rates and long term survivors of early stage HL with combined modality therapy, but with continued increased risk of long term complications from RT such as premature heart disease, lung toxicity, and secondary malignancies, many investigators have initiated randomized studies trying to omit RT in such good risk patients. Data from few randomized studies and as well few other single arm studies will be discussed briefly (these were summarized by a recent review by Straus DJ, 2011).

One of the earliest randomized studies is the prospective trial by Pavlovsky S, et al (Pavlovsky, Maschio, Santarelli, *et al*, 1988). A total of 104 patients with unfavorable clinical stages I-II HL were randomized for chemotherapy alone with 6 cycles of CVPP (cyclophosphamide, vincristine, procarbazine, and prednisone) versus 6 cycles of CVPP sandwiched with 30 Gy dose of IFRT. Combined modality treatment had higher rates of disease-free survival (75% vs. 34%) and a trend toward higher OS rates (84% vs. 66%).

Another prospective study was conducted by the Memorial Sloan Kettering Cancer Center (Straus, Portlock, Qin, *et al*, 2004) which randomized 152 patients with non-bulky stages I-II and stage IIIA disease to 6 cycles of ABVD with or without RT. There were no significant differences, but increased tendency for inferior outcomes in CR rates (87% vs. 91%), FFP rates (81 vs. 86%), and OS at 60 months (90% vs. 97%) for ABVD alone compared to the combined modality arm.

A phase II trial by the NCIC and ECOG study group (Meyer, Gospodarowicz, Connors, *et al*, 2005) randomized 399 patients with non-bulky early stage IA-IIB HL to 4-6 cycles of ABVD alone (favorable or unfavorable) vs. RT based therapy (STLI alone if favorable HL and ABVD followed by STLI if unfavorable). An interim analysis after median follow-up of 4.2 years revealed better outcomes (FFP and EFS) in the RT alone plus combined modality therapy arms compared to the chemotherapy alone arm, but no survival benefit. In a subset analysis of patients with unfavorable prognostic factors, FFP was superior for those treated with the combined modality compared to chemotherapy alone (95% vs. 88%), but with no survival differences.

The fourth 3-arm randomized study is the EORTC-GELA H9-F (Eghbali, Raemaekers & Carde, 2005) which randomized early stage favorable HL patients (total of 783 patients) to chemotherapy alone with epirubicin, bleomycin, vinblastine, and prednisone (EBVP) versus EBVP followed by 20 Gy of IF-RT versus EBVP followed by 36 Gy IF-RT. EBVP has an inferior outcome compared to the combined modality with both the 20 Gy and 36 Gy IF-RT with 4-year EFS rates of 69%, 85%, and 88%, respectively. The EBVP alone arm was then discontinued though there was no survival differences.

Of the retrospective analyses, Canellos GP et al (Canellos, Abramson, Fisher, *et al*, 2010) reported a PFS and OS of 92% and 100%, respectively, in a series of 75 patients with early stages IA-IIA and stage IIB disease (median follow-up was 52 months). Another nonrandomized study from Spain (Rueda Dominguez, Marquez, Guma, *et al*, 2004) included unselected 80 patients with early stage HL treated with 6 cycles of ABVD. The progression-free and overall survival at 7 years reported in 65 patients without B symptoms or mediastinal bulky disease were 88% and 97%, respectively.

More recently, a systematic review with meta-analysis of randomized controlled trials comparing chemotherapy alone with CMT in patients with early stage HL. Randomized studies comparing chemotherapy alone to the same chemotherapy regimen plus RT were only included. A total of 1245 patients were included. Authors concluded that adding RT to chemotherapy improves tumor control and OS in patients with early stage HL (Herbst, Rehan, Skoetz, *et al*, 2011).

Until further randomized trials are published, there will be no consensus to adopt chemotherapy alone as front line therapy for early stage HL. Enrollment in randomized clinical trials should be highly recommended. Currently, there are few ongoing randomized studies trying to answer that question. Armitage (Armitage, 2010) summarized four major randomized clinical trials which are incorporating interim PET scans to guide further therapy with or without IF-RT.

Based on available data and until further studies show convincing evidence for the opposite, we think combined modality treatment with chemotherapy and RT should remain the standard of care for early stage HL. Exceptions can be made for individual cases with either chemotherapy alone or RT alone. Of significance, and as noted by Armitage (Armitage, 2010), it appears that the actual choice of treatment modality is greatly affected by a physician's comfort with a particular treatment and by cumulative clinical experience- not just by data published in the literature.

4.4 Treatment of early stage NLPHL

4.4.1 Introduction

As discussed above, NLPHL is a rare subtype of HL with distinctive morphologic and immunophenotypic features compared to cHL. NLPHL accounts for 5% of HL cases with around 500 new diagnoses in US annually. Many retrospective analyses showed different natural history and more indolent course than cHL. Given the rarity of NLPHL, there are no randomized studies to establish standard of care for management of NLPHL. It has been managed historically similarly to cHL, however distinctive features are more recognized currently with some changes in the approach of management.

4.4.2 Presentation and prognosis

Generally, NLPHL is characterized by early presentation (stages I-II), indolent course with no constitutional symptoms, favorable prognosis, and occasional late relapses. The extremely favorable prognosis on some cases is reflected by data which showed that patients with stage IA may be treated with LN excision followed by a "watch and wait" approach or with IFRT alone (Diehl, Sextro, Franklin, *et al*, 1999; Nogova, Reineke, Eich, *et al*, 2005; Schlembach, Wilder, Jones, *et al*, 2002; Wilder, Schlembach, Jones, *et al*, 2002; Wirth, Yuen, Barton, *et al*, 2005) and that some patients with Stages IIIA-IVA may benefit as well from the "watch and wait" approach until they become symptomatic without jeopadarizing treatment outcomes.

The largest analysis to describe patients with NLPHL and identify certain prognostic factors is the recent report by Nogova , et al (Nogova, Reineke, Brillant, *et al*, 2008) who reviewed all NLPHL patients registered in the GHSG database, comparing patient characteristics and treatment outcome with cHL patients. A total of 394 patients with NLPHL were identified with 63 % having early stage favorable, 16 % has early stage unfavorable, and 21% has advanced stage. At a median follow-up of 50 months, FFTF (88% vs 82%) and OS (96% vs 92%) were found better with NLPHL compared to cHL, respectively. Among patients with NLPHL, FFTF were superior in patients with early favorable HL compared to those with early unfavorable HL and advanced HL (93% vs 87% vs 77%, respectively). The following factors were found negative prognostic factors: age (≥ 45), advanced stage, hemoglobin <10.5 g/dl, and lymphopenia. In another, but smaller series, Diehl V et al (Diehl, Sextro, Franklin, *et al*, 1999) reported similar favorable outcomes for early stage disease NLPHL compared to more advanced stages.

4.4.3 Treatment options

IF-RT or regional RT alone has been accepted by most investigators in Europe and US as a valid choice in the setting of non-bulky stage IA-IIA NLPHL, and is adopted as first line therapy by the NCCN guidelines. This is based on many retrospective analyses which showed excellent long term outcomes and no added benefit with combined modality therapy as for cHL. The Australasian Radiation Oncology Lymphoma Group (Wirth, Yuen, Barton, *et al*, 2005) described the long term outcomes of 202 patients with stage I-II NLPHL treated with RT alone. At a median follow-up of 15 years, the FFP and OS rates for the whole group were 82 % and 83 %, respectively. Various RT fields were used in this population with a median RT dose of 36 Gy. Another small series of 36 patients reported treatment outcomes with RT alone for non-bulky stage IA-IIA NLPHL (Schlembach, Wilder, Jones, *et al*, 2002). In this small series, 20 patients with stage IA received either IF-RT or EF-RT alone. At a median follow up of 8.8 years, the 5-year relapse-free and OS rates were 95% and 100%, respectively.

Treatment outcomes for early stage NLPHL with RT with or without chemotherapy have been reported in few other retrospective analyses. Chen RC et al (Chen, Chin, Ng, *et al*, 2010) reported recently the outcomes from 113 patients with stage I-II NLPHL treated with RT alone (93 patients), combined modality (13 patients), or chemotherapy alone (7 patients). Among the 106 patients treated with RT, 25 received limited-field, 35 regional-field, and 46 received EF-RT. At a median follow-up of 136 months, 10-year PFS rates were 85% (stage I) and 61% (stage II); overall survival (OS) rates were 94% and 97% for stages I and II respectively. PFS and OS did not differ among patients who received limited-field, regional-field, or extended-field RT. In contrast, six of seven patients who received chemotherapy alone developed early disease progression. In a multivariate analysis, extent of RT was not significantly associated with PFS. Addition of chemotherapy to RT didn't improve the outcomes as well.

Nogova L et al (Nogova, Reineke, Eich, *et al*, 2005) reported a retrospective analysis, from the GHSG, which included 131 patients with stage IA NLPHL treated with either IF-RT alone (45 patients), ER-FT alone (45 patients), or the RT combined with two to four cycles of ABVD chemotherapy (41 patients). At a median follow-up of 78 months for EF-RT, 17 months for the IF-RT, and 40 months for the combined modality, the estimated 24-month FFTF rates were 100, 92, and 97 percent, respectively for the three treatment groups. In another small series (48 patients), but with longer median follow-up (9.3 years), the M.D Anderson study (Wilder, Schlembach, Jones, *et al*, 2002) showed no difference in treatment outcomes for early stage NLPHL with RT alone (37 patients) compared to combined modality (11 patients).

Based on current data and until future convincing evidence is available, we think IF-RT alone is the preferred first line treatment modality for early stage favorable NLPHL. There is a general agreement for now by most investigators to treat patients with early unfavorable or advanced-stage LPHL according to the treatment protocols for cHL. However, with more data investigating the role of the monoclonal anti-CD 20 antibody (Rituximab) in patients with NLPHL, many investigators recommend incorporating rituximab alone or combined with other treatment modalities for unfavorable early stage, advanced stage, and relapsed NLPHL.

5. Special cases

5.1 Treatment of elderly patients with HL

5.1.1 Introduction

HL is a disease of relatively young patients; however, about 15-30% of patients with HL are older than 60 years according to few population-based studies. Elderly patients are mostly defined as those above ages 60-65 years. Unfortunately, the reported rates of elderly HL patients enrolled in large randomized studies is much lower than its prevalence (<5% to 10%) (Evens, Hutchings & Diehl, 2008; Klimm, Diehl & Engert, 2007). There is paucity of randomized studies that targeted the elderly HL population alone. However, many retrospective analyses derived from large studies have addressed the elderly population.

5.1.2 Presentation and prognosis

Elderly patients tend to present with increased frequency of mixed cellularity histologic subtype, advanced disease, B symptoms, and Epstein-Barr virus-positive disease. Overall, patients older than 60 years tend to have poorer outcomes than the younger population as reported by most series. Poor outcomes may be attributed to various factors including multiple co-morbidities, poor performance and/or mental status, inability to tolerate aggressive therapy, and death due to causes other than HL, among other factors as discussed below (Evens, Hutchings & Diehl, 2008; Klimm, Diehl & Engert, 2007).

Kim HK et al (Kim, Silver, Li, *et al*, 2003) reported treatment outcomes of 86 elderly patients (60-93 years) among which 52 patients had early stage disease (stages IA-IIA) and 34 patients had advanced disease (stages IIB-IV). At a median follow-up of 75 months, the 10-year FFTF and OS rates for all patients were 62% and 30%, respectively. The 10-year FFTF and OS for early stage HL were 71% and 31% and for advanced stage HL were 49% and 26%, respectively. In this study, the recurrence of HL was found to have a significant negative impact on survival. In a more recent report by Engert A et al (Engert, Ballova, Haverkamp, *et al*, 2005), a comprehensive retrospective analysis from the GHSG data base was performed and yielded poorer outcomes for elderly patients. From 4251 patients, 372 (8.8%) were 60 years or older. The 5-year OS (65% vs. 90%) and FFTF (60% vs. 80%) rates were significantly lower than those in younger patients. It was noticed in this study that the acute toxicity rate was higher in the elderly and that fewer elderly patients received the intended full dose chemotherapy. Hence, the authors concluded that the overall poorer outcome of elderly HL patients is attributed to the higher mortality during treatment and the lower dose-intensity therapy received. Of notice in this study, and as have been noticed with few other reports, adequately staged elderly patients receiving appropriate doses of therapy can achieve responses comparable to those of younger patients. However, older patients in general have a less favorable outcome which may be attributed to treatment-related deaths, shorter survival after relapse, death due to other causes, and others as mentioned above. Few other reports over the past 3-4 decades have been published with similar outcomes as above.

5.1.3 Treatment options

To date and until proven otherwise, there is an agreement among different investigators to treat the best fit elderly patients according to the management guidelines for the younger population, early stage HL with CMT and advanced stage disease with chemotherapy with or without RT as indicated. If chemotherapy is indicated, the widely used ABVD regimen would probably be the preferred regimen over the less commonly used and/or more intense-toxic regimens such as Stanford V and BEACOPP.

Over the past 10 years, attempts are being made to define the best therapeutic approach for elderly patients. Adjusting the chemotherapy and/or RT protocols to maintain high efficacy, but decrease the toxicity have been tried.

For patients with early stage unfavorable HL, Klimm et al. (Klimm, Eich, Haverkamp, *et al*, 2007) reported in 2007 the GHSC experience for the elderly early stage HL after CMT with 4 cycles of chemotherapy (COPP/ABVD) followed by EF-RT vs. IF-RT. From 1204 patients enrolled in the GHSG HD8 study, 89 patients were 60 years or older. Acute toxicity from RT was more pronounced in elderly patients receiving EF-RT compared to IF-RT. FFTF and OS rates were significantly lower in the elderly patients compared to younger population. However, more importantly, this study reported that elderly patients had poorer outcome when treated with EF-RT compared to IF-RT in terms of FFTF (58% vs. 70%) and OS (59% vs. 81%).

In regards of best chemotherapy regimen, data suggest that best outcomes in the elderly HL patients were received with adriamycin-based therapy. Weekes et al. (Weekes, Vose, Lynch, *et al*, 2002) reported that patients received anthracycline-containing regimen (ChlVPP/ABV) survived twice as long as patients given ChlVPP alone. Ballova et al. (Ballova, Ruffer, Haverkamp, *et al*, 2005), on the other hand in the HD9 elderly study, tried more intense regimen with baseline BEACOPP compared to COPP-ABVD in patients (>60 years) with advanced stage HL. Although there was better tumor control in the BEACOPP arm, that didn't translate into better outcome because of the higher toxicity.

More recently, and in an attempt to maintain dose intensity and avoid excessive toxicity, CHOP-21 regimen which is traditionally used for NHL has been studied as front line therapy for elderly HL patients with promising results (Kolstad, Nome, Delabie, *et al*, 2007).

There have been few other regimens tested in single arm phase II studies and others are being under investigation with various successes to date. Examples of such regimens include vinblastine, cyclophosphamide, procarbazine, etoposide, mitoxantrone and bleomycin (VEPEMB) (Levis, Anselmo, Ambrosetti, *et al*, 2004), vincristine, doxorubicin, bleomycin, etoposide and prednisone (ODBEP) (Macpherson, Klasa, Gascoyne, *et al*, 2002), prednisone, vinblastine, doxorubicin and gemcitabine (PVAG) (Boll, Bredenfeld, Gorgen, *et al*, 2011), and bleomycin, doxorubicin, cyclophosphamide, vincristine, procarbacine and prednisone (BACOPP) (Halbsguth, Nogova, Mueller, *et al*, 2010). However, randomized studies are highly recommended in this elderly heterogenous population in order to adopt any of the new regimens as standard of care compared to traditional regimens such as ABVD.

We do think that using a comprehensive geriatric assessment (CGA) model for elderly HL patients, addressing comorbidity and functional status prior to initiation of therapy, may guide medical providers in their decision for the intense of therapy which usually predicts treatment outcomes. A similar approach has been studied in elderly patients with diffuse large cell lymphoma (Tucci A et al, 2009) where GCA was found to be an efficient method to identify elderly patients who may benefit from a curative approach with aggressive therapy (well fit patients) compared to unfit patients who have poor outcomes. Until more data is available, treatment of well fit elderly patients should follow same guidelines as for younger population given the potentially high cure rate of HL even in advanced disease status as compared to poor outcomes with other types of cancers.

5.2 Treatment of HL during pregnancy

5.2.1 Epidemiology and prognosis

As the HL high incidence rates coincides with the female reproductive age, it is not surprising to mention that it is considered the fourth most common cancer during pregnancy (Sadural & Smith, 1995). However, as the overall incidence/prevalence of HL is low compared to other cancers the association between pregnancy and HL is low as well with only few small series describing the clinical presentation and treatment outcomes in this population. Fortunately, most reports showed that pregnancy doesn't have a negative impact on the course of HL with long term treatment outcomes comparable to those who were treated while non-pregnant (Gelb, van de Rijn, Warnke, *et al*, 1996). The challenge in managing those cases is attributed to the increased risk on the fetus with the different diagnostic and/or therapeutic interventions. Adverse teratogenic effects from chemotherapy and/or RT depend mainly on the level of fetal maturation. The highest teratogenic effects with increased risk of fetal malformation and death are noticed in the first trimester. In the second and third trimester, complications from therapy are more subtle with adverse effects such as intrauterine growth retardation, impaired functional or mental development, microcephaly, and low birth weight, among others (Fisher & Hancock, 1996).

5.2.2 Presentation and staging

Clinical presentation of HL during pregnancy is generally similar to non-pregnant patients. Staging workup approach is similar as well; however, to avoid fetus exposure to RT, CT scans should be avoided if possible. Instead, CXR and abdominal US and/or MRI may be used safely to complete staging (Nicklas & Baker, 2000).

5.2.3 Treatment options

There are no consensus guidelines to date that address standard of care. However, based on the available scattered reports there is an agreement to manage pregnant patients conservatively if possible until fetal maturation or delivery. Some authors suggested that in specialized cases (such as those with limited stage IA-IIA in their late second and third trimester), treatment may be deferred until mature fetal development and delivery, but patients should be followed then very closely for any signs of progression and proceed with delivery and/or therapy as indicated (Gelb, van de Rijn, Warnke, *et al*, 1996; Jacobs, Donaldson, Rosenberg, *et al*, 1981).

Patients who present with HL during the first trimester, in particular those with advanced disease, may be offered therapeutic abortion given the high risk of teratogenic effects associated with therapy. Data suggest that chemotherapy increases risk of fetal malformations to around 15% during the first trimester, with the greatest risk associated with the alkylatng and antimetabolite drugs, as opposed to the lowest risk with vinblastine (Doll, Ringenberg & Yarbro, 1989; Yahalom, 1990). Of notice, Doll DC et al. reported as well that there was low risk of fetal malformation in the second and third trimesters. In contrast, RT has been used more safely during pregnancy even in the first trimester. Yahalom J (Yahalom, 1990), in a series of 23 patients received supradiaphragmatic radiation therapy (five in the first trimester), reported no harm to the fetus. Based on these data and other similar reports, if treatment is indicated in the first trimester and can't be delayed for the second trimester, RT (with maximized uterine shielding) may be considered the best choice for supradiaphragmatic disease (with a dose of less than 10 Gy). However, for patients with infradiaphragmatic disease and/or advanced disease chemotherapy may be indicated with vinbastine-based therapy.

For second and third trimesters, treatment may be deferred until complete fetal development and safe delivery in specific asymptomatic localized stages. However, most patients would need treatment which may include RT alone (10 to 36 Gy in a mantle or IF-RT fashion) for supradiaphragmatic disease (with maximized uterine shielding) vs. chemotherapy for infradiaphragmatic and/or advanced disease as for the first trimester; however, in the second and third trimesters the use of chemotherapy is much safer than in the first trimester (Barnicle, 1992; Doll, Ringenberg & Yarbro, 1989), but remote side effects on long term survivor babies remain of concern.

6. Novel treatments for early stage HL

Besides the increased use of the monoclonal anti-CD20 antibody (rituximab) in NLPHL, novel targeted therapy is rarely incorporated in the management of early stage HL. This is mainly because of the high cure rates achieved with traditional chemotherapy regimens. Novel therapies are being more studied in advanced and relapsed/progressive diseases and will be discussed separately.

7. Conclusion

The treatment of early stage classical HL is mostly, today a combined modality with chemotherapy and involved field radiation. Decreasing the long-term side effects of the treatment is a goal. Decreasing the dosing of radiation and improving the radiation techniques, may demonstrate less complications in long-term follow-up. Incorporation of PET scan as a tool may select patients who will have higher risk for relapse. It is imperative to consider the acute and long-term side effects of the current therapeutic modalities in the treatment planning and future clinical trials.

8. References

Advani, R. H., Hoppe, R. T., Baer, D. M., *et al* (2009) Efficacy of Abbreviated Stanford V Chemotherapy and Involved Field Radiotherapy in Early Stage Hodgkin's Disease: Mature Results of the G4 Trial. *Blood (ASH Annual Meeting Abstracts)*, 114, 1670.

Ansell, S. M. & Armitage, J. O. (2006) Management of Hodgkin lymphoma. *Mayo Clin Proc*, 81, 419-426.

Armitage, J. O. (2010) Early-stage Hodgkin's lymphoma. *N Engl J Med*, 363, 653-662.

Ballova, V., Ruffer, J. U., Haverkamp, H., *et al* (2005) A prospectively randomized trial carried out by the German Hodgkin Study Group (GHSG) for elderly patients with advanced Hodgkin's disease comparing BEACOPP baseline and COPP-ABVD (study HD9elderly). *Ann Oncol*, 16, 124-131.

Barnicle, M. M. (1992) Chemotherapy and pregnancy. *Semin Oncol Nurs*, 8, 124-132.

Bernard, S. M., Cartwright, R. A., Darwin, C. M., *et al* (1987) Hodgkin's disease: case control epidemiological study in Yorkshire. *Br J Cancer*, 55, 85-90.

Boll, B., Bredenfeld, H., Gorgen, H., *et al* (2011) Phase II study of PVAG (prednisone, vinblastine, doxorubicin, gemcitabine) in elderly patients with early unfavorable or advanced stage Hodgkin lymphoma. *Blood*.

Bonadonna, G., Bonfante, V., Viviani, S., *et al* (2004) ABVD plus subtotal nodal versus involved-field radiotherapy in early-stage Hodgkin's disease: long-term results. *J Clin Oncol*, 22, 2835-2841.

Borchmann, P. & Engert, A. (2010) The past: what we have learned in the last decade. *Hematology Am Soc Hematol Educ Program*, 2010, 101-107.

Buchmann, I., Reinhardt, M., Elsner, K., *et al* (2001) 2-(fluorine-18)fluoro-2-deoxy-D-glucose positron emission tomography in the detection and staging of malignant lymphoma. A bicenter trial. *Cancer*, 91, 889-899.

Canellos, G. P., Abramson, J. S., Fisher, D. C., *et al* (2010) Treatment of favorable, limited-stage Hodgkin's lymphoma with chemotherapy without consolidation by radiation therapy. *J Clin Oncol*, 28, 1611-1615.

Caraway, N. P. (2005) Strategies to diagnose lymphoproliferative disorders by fine-needle aspiration by using ancillary studies. *Cancer*, 105, 432-442.

Carbone, P. P., Kaplan, H. S., Musshoff, K., *et al* (1971) Report of the Committee on Hodgkin's Disease Staging Classification. *Cancer Res*, 31, 1860-1861.

Carde, P., Burgers, J. M., Henry-Amar, M., *et al* (1988) Clinical stages I and II Hodgkin's disease: a specifically tailored therapy according to prognostic factors. *J Clin Oncol*, 6, 239-252.

Chen, R. C., Chin, M. S., Ng, A. K., *et al* (2010) Early-stage, lymphocyte-predominant Hodgkin's lymphoma: patient outcomes from a large, single-institution series with long follow-up. *J Clin Oncol*, 28, 136-141.

Cheson, B. D., Horning, S. J., Coiffier, B., *et al* (1999) Report of an international workshop to standardize response criteria for non-Hodgkin's lymphomas. NCI Sponsored International Working Group. *J Clin Oncol*, 17, 1244.

Cheson, B. D., Pfistner, B., Juweid, M. E., *et al* (2007) Revised response criteria for malignant lymphoma. *J Clin Oncol*, 25, 579-586.

Correa, P., O'Conor, G. T., Berard, C. W., *et al* (1973) International comparability and reproducibility in histologic subclassification of Hodgkin's disease. *J Natl Cancer Inst*, 50, 1429-1435.

Cosset, J. M., Ferme, C., Noordijk, E. M., *et al* (1996) Combined Modality Treatment for Poor Prognosis Stages I and II Hodgkin's Disease. *Semin Radiat Oncol*, 6, 185-195.

de Wit, M., Bohuslavizki, K. H., Buchert, R., *et al* (2001) 18FDG-PET following treatment as valid predictor for disease-free survival in Hodgkin's lymphoma. *Ann Oncol*, 12, 29-37.

Diehl, V. (2007) Hodgkin's disease--from pathology specimen to cure. *N Engl J Med*, 357, 1968-1971.

Diehl V, E. A., Mueller RP, et al (2005a) HD10: investigating reduction of combined modality treatment intensity in early stage Hodgkin's lymphoma. Interim analysis of a randomized trial of the German Hodgkin Study Group. *J Clin Oncol*, 23, 561S.

Diehl V, H. N., Mauch PM (2005b) *Hodgkin's disease* (7th edn). Philadelphia: Lippincott Williams & Wilkins.

Diehl, V., Sextro, M., Franklin, J., *et al* (1999) Clinical presentation, course, and prognostic factors in lymphocyte-predominant Hodgkin's disease and lymphocyte-rich classical Hodgkin's disease: report from the European Task Force on Lymphoma Project on Lymphocyte-Predominant Hodgkin's Disease. *J Clin Oncol*, 17, 776-783.

Doll, D. C., Ringenberg, Q. S. & Yarbro, J. W. (1989) Antineoplastic agents and pregnancy. *Semin Oncol*, 16, 337-346.

Edwards-Bennett, S. M., Jacks, L. M., Moskowitz, C. H., *et al* (2010) Stanford V program for locally extensive and advanced Hodgkin lymphoma: the Memorial Sloan-Kettering Cancer Center experience. *Ann Oncol*, 21, 574-581.

Eghbali, H., Raemaekers, J. & Carde, P. (2005) The EORTC strategy in the treatment of Hodgkin's lymphoma. *Eur J Haematol Suppl*, 135-140.

Eich, H. T., Diehl, V., Gorgen, H., *et al* (2010) Intensified chemotherapy and dose-reduced involved-field radiotherapy in patients with early unfavorable Hodgkin's lymphoma: final analysis of the German Hodgkin Study Group HD11 trial. *J Clin Oncol*, 28, 4199-4206.

Engert, A., Ballova, V., Haverkamp, H., *et al* (2005) Hodgkin's lymphoma in elderly patients: a comprehensive retrospective analysis from the German Hodgkin's Study Group. *J Clin Oncol*, 23, 5052-5060.

Engert, A., Franklin, J., Eich, H. T., *et al* (2007) Two cycles of doxorubicin, bleomycin, vinblastine, and dacarbazine plus extended-field radiotherapy is superior to radiotherapy alone in early favorable Hodgkin's lymphoma: final results of the GHSG HD7 trial. *J Clin Oncol*, 25, 3495-3502.

Engert, A., Plutschow, A., Eich, H. T., *et al* (2010) Reduced treatment intensity in patients with early-stage Hodgkin's lymphoma. *N Engl J Med*, 363, 640-652.

Engert, A., Schiller, P., Josting, A., *et al* (2003) Involved-field radiotherapy is equally effective and less toxic compared with extended-field radiotherapy after four cycles of chemotherapy in patients with early-stage unfavorable Hodgkin's lymphoma: results of the HD8 trial of the German Hodgkin's Lymphoma Study Group. *J Clin Oncol*, 21, 3601-3608.

Evens, A. M., Hutchings, M. & Diehl, V. (2008) Treatment of Hodgkin lymphoma: the past, present, and future. *Nat Clin Pract Oncol*, 5, 543-556.

Falini B, D. F. R., Pileri S (1995) BCL-6 gene rearrangement and expression in Hodgkin's disease. In *Third International Symposium on Hodgkin's Lymphoma.* Cologne, Germany.

Ferme, C., Eghbali, H., Meerwaldt, J. H., *et al* (2007) Chemotherapy plus involved-field radiation in early-stage Hodgkin's disease. *N Engl J Med*, 357, 1916-1927.

Fisher, P. & Hancock, B. (1996) Hodgkin's disease in the pregnant patient. *Br J Hosp Med* 56, 529.

Fuchs, M., Diehl, V. & Re, D. (2006) Current strategies and new approaches in the treatment of Hodgkin's lymphoma. *Pathobiology*, 73, 126-140.

Gelb, A. B., van de Rijn, M., Warnke, R. A., *et al* (1996) Pregnancy-associated lymphomas. A clinicopathologic study. *Cancer*, 78, 304-310.

Glaser, S. L. & Jarrett, R. F. (1996) The epidemiology of Hodgkin's disease. *Baillieres Clin Haematol*, 9, 401-416.

Gustavsson, A., Osterman, B. & Cavallin-Stahl, E. (2003) A systematic overview of radiation therapy effects in Hodgkin's lymphoma. *Acta Oncol*, 42, 589-604.

Hagenbeek A, E. H., Fermé C, et al (2000) Three cycles of MOPP/ABV hybrid and involved-field irradiation is more effective than subtotal nodal irradiation in favorable supra-diaphragmatic clinical stages I-II Hodgkin's disease: preliminary results of the EORTC-GELA H8-F randomized trial in 543 patients. *Blood*, 575a.

Halbsguth, T. V., Nogova, L., Mueller, H., *et al* (2010) Phase 2 study of BACOPP (bleomycin, adriamycin, cyclophosphamide, vincristine, procarbazine, and prednisone) in older patients with Hodgkin lymphoma: a report from the German Hodgkin Study Group (GHSG). *Blood*, 116, 2026-2032.

Harris, N. L., Jaffe, E. S., Diebold, J., *et al* (1999) World Health Organization classification of neoplastic diseases of the hematopoietic and lymphoid tissues: report of the Clinical Advisory Committee meeting-Airlie House, Virginia, November 1997. *J Clin Oncol*, 17, 3835-3849.

Hehn, S. T., Grogan, T. M. & Miller, T. P. (2004) Utility of fine-needle aspiration as a diagnostic technique in lymphoma. *J Clin Oncol*, 22, 3046-3052.

Herbst, C., Rehan, F. A., Skoetz, N., *et al* (2011) Chemotherapy alone versus chemotherapy plus radiotherapy for early stage Hodgkin lymphoma. *Cochrane Database Syst Rev*, CD007110.

Hoppe, R. T., Advani, R. H., Ai, W. Z., *et al* (2011) Hodgkin lymphoma. *J Natl Compr Canc Netw*, 9, 1020-1058.

Horning SJ, H. R., Advani RH, et al (2004) Efficacy and late effects of Stanford V chemotherapy and radiotherapy in untreated Hodgkin's disease: mature data in early and advanced stage patients [abstract]. *Blood*, Abstract 308.

Horwich, A., Specht, L. & Ashley, S. (1997) Survival analysis of patients with clinical stages I or II Hodgkin's disease who have relapsed after initial treatment with radiotherapy alone. *Eur J Cancer*, 33, 848-853.

Isasi, C. R., Lu, P. & Blaufox, M. D. (2005) A metaanalysis of 18F-2-deoxy-2-fluoro-D-glucose positron emission tomography in the staging and restaging of patients with lymphoma. *Cancer*, 104, 1066-1074.

Jacobs, C., Donaldson, S. S., Rosenberg, S. A., *et al* (1981) Management of the pregnant patient with Hodgkin's disease. *Ann Intern Med*, 95, 669-675.

Jaffe ES, H. N., Stein H (2001) Tumors of Hematopoietic and Lymphoid Tissues. *Lyon: IARC Press*.

Jemal, A., Siegel, R., Xu, J., *et al* (2010) Cancer statistics, 2010. *CA Cancer J Clin*, 60, 277-300.

Jerusalem, G., Beguin, Y., Fassotte, M. F., *et al* (2003) Early detection of relapse by whole-body positron emission tomography in the follow-up of patients with Hodgkin's disease. *Ann Oncol*, 14, 123-130.

Jerusalem, G., Beguin, Y., Fassotte, M. F., *et al* (1999) Whole-body positron emission tomography using 18F-fluorodeoxyglucose for posttreatment evaluation in Hodgkin's disease and non-Hodgkin's lymphoma has higher diagnostic and prognostic value than classical computed tomography scan imaging. *Blood*, 94, 429-433.

Jerusalem, G., Warland, V., Najjar, F., *et al* (1999) Whole-body 18F-FDG PET for the evaluation of patients with Hodgkin's disease and non-Hodgkin's lymphoma. *Nucl Med Commun*, 20, 13-20.

Josting, A., Wolf, J. & Diehl, V. (2000) Hodgkin disease: prognostic factors and treatment strategies. *Curr Opin Oncol*, 12, 403-411.

Juweid, M. E. (2006a) Utility of positron emission tomography (PET) scanning in managing patients with Hodgkin lymphoma. *Hematology Am Soc Hematol Educ Program*, 259-265, 510-251.

Juweid, M. E., Stroobants, S., Mottaghy, F.M. (2006b) Recommendations of the imaging committee of the International Harmonization Project (IHP) for FDG-PET (PET) use in patients with lymphoma. *J Nucl Med*, 452.

Kim, H. K., Silver, B., Li, S., *et al* (2003) Hodgkin's disease in elderly patients (> or =60): clinical outcome and treatment strategies. *Int J Radiat Oncol Biol Phys*, 56, 556-560.

Klimm, B., Diehl, V. & Engert, A. (2007) Hodgkin's lymphoma in the elderly: a different disease in patients over 60. *Oncology (Williston Park)*, 21, 982-990; discussion 990, 996, 998 passim.

Klimm, B., Eich, H. T., Haverkamp, H., *et al* (2007) Poorer outcome of elderly patients treated with extended-field radiotherapy compared with involved-field radiotherapy after chemotherapy for Hodgkin's lymphoma: an analysis from the German Hodgkin Study Group. *Ann Oncol*, 18, 357-363.

Kolstad, A., Nome, O., Delabie, J., *et al* (2007) Standard CHOP-21 as first line therapy for elderly patients with Hodgkin's lymphoma. *Leuk Lymphoma*, 48, 570-576.

Levis, A., Anselmo, A. P., Ambrosetti, A., *et al* (2004) VEPEMB in elderly Hodgkin's lymphoma patients. Results from an Intergruppo Italiano Linfomi (IIL) study. *Ann Oncol*, 15, 123-128.

Levy, R., Colonna, P., Tourani, J. M., *et al* (1995) Human immunodeficiency virus associated Hodgkin's disease: report of 45 cases from the French Registry of HIV-Associated Tumors. *Leuk Lymphoma*, 16, 451-456.

Lister, T. A., Crowther, D., Sutcliffe, S. B., *et al* (1989) Report of a committee convened to discuss the evaluation and staging of patients with Hodgkin's disease: Cotswolds meeting. *J Clin Oncol*, 7, 1630-1636.

Loeffler, M., Pfreundschuh, M., Ruhl, U., *et al* (1989) Risk factor adapted treatment of Hodgkin's lymphoma: strategies and perspectives. *Recent Results Cancer Res*, 117, 142-162.

Lynch, H. T., Marcus, J. N. & Lynch, J. F. (1992) Genetics of Hodgkin's and non-Hodgkin's lymphoma: a review. *Cancer Invest*, 10, 247-256.

Mack, T. M., Cozen, W., Shibata, D. K., *et al* (1995) Concordance for Hodgkin's disease in identical twins suggesting genetic susceptibility to the young-adult form of the disease. *N Engl J Med*, 332, 413-418.

Macpherson, N., Klasa, R. J., Gascoyne, R., *et al* (2002) Treatment of elderly Hodgkin's lymphoma patients with a novel 5-drug regimen (ODBEP): a phase II study. *Leuk Lymphoma*, 43, 1395-1402.

Mauch, P., Tarbell, N., Weinstein, H., *et al* (1988) Stage IA and IIA supradiaphragmatic Hodgkin's disease: prognostic factors in surgically staged patients treated with mantle and paraaortic irradiation. *J Clin Oncol*, 6, 1576-1583.

Meda, B. A., Buss, D. H., Woodruff, R. D., *et al* (2000) Diagnosis and subclassification of primary and recurrent lymphoma. The usefulness and limitations of combined fine-needle aspiration cytomorphology and flow cytometry. *Am J Clin Pathol*, 113, 688-699.

Meyer, R. M., Gospodarowicz, M. K., Connors, J. M., *et al* (2005) Randomized comparison of ABVD chemotherapy with a strategy that includes radiation therapy in patients with limited-stage Hodgkin's lymphoma: National Cancer Institute of Canada Clinical Trials Group and the Eastern Cooperative Oncology Group. *J Clin Oncol*, 23, 4634-4642.

Nicklas, A. H. & Baker, M. E. (2000) Imaging strategies in the pregnant cancer patient. *Semin Oncol*, 27, 623-632.

Nogova, L., Reineke, T., Brillant, C., *et al* (2008) Lymphocyte-predominant and classical Hodgkin's lymphoma: a comprehensive analysis from the German Hodgkin Study Group. *J Clin Oncol*, 26, 434-439.

Nogova, L., Reineke, T., Eich, H. T., *et al* (2005) Extended field radiotherapy, combined modality treatment or involved field radiotherapy for patients with stage IA lymphocyte-predominant Hodgkin's lymphoma: a retrospective analysis from the German Hodgkin Study Group (GHSG). *Ann Oncol*, 16, 1683-1687.

Noordijk, E. M., Carde, P., Dupouy, N., *et al* (2006) Combined-modality therapy for clinical stage I or II Hodgkin's lymphoma: long-term results of the European Organisation for Research and Treatment of Cancer H7 randomized controlled trials. *J Clin Oncol*, 24, 3128-3135.

Noordijk EM, T. J., Fermé C, et al (2005) First results of the EORTC-GELA H9 randomized trials: the H9-F trial (comparing 3 radiation dose levels) and H9-U trial (comparing 3 chemotherapy schemes) in patients with favorable or unfavorable early stage Hodgkin's lymphoma. *J Clin Oncol*, 23, 561S.

Pavlovsky, S., Maschio, M., Santarelli, M. T., *et al* (1988) Randomized trial of chemotherapy versus chemotherapy plus radiotherapy for stage I-II Hodgkin's disease. *J Natl Cancer Inst*, 80, 1466-1473.

Peters, M. (1950) A study of survivals in Hodgkin's disease treated radiologically. *Am J Roentgenol*, 63, 299.

Press, O. W., LeBlanc, M., Lichter, A. S., *et al* (2001) Phase III randomized intergroup trial of subtotal lymphoid irradiation versus doxorubicin, vinblastine, and subtotal lymphoid irradiation for stage IA to IIA Hodgkin's disease. *J Clin Oncol*, 19, 4238-4244.

Rueda Dominguez, A., Marquez, A., Guma, J., *et al* (2004) Treatment of stage I and II Hodgkin's lymphoma with ABVD chemotherapy: results after 7 years of a prospective study. *Ann Oncol*, 15, 1798-1804.

Sadural, E. & Smith, L. G., Jr. (1995) Hematologic malignancies during pregnancy. *Clin Obstet Gynecol*, 38, 535-546.

Santoro, A., Bonadonna, G., Valagussa, P., *et al* (1987) Long-term results of combined chemotherapy-radiotherapy approach in Hodgkin's disease: superiority of ABVD plus radiotherapy versus MOPP plus radiotherapy. *J Clin Oncol*, 5, 27-37.

Santoro, A., Viviani, S. & Zucali, R. (1983) Comparative results and toxicity of MOPP vs ABVD com-bined with radiotherapy (RT) in PS IIB, III (A,B) Hodgkin's disease (HD). *Annual Meeting American Society of Clinical Oncology, San Diego, CA*.

Schlembach, P. J., Wilder, R. B., Jones, D., *et al* (2002) Radiotherapy alone for lymphocyte-predominant Hodgkin's disease. *Cancer J*, 8, 377-383.

Seam, P., Juweid, M. E. & Cheson, B. D. (2007) The role of FDG-PET scans in patients with lymphoma. *Blood*, 110, 3507-3516.

Srour, S. A. & Fayad, L. E. (2010) Treatment of Hodgkin Lymphoma. In *Neoplastic Hematopathology: Experimental and Clinical Approaches* (ed D. Jones), pp. 367-390: Humana Press.

Straus, D. J., Portlock, C. S., Qin, J., *et al* (2004) Results of a prospective randomized clinical trial of doxorubicin, bleomycin, vinblastine, and dacarbazine (ABVD) followed by radiation therapy (RT) versus ABVD alone for stages I, II, and IIIA nonbulky Hodgkin disease. *Blood*, 104, 3483-3489.

Tirelli, U., Errante, D., Dolcetti, R., *et al* (1995) Hodgkin's disease and human immunodeficiency virus infection: clinicopathologic and virologic features of 114 patients from the Italian Cooperative Group on AIDS and Tumors. *J Clin Oncol*, 13, 1758-1767.

Tubiana, M., Henry-Amar, M., Carde, P., *et al* (1989) Toward comprehensive management tailored to prognostic factors of patients with clinical stages I and II in Hodgkin's disease. The EORTC Lymphoma Group controlled clinical trials: 1964-1987. *Blood*, 73, 47-56.

Wasserman, T. H., Petroni, G. R., Millard, F. E., *et al* (1999) Sequential chemotherapy (etoposide, vinblastine, and doxorubicin) and subtotal lymph node radiation for patients with localized Hodgkin disease and unfavorable prognostic features: A phase II Cancer and Leukemia Group B Study (9051). *Cancer*, 86, 1590-1595.

Weekes, C. D., Vose, J. M., Lynch, J. C., *et al* (2002) Hodgkin's disease in the elderly: improved treatment outcome with a doxorubicin-containing regimen. *J Clin Oncol*, 20, 1087-1093.

Weihrauch, M. R., Re, D., Scheidhauer, K., *et al* (2001) Thoracic positron emission tomography using 18F-fluorodeoxyglucose for the evaluation of residual mediastinal Hodgkin disease. *Blood*, 98, 2930-2934.

Weiss, L. M., Strickler, J. G., Warnke, R. A., *et al* (1987) Epstein-Barr viral DNA in tissues of Hodgkin's disease. *Am J Pathol*, 129, 86-91.

Wilder, R. B., Schlembach, P. J., Jones, D., *et al* (2002) European Organization for Research and Treatment of Cancer and Groupe d'Etude des Lymphomes de l'Adulte very favorable and favorable, lymphocyte-predominant Hodgkin disease. *Cancer*, 94, 1731-1738.

Wirth, A., Grigg, A., Wolf, M., *et al* (2011) Risk and response adapted therapy for early stage Hodgkin lymphoma: a prospective multicenter study of the Australasian Leukaemia and Lymphoma Group/Trans-Tasman Radiation Oncology Group. *Leuk Lymphoma*, 52, 786-795.

Wirth, A., Seymour, J. F., Hicks, R. J., *et al* (2002) Fluorine-18 fluorodeoxyglucose positron emission tomography, gallium-67 scintigraphy, and conventional staging for Hodgkin's disease and non-Hodgkin's lymphoma. *Am J Med*, 112, 262-268.

Wirth, A., Yuen, K., Barton, M., *et al* (2005) Long-term outcome after radiotherapy alone for lymphocyte-predominant Hodgkin lymphoma: a retrospective multicenter study of the Australasian Radiation Oncology Lymphoma Group. *Cancer*, 104, 1221-1229.

Yahalom, J. (1990) Treatment options for Hodgkin's disease during pregnancy. *Leuk Lymphoma*, 2, 151.

Yahalom, J. (2006) Favorable early-stage Hodgkin lymphoma. *J Natl Compr Canc Netw*, 4, 233-240.

Part 6

State of the Art Therapy of Advanced Hodgkin's Lymphoma

6

State of the Art Therapy of Advanced Hodgkin Lymphoma

Mark J. Fesler
Saint Louis University, USA

1. Introduction

Given that a clear, universal definition of advanced Hodgkin lymphoma does not exist, it comes as no surprise that the treatment of this disease is a controversial subject. Currently, the cure rate of advanced Hodgkin lymphoma is relatively high, although most physicians and patients confronting this disease recognize that the cure rate is less than ideal and the costs of treatment are substantial in terms of morbidity and mortality. The current research focus in this disease, as with any oncologic disorder, is to maximize the curative potential of treatment while minimizing patient suffering.

In this chapter, the following topics will be discussed: the definition of advanced Hodgkin lymphoma, the development of combination chemotherapy for this disease, the important clinical trials that led to ABVD (a combination chemotherapy regimen consisting of: adriamycin, bleomycin, vinblastine, and dacarbazine) becoming the gold standard, the emergence of escalated BEACOPP (a combination chemotherapy regimen consisting of: bleomycin, etoposide, adriamycin, cyclophosphamide, oncovin, procarbazine, and prednisone), as a challenger to ABVD therapy, utilization and role of other combination chemotherapy regimens, the controversial role of radiotherapy, the roles of autologous and allogeneic hematopoietic stem cell transplantation, prognostic factors in both untreated and relapsed patients, promising therapies of the future, and case studies.

As a young physician and investigator, the two most exciting areas of research currently involve the use of fusion positron emission tomography/ computed tomography (PET/CT) imaging and the continued expansion of targeted treatment strategies, such as brentuximab vedotin and rituximab, which will hopefully allow both improved treatment tailoring and subsequent outcome for patients.

2. Definition of "advanced" Hodgkin Lymphoma

Applying the term "advanced" to a patient with Hodgkin lymphoma implies that there is a clear definition of the opposite term, or "limited" disease. Precise, universally accepted definitions do not exist for either term as applied to Hodgkin lymphoma.

Eligibility criteria for clinical trial enrollment are an important source of definitions in clinical medicine. For example, the international leaders of Hodgkin lymphoma, the German

Hodgkin Study Group (GHSG), included all patients with stage IIIB-IV disease in the HD9 trial (Diehl et al. 1998), but required that patients with stage IIB disease have one of the following: an extralymphatic site, a bulky spleen (diffuse infiltration or > 5 focal lesions), or a bulky mediastinum (more than one third of the maximum thoracic diameter). Patients with stage IIIA disease were required to have either an erythrocyte sedimentation rate >50 mm/hr or ≥ 3 affected lymph node areas. Similarly, two major Italian studies, each comparing ABVD with other regimens, enrolled patients with stage IIB along with stage III-IV disease, although one study uses the term "intermediate and advanced" (Gobbi et al. 2005) and the other "unfavorable" rather than "advanced"(Viviani et al. 2011). Studies comparing MOPP with ABVD (Canellos et al. 1992) or ABVD with hybrid regimens (Duggan et al. 2003) in North America have included only stage III and IV patients.

In order to more easily compare results of studies performed all over the globe, the Hodgkin lymphoma community should insist upon homogeneity across clinical trials. In spite of the fact that there may be prognostic rationale for including patients with "B" symptoms or bulky disease with stage III and IV patients, it is probably more important to have uniformity across clinical trials internationally. It is reasonable to reserve the term "advanced" Hodgkin lymphoma for stage III and IV patients regardless of disease bulk, B symptoms, or any other adverse prognostic factor. Patients with adverse features and stage I or II disease would fall into a category of "limited unfavorable".

3. Role of combination chemotherapy

Combination chemotherapy for advanced Hodgkin lymphoma was initially developed by Vincent DeVita at the National Cancer Institute (NCI) in response to the initial successes in childhood leukemia treatment with combinations of agents. MOMP (mechlorethamine, vincristine, methotrexate, prednisone) was the initial combination regimen developed. Once procarbazine was developed sufficiently, it replaced methotrexate and the regimen was termed MOPP (DeVita et al. 1978). In a landmark study on the results of MOPP, 81 percent of stage III/IV Hodgkin lymphoma patients achieved a complete remission, a roughly four-fold higher response rate than with single agents, and the remission duration, when compared retrospectively, was increased approximately ten-fold over single agents alone (Devita, Serpick, and Carbone 1970). Ultimately, MOPP was shown in a prospective fashion to be superior to single agent nitrogen mustard in a small, randomized trial conducted by the Southeastern Cancer Group. One hundred eight patients with stage III or IV Hodgkin lymphoma were randomized between MOPP and mechlorethamine given biweekly, and patients receiving MOPP were found to have superior complete remission rates and overall survival (Huguley et al. 1975). From that time on, combination chemotherapy for advanced Hodgkin lymphoma became standard, and comparisons between various combination regimens ensued.

The Cancer and Leukemia Group B (CALGB) performed a randomized comparison amongst four different combination chemotherapy regimens: the four-drug combinations were BOPP (mechlorethamine substituted with BCNU) and MOPP, and the three-drug combinations were BOP (procarbazine eliminated) and OPP (BCNU or mechlorethamine eliminated). This study demonstrated superiority of four-drug over three-drug combinations, it highlighted the importance of the alkylating agents mechlorethamine and procarbazine, and it further solidified the role of four-drug combinations for treating Hodgkin lymphoma (Nissen et al.

1979). Interestingly, MOPP and BOPP were equivalent regimens, which demonstrated that BCNU and mechlorethamine may have equivalent efficacy. Similarly, a comparison of LOPP (lomustine replaces mechlorethamine) with MOPP demonstrated equal efficacy as well, further demonstrating that nitrosureas could substitute for alkylating agents in treatment of this disease (Hancock 1986).

In summary, combination chemotherapy became standard on the basis a landmark study of MOPP therapy developed at the NCI, with formal confirmation of superiority over single agents in one randomized trial. Combination chemotherapy with four drugs was superior to three drugs. MOPP, with an alkylating agent meclorethamine, although equivalent in efficacy to nitrosurea-containing combinations, was likely favored by most experts in the field due to the short and long-term side effects associated with nitrosureas.

4. ABVD as gold standard

MOPP combination chemotherapy for advanced Hodgkin lymphoma resulted in twenty to thirty percent of patients failing to achieve a complete remission and only fifty percent of patients being cured with risks of both sterility and secondary malignancies such as acute leukemia (Bonadonna, Valagussa, and Santoro 1986; Longo et al. 1991). Bonadonna Gianni developed the ABVD (adriamycin, bleomycin, vinblastine, dacarbazine) regimen in order to salvage MOPP failures (Bonadonna et al. 1975). In an initial Italian study comparing three cycles of ABVD or MOPP with receipt of radiotherapy in both arms, ABVD was superior with a seven-year overall survival of 77.4 percent versus 67.9 percent for MOPP (Santoro et al. 1987). ABVD therapy became solidified as the gold standard after a landmark three-arm CALGB study, which compared ABVD with MOPP and an alternating regimen, MOPP/ABVD. The study demonstrated five-year failure-free survival rates of 61 percent for ABVD, 50 percent with MOPP, and 65 percent for alternating MOPP/ABVD (Canellos et al. 1992). The toxicity profile of ABVD was more favorable than either the alternating regimen or MOPP, and therefore ABVD became the standard combination chemotherapy regimen for advanced Hodgkin lymphoma.

Interest in the Goldie and Coldman hypothesis (Goldie and Coldman 1979), which hypothesized that early introduction of all active agents for a disease would prevent the development of resistant clones, led to three major studies comparing hybrid and alternating regimens of MOPP and ABVD. No advantage in overall survival was found with the hybrid regimens (Connors et al. 1997; Sieber et al. 2002; Viviani et al. 1996). An important US Intergroup trial dampened further interest in hybrid regimens by demonstrating equivalent efficacy ABVD over a MOPP/ABV hybrid, with a similar failure-free survival and overall survival at five years but a better toxicity profile of the ABVD regimen (Duggan et al. 2003). The solidification of ABVD as the true gold standard would take place in the 1990 and 2000's, in which ABVD became the comparator arm for most randomized clinical trials.

5. The emergence of escalated BEACOPP

The group with a lead role in the advancement of Hodgkin therapy, the GHSG, developed the escalated BEACOPP regimen initially through mathematical modeling of tumor growth and chemotherapy effects, (Hasenclever, Loeffler, and Diehl 1996) which led to a pilot clinical trial in which doses of cytotoxic agents were increased in a stepwise fashion (Tesch et al. 1998). Escalated BEACOPP, the new dose dense regimen relative to COPP/ABVD and dose intense regimen relative to standard BEACOPP, was tested against these two regimens in the HD9 clinical trial. Ten year follow-up of that study, in which seventy percent of patients received additional radiotherapy, demonstrated statistically and clinically significant superiority of escalated BEACOPP over COPP/ABVD and standard BEACOPP in terms of freedom from treatment failure rate (82, 70, and 64 percent, respectively) and overall survival rate (86, 80, and 75 percent, respectively) (Engert et al. 2009).

BEACOPP, given in different schedules than the German standard of eight escalated cycles, has also been compared with other regimens in two prospective, randomized, Italian studies. The HD2000 Gruppo Italiano per lo Studio dei Linfomi Trial was initially designed as a toxicity trial to compare rates of leucopenia between three arms: a BEACOPP regimen (consisting of four escalated cycles and two standard cycles), a CEC regimen, and ABVD (Federico et al. 2009). Once the study centers became comfortable with BEACOPP administration, which requires the greatest attention and familiarity in the initial cycles, the trial was changed to a primary endpoint of failure-free survival. With a median follow-up of forty-one months and a suggestion of lower median dose intensity of BEACOPP delivered and resulting lower rates of grade III/IV hematologic toxicity compared with the escalated BEACOPP arm of the HD9 trial, the five-year estimated rates of failure-free survival were 78 and 65 percent in the arms of interest, BEACOPP and ABVD, respectively, which reached both clinical and statistical significance. The five-year estimated overall survival demonstrated numerical superiority of BEACOPP over ABVD with rates of 92 versus 84 percent, although this failed to meet statistical significance. In a second recently published Italian study, conducted in a similar time period as the HD2000 study, four cycles of escalated BEACOPP plus four cycles of standard BEACOPP were compared with ABVD with a primary endpoint of freedom from first progression (Viviani et al. 2011). With a median follow-up of sixty-one months, the estimated seven-year rate of freedom from first progression was 85 percent in the BEACOPP group versus 73 percent in the ABVD group. The primary endpoint importantly achieved both statistical and clinical significance. Counter to this, the secondary endpoints, which did not have statistical power, were overall survival and rate of freedom from second progression. These endpoints were 84 and 82 percent in the ABVD arm, respectively, versus 89 and 88 percent in the BEACOPP arm, and they did not reach statistical significance. Details of exact dose intensity were not provided, and one could certainly debate, in spite of the author's conclusions, the relevance of a five percent difference in overall survival, which numerically favored the BEACOPP program. The final analysis of the HD12 trial (Diehl et al. 2008), a comparison of eight cycles of escalated BEACOPP with four escalated cycles followed by four standard cycles of BEACOPP, demonstrates statistical equivalence at five year follow-up between the arms, with the eight escalated cycles being numerically superior and still the gold standard comparator arm for the HD15 study. The HD15 trial (Kobe et al. 2008) compares eight escalated cycles of BEACOPP with six escalated cycles of BEACOPP or eight cycles of fourteen day compressed BEACOPP. The results of this study, as well as the results of a global study comparing four cycles of escalated BEACOPP followed by four cycles of baseline BEACOPP with eight cycles of ABVD (European Organization for Research and Treatment of Cancer 2002), are eagerly anticipated.

6. Other chemotherapy regimens

Stanford V is a regimen incorporating twelve total weeks of alternating weekly cycles of myelotoxic and nonmyelotoxic polychemotherapy followed by liberal irradiation of 36 Gy to sites > 5 cm or macroscopic splenic disease (Bartlett et al. 1995). It was originally designed at Stanford although the chemotherapy backbone was likely drawn from the VACOPB regimen designed in Vancouver for non-Hodgkin lymphoma (O'Reilly et al. 1991). Stanford V was initially compared with ABVD and a regimen called MOPPEBVCAD by the Intergruppo Italiano Linfomi. Focusing on the Stanford V and ABVD arms, the primary endpoint of failure-free survival at five years was 76 perecent with Stanford V versus 89 percent with ABVD, with overall survival of 82 percent versus 90 percent, respectively (Gobbi et al. 2005). The trial has been criticized for utilizing radiotherapy differently than the original Stanford V report, as 66 versus 89 percent of patients, respectively, received radiotherapy. Sites > 6 cm rather than >5 cm were irradiated, and radiotherapy occurred 4-6 weeks rather than 2-4 weeks post-chemotherapy (so called optional versus adjuvant radiotherapy). More recently, a large Intergroup study was reported which compared Stanford V with six to eight cycles of ABVD. Somewhat unrealistically, the trial was designed to detect a 33 percent reduction in the failure-free survival hazard rate with Stanford V versus ABVD, and the failure-free survival at five years with Stanford V was 71 versus 73 percent with ABVD with 87 and 88 percent overall survival rates, respectively (Gordon et al. 2010). This trial further solidifies ABVD as the standard polychemotherapy regimen in advanced Hodgkin lymphoma, and is still the comparator arm for further investigational work.

Other polychemotherapy regimens which have been the subject of prospective, randomized investigation in advanced Hodgkin lymphoma which have not gained widespread appeal include: MEC, CHLVPP/EVA, and VAPEC-B. MEC, or MOPPEBVCAD (a regimen consisting of: mechlorethamine, lomustine, vindesine, melphalan, prednisone, epidoxorubicin, vincristine, procarbazine, vinblastine, and bleomycin), was compared with Stanford V and ABVD in an Italian study, with all arms receiving optional radiotherapy. MEC provided similar disease control as ABVD with similar rates of freedom from first progression, although the grade III-IV toxicity rates, particularly hematologic toxicity, were higher with MEC than ABVD (Gobbi et al. 2005). Therefore, given the better balance of efficacy and toxicity afforded by ABVD, MEC fell out of favor. A United Kingdom/Italian study compared the hybrid regimen CHLVPP/EVA to VAPEC-B (Radford et al. 1997), an abbreviated 11 week polychemotherapy regimen similar to VACOP-B or Stanford V. CHLVPP/EVA resulted in a superior three year disease-free and overall survival, with rates of 82 and 89 percent versus 62 and 79 percent, respectively for VAPEC-B. When British investigators compared ABVD with CHLVPP/EVA or a similar regimen, CHLVPP/PABLOE, the three year event-free survival and overall survival were similar, and ABVD was better tolerated (Johnson et al. 2005). Since that study, these hybrid polychemotherapy regimens have not been utilized.

In summary of chapters five and six, there is still controversy regarding the optimal chemotherapy approach in untreated Hodgkin lymphoma patients. In spite of the two "negative" Italian studies, and considering the difference in patient numbers between those studies and HD9, it is reasonable to treat patients with advanced Hodgkin lymphoma with either escalated BEACOPP or ABVD. Stanford V can be considered in selected patients, recognizing that it has never shown superiority over ABVD or a similar regimen. Further refinement of chemotherapy for advanced Hodgkin lymphoma, utilizing both PET/CT guidance and monoclonal antibodies, is likely to occur in the future.

7. Role of radiotherapy

Radiotherapy is a treatment modality that is believed to be non-crossresistant with standard combination chemotherapy (DeVita 2008). Its use can be considered in several contexts in advanced Hodgkin lymphoma: as an adjuvant therapy after complete remission is obtained with chemotherapy, integrated as combined modality therapy, or utilized as a definitive modality when response to chemotherapy is unsatisfactory.

The first use, as an adjuvant after complete response with polychemotherapy, was assessed in four randomized studies. Two studies compared radiotherapy with observation, and two studies compared radiotherapy with two additional cycles of chemotherapy. The Southwest Oncology Group randomized three hundred and twenty two patients with stage III or IV Hodgkin lymphoma who achieved a complete remission by computed tomographic assessment after six cycles of MOP-BAP between observation or low-dose (2000 cGy to lymph nodes, 1000-1500 cGy to other organs) involved field radiotherapy (IFRT). With a median follow-up of eight years, there were no statistically significant differences in relapse-free or overall survival (Fabian et al. 1994). The GHSG randomized patients with stage III or IV disease in complete remission by computed tomographic assessment after six cycles of COPP/ABVD to two more cycles of chemotherapy or low-dose (20 Gy) IFRT, and this study demonstrated no difference in relapse rate between the two arms (Diehl et al. 1995). A GELA study assessed the role of more extensive radiotherapy (subtotal nodal or total) versus two more cycles of chemotherapy in stage III/IV patients having achieved a complete or very good partial remission (≥ 75% size reduction) with six cycles of either MOPP/ABV or ABVPP. With a median follow-up of forty-eight months, the five year disease-free survival was 79 percent for the radiotherapy versus 74 percent for continued chemotherapy (Ferme et al. 2000). In the largest trial to determine the role of IFRT in stage III/IV Hodgkin lymphoma, four hundred twenty-one patients with computed tomogram complete remission after MOPP/ABV polychemotherapy were randomly assigned to observation versus IFRT. With a median follow-up of seventy-nine months, the five year event-free and overall survival rates were 84 percent and 91 percent in the observation group, respectively versus 79 percent and 85 percent in the IFRT group, which demonstrated that there is no role for IFRT in advanced Hodgkin lymphoma patients who achieve a complete remission with polychemotherapy (Aleman et al. 2003).

The second use, as an integrated therapy with chemotherapy, implies that radiotherapy is a pre-planned treatment regardless of response. The most common example of this is the administration of 36 Gy radiotherapy to patients receiving the Stanford V regimen who have sites of disease > 5cm or macroscopic splenic involvement. Unfortunately, radiotherapy administered in this context is completely of unproven value, and the harms are certain. For example, with intense polychemotherapy such as escalated BEACOPP, the GHSG has been able to reduce the percentage of patients on their studies receiving pre-planned radiotherapy from nearly 70 percent to approximately 10 percent without loss of efficacy and with a clear-cut reduction in the rate of secondary leukemia, from 1.7 to 0.6 percent comparing HD9 data with HD12 data (Diehl et al. 1998; Diehl et al. 2008). Unfortunately, many recently completed clinical trials still include pre-planned radiotherapy, such as the ECOG 2496 Intergroup study comparing ABVD with Stanford V, which provided radiotherapy to all patients on the ABVD arm with bulky mediastinal disease (Gordon et al. 2010). Fortunately, most of the new generation of clinical trials, such as SWOG 0816 and CALGB 50604, which utilize PET/CT to risk stratify patients for subsequent therapeutic strategy, only include radiotherapy to patients categorized as high risk with a positive PET/CT after a certain number of chemotherapy cycles (Southwest Oncology Group 2011; Cancer and Leukemia Group B 2011).

The third use, with utilization based on an unsatisfactory response to chemotherapy, certainly has theoretical appeal in order to improve outcomes of those patients with partial response to combination chemotherapy. Many studies include involved field radiotherapy for those patients with "residual tumor", which again has various definitions. Indirect justification for this approach is made by analysis of the Aleman study. The cohort of patients who were irradiated after achievement of a partial response with chemotherapy had five year event-free and overall survivals of 79 and 87 percent, respectively, which compared favorably with those patients having achieved a complete response with chemotherapy alone, with event-free and overall survivals of 84 and 91 percent, respectively (Aleman et al. 2003). An important question is whether a subset of the patients in partial response can be spared the additional toxicity of radiotherapy. In a recent analysis of the HD15 trial, in which eight cycles of escalated BEACOPP was compared with six cycles of escalated BEACOPP or 14 day compressed BEACOPP, thirty-eight percent of patients had residual tumor > 2.5 cm at the completion of chemotherapy. Of this patient group, twenty-one percent had a positive post-therapy PET/CT and seventy-nine percent had a negative PET/CT. The patients with a negative PET/CT were observed, and patients with a positive PET/CT received IFRT. The 18 month progression-free survival was 95 percent for patients who achieved a CR with chemotherapy, 96 percent for patients with > 2.5 cm residual tumor with PET/CT negativity who were observed, and 85 percent for PET/CT positive patients who received additional IFRT (Kobe et al. 2008). The authors recommend additional study, but in the meantime, a reasonable clinical practice would be to omit radiotherapy in those patients in complete metabolic remission post-therapy regardless of the initial disease features.

In summary, there is no role for adjuvant radiotherapy in patients who achieve a computed tomography defined complete remission based on several randomized studies. There is no clear role of a pre-planned chemotherapy plus radiotherapy approach in advanced Hodgkin lymphoma, and although preliminary, it appears reasonable to defer decisions about radiotherapy until the post-therapy PET/CT is completed. It appears that patients with non-FDG avid residual tumors can be safely observed, and based on indirect evidence, radiotherapy may benefit those with remaining FDG avidity in tumor masses.

8. Role of autologous hematopoietic stem cell transplantation

Autologous hematopoietic stem cell transplant has been studied in four separate prospective, randomized controlled clinical trials in Hodgkin lymphoma, in two instances in upfront consolidation and in two instances in the relapsed setting.

First, two studies utilizing transplant as consolidation of upfront polychemotherapy of Hodgkin lymphoma will be discussed. In a Scottish and Newcastle Lymphoma Group Study, sixty-five patients with "poor risk" disease were administered three cycles of PVACE-BOP chemotherapy with or without XRT. Those patients with a good partial or complete response were randomized to a melphalan/etoposide-conditioned autologous hematopoietic stem cell transplant versus 2 additional cycles of PVACE-BOP chemotherapy (Proctor et al. 2002). With a median follow-up of six years, the arms had a similar time to treatment failure, 79 percent in the transplant arm versus 85 percent in the non-transplant arm. The major conclusion of this study is that for a subset of patients with "poor risk" features derived by calculation of a Scottish Newcastle Lymphoma Group prognostic index, autologous hematopoietic stem cell transplantation offers no benefit over standard chemotherapy if a very good response on computed tomography is obtained after three cycles of polychemotherapy. In a second European Intergroup study, the HD 01 trial, one hundred sixty-three patients with "poor risk" disease at baseline were randomized after four cycles of ABVD or ABVD-like therapy in complete or partial response to a BEAM or CVB-conditioned autologous transplant or four additional cycles of chemotherapy (Federico et al. 2003). With a median follow-up of 48 months, the five year failure-free survival was 75 percent in the transplant arm versus 82 percent in the chemotherapy arm. Rates of overall survival were 88 percent in each arm. Although the transplant conditioning regimens utilized were different, both trials have similar features, such as attempting to identify a poor-risk subset of patients in spite of different criteria used. Additionally, an abbreviated course of chemotherapy was utilized prior to the randomization of continued chemotherapy versus transplant. Both trials only randomized patients with a response to chemotherapy, were small in number, and obtained similar results. Based on these data, there appears to be no role for performing autologous transplantation in previously untreated Hodgkin lymphoma patients with poor risk features who achieve a response on computed tomography imaging.

Two prospective randomized trials of autologous transplant have been conducted in patients with relapsed Hodgkin lymphoma. In the first trial, British investigators randomized forty patients with both relapsed and refractory "high risk" disease to either a chemotherapy regimen, mini-BEAM, or a BEAM-conditioned autologous transplant without details of exact number of chemotherapy courses given. The event-free survival at three years was 53 percent in the BEAM group versus 10 percent in the mini-BEAM group (Linch et al. 1993). The three year overall survival rate favored the BEAM group but did not achieve statistical significance. In the second study, German investigators randomized one hundred sixty-one patients with relapsed Hodgkin lymphoma to four cycles of Dexa-BEAM versus 2 cycles of Dexa-BEAM followed by a BEAM-conditioned autologous transplant (Schmitz et al. 2002). The three year estimated freedom from treatment failure was significantly better at 55 percent in the transplant arm versus 34 percent in the chemotherapy alone arm, while the overall survival did not reach statistical significance, with a rate of 71 percent in the transplant arm versus 65 percent in the chemotherapy alone arm. In spite of the lack of overall survival improvement, the disease-free survival improvement demonstrated in the above studies has lead to international acceptance that relapsed Hodgkin lymphoma is a definite indication for autologous hematopoietic stem cell transplantation.

A small number of refractory patients were included in the British transplant trial, and based on their inclusion in that study plus retrospective datasets indicating possible benefit of autologous transplant, (Lazarus et al. 1999; Andre et al. 1999; Josting et al. 2000) patients with refractory Hodgkin lymphoma who achieve a response or even disease stabilization with a salvage chemotherapy regimen can be considered for autologous transplantation.

Various conditioning regimens for autologous transplantation exist, and the BEAM (BCNU, etoposide,cytarabine, melphalan) regimen has been utilized in both randomized trials for relapsed/refractory disease. Other reported high-dose chemotherapy regimens include: CBV (cyclophosphamide, BCNU, VP-16), CBVP (CBV + cisplatin), Etoposide/Melphalan, high dose Melphalan, CCV (cyclophosphamide, CCNU, VP-16), and TLI (total lymphoid irradiation)+VP-16/cyclophosphamide). No prospective comparative trials of these regimens exist, and due to heterogeneity in parameters reported, even indirect comparison is challenging. In a retrospective comparison of two different condidtioning regimens, one radiation based with TBI/ cyclophosphamide/etoposide versus a chemotherapy regimen of busulfan/melphalan/ thiotepa (Bu/Mel/T), investigators at Fred Hutchinson Cancer Center found no difference in efficacy or toxicity of either preparative regimen. Patients who had a history of dose-limiting irradiation were treated with the Bu/Mel/T regimen preferentially (Gutierrez-Delgado et al. 2003). The BEAM regimen, given its use in the randomized trials, is a reasonable choice in the absence of comparative data, and the primary clinical issues with use of this regimen are melphalan-related gastrointestinal toxicity and BCNU-related pulmonary toxicity, the latter of which requires corticosteroid initiation at recognition.

Further intensification of a single autologous transplant for relapsed/refractory patients has been studied, both by utilizing higher doses of standard chemotherapy pre-transplant and by the addition of a planned second, or tandem transplant. In the HD-R2 trial, a European multicenter (GHSG, EORTC, EBMT, and GEL/TAMO) study for relapsed Hodgkin lymphoma, investigators randomized two hundred forty one patients without progressive disease after two cycles of DHAP to either a BEAM conditioned autologous transplant or sequential high dose chemotherapy with cyclophosphamide 4gm/m^2, methotrexate 8gm/m^2, and etoposide 500mg/m^2, followed by a BEAM conditioned autologous transplant, with IFRT to residual masses > 1.5cm in both arms. With a median follow-up of 42 months, the three year OS was 87 percent in the standard arm versus 83 percent in the high dose sequential arm, with corresponding rates of freedom from treatment failure of 71 percent and 65 percent, respectively (Josting et al. 2010). The conclusions of the authors, based on the largest randomized trial in relapsed Hodgkin lymphoma to date, is that sequential high dose chemotherapy has no role and that patient outcomes were quite good with two cycles of DHAP followed by a BEAM conditioned transplant. In the prospective, multicenter H96 trial conducted by the GELA/SFGM group, investigators studied the role of tandem autologous transplant for relapsed/refractory Hodgkin lymphoma patients with poor risk disease, defined as primary refractoriness to initial chemotherapy or ≥ 2 risk factors of the following: relapse < 12 months from primary therapy, stage III/IV disease at relapse, and relapse within a previously irradiated site with combined modality therapy. These poor-risk patients received two cycles of chemotherapy followed by a CBV plus mitoxantrone or BEAM-conditioned first transplant, with a second transplant with TAM (total-body irradiation, cytarabine, melphalan) or BAM (busulfan, cytarabine, melphalan)

45-90 days later. On an intent-to-treat basis, with a median follow-up of fifty one months, the five year freedom treatment failure and overall survival rates were 46 percent and 57 percent, respectively (Morschhauser et al. 2008). Seventy percent of poor risk patients received a second transplant with a transplant-related mortality of four percent. The authors concluded that tandem transplant was an advance in the treatment of poor risk patients with partial response to salvage chemotherapy and in those with primary refractory disease, given the superior results to historical data of single transplant in those populations.

In summary, autologous hematopoietic stem cell transplant has no role in the upfront treatment of patients with Hodgkin lymphoma. For patients with relapsed disease, it is considered the standard of care if chemotherapy sensitivity can be demonstrated. For patients with primary refractory disease, autologous transplantation is controversial but a small amount of retrospective data indicates a possible benefit. Chemotherapy intensification over traditional salvage regimens for relapsed/refractory patients appears to have no role, and there is possible benefit in tandem transplant for patients who are at high risk for poor outcome with a single autologous transplant.

9. Salvage therapy for relapsed/refractory disease

For patients who experience relapse after achievement of a complete response or who do not achieve a complete response and have biopsy proven residual Hodgkin lymphoma, conventional treatment consists of several cycles of non-crossresistant chemotherapy followed by autologous hematopoietic stem cell transplantation. In this chapter, the roles of radiotherapy and chemotherapy specifically for relapsed disease will be discussed.

The use of radiotherapy alone or in combination with salvage chemotherapy in relapsed/refractory Hodgkin lymphoma is controversial. Several retrospective reports exist on utilizing isolated radiotherapy for patients with relapsed/refractory disease after failure of combination chemotherapy. In the largest study, the GHSG found that of the one hundred patients in their database treated with radiotherapy alone after failure of anthracycline-based chemotherapy, the five-year freedom from treatment failure was 28 percent with an overall survival of 51 percent (Josting et al. 2005). The authors conclude that salvage radiotherapy is a treatment option for a subset of patients without B symptoms but with good performance status, limited stage, and late relapses, which effectively excludes the majority of Hodgkin lymphoma patients with relapsed disease and all patients with refractory disease.

No reports have compared outcomes of patients who do and do not receive radiotherapy as a component of salvage chemotherapy with autologous transplantation, and therefore the balance of efficacy and toxicity in this scenario is uncertain. Radiotherapy to "residual lesions" after the BEAM-conditioned autologous transplant was recommended in the German transplant study in relapsed disease, although too few patients received radiotherapy to allow comparison of outcomes to those without radiotherapy. Given that the opportunity for cure is greatly diminished in relapsed/refractory Hodgkin lymphoma, in spite of an absence of evidence of a definite benefit of radiotherapy, it is reasonable to include radiotherapy as part of a treatment regimen that includes salvage chemotherapy and autologous transplantation, particularly if the relapse is localized on imaging. Based on retrospective information regarding high rates of toxicity when radiotherapy is utilized pre-transplant (Tsang et al. 1999), it may be most reasonable to use this modality post-transplant.

Salvage chemotherapy is administered to the majority of patients with relapsed/refractory Hodgkin lymphoma with the goal of disease reduction or eradication prior to autologous transplantation. In fact, in the era of computed tomography, multiple reports document that the response to salvage chemotherapy is a major determinant of the outcome of autologous transplant (Sureda et al. 2001; Gutierrez-Delgado et al. 2003; Martin et al. 2001) and that the degree of response is associated with the progression-free survival at five years (Sirohi et al. 2008).

An ideal salvage regimen has an excellent response rate, non-overlapping organ toxicities with the primary regimen, and preserves the ability to mobilize and collect hematopoietic stem cells. Because initial treatment of Hodgkin lymphoma nearly always consists of anthracycline and bleomycin therapy, and because autologous transplant is the usual goal, which is a stress on the cardiopulmonary system, salvage therapy choices are typically made to limit cardiopulmonary toxicity.

Many different salvage polychemotherapy regimens have been utilized in the past, and all studies have been phase II investigations with heterogeneous patient populations with relapsed/refractory disease. See Table 1. Because only DEXA-BEAM and mini-BEAM regimens have been used pre-transplant in randomized clinical trials, the purist would utilize these regimens at the exclusion of other choices in spite of a toxic death rate between two to five percent. In one-hundred forty four patients, the DEXA-BEAM regimen resulted in a complete response rate of 27 percent, a partial response rate of 54 percent, and a toxic death rate of 5 percent (Schmitz, 2002). In fifty-five patients, the mini-BEAM regimen produced a complete response rate of 49 percent, a partial response rate of 33 percent, a toxic death rate of 2 percent, and in another cohort of patients, 82 percent collected $\geq 2 \times 10^6$ CD34 cells/kg (Martin et al. 2001; Kuruvilla et al. 2006).

The platinum-based salvage regimens include ESHAP (etoposide, solumedrol, high-dose cytarabine, and cisplatin), ASHAP (doxorubicin, solumedrol, high-dose cytarabine, and cisplatin), DHAP (dexamethasone, cytarabine, and cisplatin), and GDP (gemcitabine, dexamethasone, and cisplatin). ASHAP as a salvage regimen has limited applicability given that most patients will have anthracycline exposure during initial treatment. In twenty-three patients, the GDP regimen was reported to have a complete response rate of 17 percent, partial response rate of 52 percent, no toxic deaths, and 97 percent of patients collected $\geq 2 \times 10^6$ CD34 cells/kg. (Baetz et al. 2003; Kuruvilla et al. 2006). In twenty-two patients given the ESHAP regimen, the complete response rate was 41 percent, partial response rate 32 percent, toxic death rate 4 percent, with no stem cell collection data provided (Aparicio et al. 1999). In a report on one hundred two patients administered DHAP on an every two week schedule, the complete response rate was 21 percent, partial response rate 68 percent, and toxic death rate zero without collection data provided (Josting, Rudolph, et al. 2002).

Of the ifosfamide-based salvage regimens, two of the regimens are worth mention, ICE (ifosfamide, carboplatin, etoposide) and IGEV (ifosfamide, gemcitabine, vinorelbine, prednisolone). The ICE regimen, developed at Memorial Sloan-Kettering in an effort to reduce the nonhematologic toxicity of cisplatin-based regimens, resulted in a complete response rate of 26 percent, partial response rate of 59 percent, a toxic death rate of zero, and 86 percent of the sixty-five patients studied achieved a collection of $\geq 2 \times 10^6$ CD34 cells/kg (Moskowitz et al. 2001). In a report of ninety-one patients given the IGEV regimen, the complete response rate was 54 percent, partial response rate 37 percent, a toxic death rate of zero, and 98.7 percent achieved a stem cell collection of ≥ 3 x 10^6 CD34 cells/kg (Santoro, 2007).

In spite of the lack of comparative data, the ICE, IGEV, and GDP regimens appear to have the most favorable balance of the three key factors of response, low toxic death rate, and stem cell preservation. The ICE regimen is typically administered in the inpatient setting with the other two regimens given in an outpatient setting. Individual patient factors, such as pre-existing neuropathy or renal dysfunction, do play an important role in the final choice of a salvage combination chemotherapy regimen.

In summary, the role of radiotherapy, particularly isolated radiotherapy, in the management of relapsed Hodgkin lymphoma remains uncertain, and the standard of care is salvage combination chemotherapy for an arbitrary number of cycles followed by high dose preparative chemotherapy with autologous hematopoietic stem cell transplantation. Given the poorer results in salvage than upfront treatment, and the belief that disease is ultimately the greater problem than therapy toxicity in this younger patient population, erring on the side of consolidative radiotherapy post-transplant in those with limited stage relapse is reasonable.

Regimen	Composition	CR, ORR%	Toxic Death Rate	Stem Cell Colllection
DEXA-BEAM	Dexamethasone, BCNU, Etoposide, Ara-C, Melphalan	27, 81	5	NR
Mini-BEAM	BCNU, Etoposide, Ara-C, Melphalan	49, 82	2	82 percent ≥ 2 x 10^6 CD34+ cells/kg
GDP	Gemcitabine, Dexamethasone, Cisplatin	17, 69	0	97 percent ≥ 2 x 10^6 CD34+ cells/kg
ESHAP	Etoposide, SoluMedrol, Ara-C, Cisplatin	41, 73	4	NR
DHAP	Dexamethasone, Ara-C, Cisplatin	21, 89	0	NR
ICE	Ifosfamide, Carboplatin, Etoposide	26, 85	0	86 percent ≥ 2 x 10^6 CD34+ cells/kg
IGEV	Ifosfamide, Gemcitabine, Vinorelbine, Prednisone	54, 91	0	98 percent ≥ 3 x 10^6 CD34+ cells/kg

Table 1. Comparison of salvage chemotherapy regimens for relapsed/refractory Hodgkin lymphoma.

10. Role of allogeneic hematopoietic stem cell transplantation

Patients with Hodgkin lymphoma who relapse after autologous hematopoietic stem cell transplantation have a very poor long term outlook, with several series documenting a low rate of long term survivors (Crump 2008; Constans et al. 2004). In a retrospective Spanish analysis of patients who relapsed after autologous transplant, the progression free survival and overall survival were 23 percent and 35 percent at three years, respectively. Investigators at Wayne State retrospectively studied this patient population, and found an approximate 10 percent survival rate at four years post autologous transplant, and similar results were found in a series of patients from Memorial Sloan Kettering (Varterasian et al. 1995). Two findings were interesting in the Memorial series: one, nearly all of the long term survivors received a reduced-intensity allogeneic hematopoietic stem cell transplant, and second, the reduced-intensity allogeneic transplant appeared to be of little benefit to patients who relapsed within six months of the autologous transplant (Moskowitz et al. 2009).

Allogeneic transplants are typically divided into myeloablative versus reduced-intensity or nonmyeloablative depending on the intensity of the preparative regimen. Multiple reports on the efficacy and toxicity of myeloablative transplants for Hodgkin Lymphoma exist in the literature, and all are consistent in demonstrating an unacceptably high rate of treatment-related mortality. In a retrospective assessment of one hundred patients in the International Bone Marrow Transplant Registry (IBMTR), eighty-nine percent of the patients had active disease at the time of transplant, with a resulting three year disease-free survival rate of 15 percent, overall survival of 21 percent, and probabilities of acute and chronic graft-versus-host disease of 35 and 45 percent, respectively (Gajewski et al. 1996). The authors appropriately concluded that myeloablative sibling transplants have little role in the treatment of Hodgkin lymphoma. In a similar retrospective analysis, the European Bone Marrow Transplant (EBMT) registry retrospectively analyzed the outcomes of one hundred sixty-seven allogeneic transplants in patients with Hodgkin lymphoma, and found an actuarial overall survival of 24 percent at four years, primarily related to a 52 percent procedure-related mortality at four years (Peniket et al. 2003). Again, the authors appropriately concluded that the toxicity of allogeneic procedures would have to be reduced before broader applicability would be realized. In a retrospective matched case analysis by the EBMT of forty five allogeneic and forty five autologous transplants, it was found that the four year probability of survival, progression-free survival, relapse, and non-relapse mortality were 25, 15, 61, and 48 percent after allogeneic transplant with corresponding figures of 37, 24, 81, and 27 percent after autologous transplant (Milpied et al. 1996). The authors concluded that the positive effect of a decreased relapse rate with allogeneic transplant is offset by the toxicity and transplant-related mortality. Hence, multiple retrospective series of myeloablative allogeneic transplantation in Hodgkin lymphoma reached the same conclusion, namely the toxicity outweighs the small benefit from the treatment.

The applicability of allogeneic hematopoietic stem cell transplantation in a wide spectrum of hematologic disorders has been broadened by the advent of reduced-intensity conditioning, in which lower, non or partially myeloablative doses of chemotherapy either with or without radiotherapy are administered prior to infusion of allogeneic stem cells.

A convincing graft versus Hodgkin lymphoma effect was demonstrated after reduced-intensity allogeneic transplantation (Peggs et al. 2005). Several reports of long term follow-up of reduced-intensity allogeneic transplant demonstrate the curative potential of this procedure. In an EBMT retrospective analysis, with a median follow-up of seventy-five months for survivors, 18 percent were progression free at five years with an overall survival rate of 20 percent (Sureda et al. 2008). In another report with a median follow-up of forty-nine months, the estimated progression-free survival was 34 percent and overall survival 51 percent at five years.

In summary, myeloablative allogeneic transplantation appears to have little role in the treatment of Hodgkin lymphoma given the morbidity and mortality associated with the procedure. However, reduced-intensity allogeneic transplantation is a reasonable consideration in patients with a matched donor who have relapsed following an autologous transplant given the curative potential of the procedure in a desperate clinical situation.

11. Prognostic factors along the disease spectrum of advanced disease

Prognostic factors are measurements on individuals performed at or soon after diagnosis which gives likely outcome of the disease. Although far less useful to the clinician than predictive factors, which are directly influenced by treatment, prognostic factors can be used as guides in choosing an appropriate treatment strategy. Prognostic factors for advanced Hodgkin lymphoma are fairly well established because treatment over time has been more uniform and relapses are higher in frequency than for limited stage Hodgkin lymphoma.

The most useful information for prognosis in advanced Hodgkin lymphoma comes from a large retrospective analysis, a so-called tour de force, performed by German investigators (Hasenclever and Diehl 1998). They analyzed baseline characteristics and determined the outcomes of five thousand one hundred forty-one patients with primarily stage III/IV disease treated with ABVD or similar regimens in multiple centers. The authors found, on multivariate analysis that the prognosis of patients with advanced Hodgkin lymphoma depended on seven baseline characteristics including: age, gender, total leukocyte count, lymphocyte percentage or absolute number, albumin, hemoglobin, and stage. Because the relative risk for poorer outcome was similar between factors, the authors created the International Prognostic Score (IPS) for advanced Hodgkin lymphoma by simply adding each factor for a total score of 0-7: 1 point for age>45, male gender, total leukocyte count >15,000 cells/mcL, absolute lymphocyte count <600 cells/mcL or lymphocyte percentage <8%, albumin <4 g/dL, hemoglobin <10.5 g/dL, and stage IV. Higher scores indicate a worse prognosis, and this information was confirmed in an independent data set. Although many other reports exist describing other adverse prognostic features in advanced Hodgkin lymphoma, the significance of other factors in relation to the IPS is uncertain, and the IPS appears to be the principal prognostic tool for patients at baseline.

The risk factors in relapsed Hodgkin lymphoma are more controversial than in untreated disease, but the GHSG contributed a large retrospective study analyzing the risk factors for poor outcome in four hundred twenty-two relapsed patients. They developed a prognostic score based on three factors: time to relapse, clinical stage, and presence of anemia (Josting, Franklin, et al. 2002).

More recently, interest has grown to better refine baseline prognosis with information on disease response with therapy, which has consistently shown to be an important factor when degree of response in untreated or relapsed patients is considered. In other words, attainment of complete response, as is the case for most hematologic malignancies, is the name of the game for Hodgkin lymphoma. Computed tomography, an extremely valuable tool for assessment of anatomic structures, has been the traditional assessment tool for response in lymphomas, with criteria for definition of complete and partial response clearly delineated (Cheson et al. 1999). Given that lymph node size may correlate less well with viable cancer than functional imaging with positron emission tomography, it is now generally accepted that either fusion PET/CT or PET and CT are superior to CT alone at baseline and post-therapy restaging. Given the superiority in re-staging, interest grew in obtaining information from PET at earlier and earlier timepoints, in order to utilize that information, the so-called interim PET, for treatment decisions. A major report in this arena was a retrospective study by an Italian group of patients with advanced Hodgkin lymphoma treated with ABVD or similar regimens, who underwent PET scanning after two cycles of treatment, and outcomes were compared between PET positive and negative patients, with a comparison with IPS to delineate the most robust prognostic factor. The results of PET essentially made results of IPS inconsequential, with a clear difference between patients with positive and negative PET, with progression-free survivals of 12.8 versus 95 percent, respectively, and only PET was significant for prognosis in multivariate analysis, which included the IPS (Gallamini et al. 2007). Based on this result and promising information from other similar yet smaller reports, most current clinical trials in Hodgkin lymphoma are determining in a prospective fashion the prognostic value of PET/CT. Additionally, many are also testing risk-adapted therapeutic strategies to improve outcomes.

Not only has PET scanning been found to be prognostic in untreated patients as a re-staging strategy, but it has been utilized prior to autologous or allogeneic transplant (Svoboda et al. 2006; Jabbour et al. 2007), with a clear improvement in transplant outcome in those patients with negative functional imaging prior to transplant.

12. Promising therapies of the future

There are many exciting therapies on the horizon for patients with advanced Hodgkin lymphoma. Although none of the treatments discussed below have made their way into the armamentarium for the newly diagnosed patient, the treatments below have been selected as they appear to be associated with the most promise and are furthest in development in relapsed/refractory Hodgkin lymphoma. The most important future therapies, in the opinion of the author, are brentuximab vedotin, rituximab, bendamustine, panobinostat, and lenalidomide. See Table 2. Each will be discussed in further detail in this section.

Brentuximab vedotin, long known as SGN-35, and now known as Adcetris after the United States Food & Drug Administration granted accelerated approval of this antibody-drug conjugate on August 19, 2011, appears to be an important new treatment option in Hodgkin lymphoma. The approval was long awaited by those who had seen multiple failures of unconjugated monoclonal antibodies to CD30, a protein expressed on the surface of Reed Sternberg cells. To specifically enhance clinical anti-tumor activity, the antitubulin agent monomethyl auristatin E was attached to the CD30-specific monoclonal antibody cAC10 by an enzyme-cleavable dipeptide linker (Hamblett et al. 2004). It is indicated for patients with relapsed or refractory Hodgkin's lymphoma after failure of autologous stem cell transplant or at least two prior multi-agent chemotherapy regimens in patients who are not transplant candidates. The accelerated approval was based on a single-arm, multicenter clinical trial in one hundred two patients with multiply relapsed or refractory Hodgkin lymphoma to evaluate the objective response rate as a single agent. Patients were treated with 1.8 mg/kg intravenously over thirty minutes every three weeks. The primary efficacy endpoint, the overall response rate, was achieved in 73 percent of patients with a complete remission rate of 32 percent. The median duration of response was 6.7 months (Chen et al. 2010). The most common adverse events were peripheral sensory neuropathy, fatigue, nausea, neutropenia, diarrhea, and pyrexia, with most events being grade 1 or 2, and no grade 5 events occurred on treatment. The response rate associated with this agent given as monotherapy is highly encouraging, and further study of this compound is anxiously anticipated. Currently, it is being investigated in a phase I clinical trial in combination with ABVD chemotherapy (Seattle Genetics 2011), and in a phase III randomized clinical trial, AETHERA, in which its use is compared with placebo in "high risk" Hodgkin lymphoma patients post-autologous transplant (Seattle Genetics 2011). This compound appears to represent a major advance in the treatment of Hodgkin lymphoma given the unprecedented response rates in multiply relapsed and highly refractory patient populations.

Rituximab is an intravenous chimeric monoclonal antibody directed at the CD20 antigen, which is present only on a minority of Reed Sternberg or Hodgkin cells of classic Hodgkin lymphoma (Schmid et al. 1991). In spite of this, a pilot study of rituximab was performed in patients with relapsed/refractory classic Hodgkin lymphoma regardless of CD20 status (Younes et al. 2003). In that study, five of twenty-two patients (22 percent) responded with 36 percent achieving stable disease with expected excellent tolerability. Further study by the same investigators at MD Anderson focused on the addition of rituximab to ABVD therapy. One hundred four patients with newly diagnosed advanced disease were treated with six weekly doses of rituximab during ABVD chemotherapy, and their outcomes were compared with historical patients treated with ABVD. The five year event-free survival with ABVD was 66 percent versus a projected 87 percent for R-ABVD with a median follow-up time of five years, and all IPS risk groups seemed to benefit from the addition of rituximab (Copeland et al. 2009). This study generated great excitement, and it is the springboard for two major ongoing advanced Hodgkin lymphoma studies. In the HD18 trial of the GHSG, patients with PET positivity after two cycles of escalated BEACOPP are randomly assigned to further chemotherapy with or without rituximab (University of Cologne 2011). The second trial is a phase II study randomizing patients to R-ABVD versus ABVD at a single institution (M.D. Anderson Cancer Center 2011). In summary, rituximab appears to be a promising step forward with little toxicity in the treatment of advanced classic Hodgkin lymphoma, and the results of the above studies are eagerly anticipated.

In contrast to classic Hodgkin lymphoma, the neoplastic cells, known as the lymphocyte predominant cells of nodular lymphocyte predominant Hodgkin lymphoma, express CD20 strongly. Importantly, several studies indicate that rituximab as a single agent in both previously treated and untreated patients carries a very high response rate in this subtype of Hodgkin lymphoma (Ekstrand et al. 2003; Schulz et al. 2008), and it is reasonable, given the rarity of advanced disease with nodular lymphocyte predominant Hodgkin lymphoma, to utilize rituximab in combination with chemotherapy for patients with this disease.

Bendamustine, an intravenous bifunctional alkylator and nucleoside analogue, was synthesized in East Germany in 1963 but only recently its use has become popularized in the United States with FDA approval for CLL and indolent NHL occurring in 2008. Its activity in Hodgkin lymphoma was well known to the East Germans, and recently Memorial Sloan Kettering investigators put this compound on the international map in Hodgkin lymphoma. Benadmustine was administered at a dose of 120mg/m^2 day one and two of twenty-eight day cycles with pegylated filgrastim support in a single center phase II study of relapsed Hodgkin lymphoma patients post-transplant or transplant-ineligible. Although major conclusions are limited by the small evaluable patient number of sixteen, the overall response rate of 75 percent and CR rate of 38 percent are encouraging, along with twelve of sixteen patients with response becoming eligible for a non-myeloablative allogeneic transplant. Currently, an Italian study is investigating in a phase I/II trial its efficacy and toxicity combined with another promising agent for Hodgkin lymphoma, lenalidomide (Fondazione Giovanni Pascale).

Another promising new compound in the treatment of advanced Hodgkin lymphoma is the oral histone deacetylase inhibitor, panobinostat. Preliminary evidence of activity in refractory Hodgkin lymphoma was demonstrated in a small phase I/II prospective, multicenter study of thirteen patients, and a remarkable response rate of 38 percent was found with computed tomography criteria, with 58 percent of patients responding by positron emission tomography criteria (Dickinson et al. 2009). The principal dose-limiting toxicity with panobinostat is thrombocytopenia, unfortunately, as many patients with relapsed disease have impaired bone marrow reserve. Forty percent of patients in this study developed grade 3/4 thrombocytopenia. In a large multicenter, prospective, phase II study, 40 mg of panobinostat was administered orally three times per week every week in 21 day cycles to one hundred twenty-nine relapsed/refractory patients (Sureda et al. 2010). Responses were observed in 27 percent of patients with 82 percent of patients having stable disease or better. This phase II study, with very promising response rates in a large number of heavily pre-treated patients, has led to a number of current studies in Hodgkin lymphoma, including a phase III study of panobinostat versus placebo for maintenance therapy (Novartis Pharmaceuticals 2011), and a phase I study in combination with ICE and a planned follow-on phase II study of panobinostat plus ICE versus ICE alone (M.D. Anderson Cancer Center 2011).

Lenalidomide is an oral immunomodulatory agent with an uncertain mechanism of action that appears to have activity in a broad range of hematopoietic malignancies. The use of lenalidomide was empiric, and in an initial small cohort of twelve patients with multiply relapsed Hodgkin lymphoma treated in Germany, it was found to be safe with no toxicity greater than grade two. Additionally, it was efficacious with a response rate of fifty percent with at least disease stabilization in all patients (Boll et al. 2010). In a prospective phase II Canadian study, fifteen patients with relapsed/refractory disease were enrolled and given lenalidomide 25 mg orally day 1-21 of 28 day cycles. The overall response rate was 14 percent with at least disease stabilization in 64 percent of patients. Hematologic toxicity was the predominant toxicity seen, with 29 percent of patients with grade 3/4 neutropenia and thrombocytopenia (Kuruvilla et al. 2008). In a similar study conducted by United States investigators, thirty-eight patients were enrolled on a prospective phase II study of relapsed/refractory patients with lenalidomide administered in the same fashion as the prior study (Fehniger et al. 2009). Of thirty-five evaluable patients, the overall response rate was 17 percent with stabilization of disease for greater than six months in 34 percent. Grade 3/4 toxicity was primarily hematologic, with neutropenia being the most common at 40 percent of patients. The authors concluded that activity was seen and continuous dosing and utilization in combinations would be reasonable in the future. Currently, lenalidomide is under evaluation in phase I studies in combination with benadmustine (Fondazione Giovanni Pascale 2011), AVD (University of Cologne 2011), and as maintenance post-autologous transplant (Washington University School of Medicine).

In summary, there are a number of agents with promising activity in relapsed Hodgkin lymphoma currently in development. Further study will define their ultimate role, but the favorable toxicity profile and encouraging reports of activity of the monoclonal antibodies make these compounds of high interest for further investigation.

Compound	Mechanism	Route	CR, ORR% Median Response Duration	Current Status
Brentuximab Vedotin	Monoclonal Antibody-drug conjugate (anti-CD30)	Intravenous	32%, 78% 6.7 months	FDA approved, relapsed/ refractory Ongoing phase I, III studies
Rituximab	Chimeric monoclonal antibody (anti-CD20)	Intravenous	5%, 22% 7.8 months	Ongoing phase II, III studies
Bendamustine	Bifunctional Alkylator/ nucleoside analog	Intravenous	38%, 75% 2.6 months	Ongoing phase I/II study
Panobinostat	Histone deacetylase inhibitor	Oral	4%, 27% 6.9 months	Ongoing phase I, III studies
Lenalidomide	Immunomodulator (many mechanisms)	Oral	3%, 17% 4.5 months	Ongoing phase I/II studies

Table 2. Promising Drugs in Development for Hodgkin lymphoma.

13. Case studies

In this section, several case scenarios will be presented, and management will be discussed, which integrates material covered in prior sections.

Case 1. A twenty-three year old otherwise healthy Caucasian female was diagnosed with stage IIIB nodular sclerosis Hodgkin lymphoma after an excisional biopsy was performed due to left neck adenopathy. The mediastinum was bulky at diagnosis. The IPS was 1 for anemia. She was treated with six cycles of ABVD at full dose and schedule and achieved a complete metabolic remission on PET/CT. Fifteen months later, PET/CT revealed asymptomatic FDG avid mediastinal adenopathy, and thoracotomy with excisional biopsy revealed a relapse of nodular sclerosis Hodgkin lymphoma. Hemoglobin was normal. She was treated with ICE for three cycles followed by stem cell mobilization and collection and autologous hematopoietic stem cell transplantation with BEAM conditioning. She receives 36 Gy to the mediastinum two months post-transplant and is alive and well seven years post-transplant.

Case 1 Discussion. This young woman was given a standard of care for advanced Hodgkin lymphoma at diagnosis, and ABVD was favored in this instance over escalated BEACOPP for fertility preservation, as the patient expressed interest in maintaining fertility. The author's preference is to enroll patients with advanced Hodgkin lymphoma on a clinical trial if possible, and currently this would be the SWOG 0816 at the author's institution. The lack of thoracic radiotherapy was reasonable given the PET/CT defined complete remission. This patient's relapse can be classified as low risk by the Josting score as she had none of the the adverse factors which include: early relapse, advanced stage at relapse, and anemia. Therefore, she again received a standard of care including: choice of salvage regimen, decision for autologous transplant, and choice of preparative regimen. The exact value of thoracic radiotherapy administration post-transplant is uncertain but reasonable given the bulky disease of mediastinum initially and the limited stage relapse. The increased risk of solid cancers including breast and lung with thoracic radiotherapy should be discussed with the patient, and long term follow-up should include counseling on smoking cessation, breast and skin examination regularly, breast mammography, and vaccinations yearly for influenza, every five years for pneumococcus, and every ten years for tetanus/diphtheria (Connors 2005).

Case 2. A thirty-five year old otherwise healthy African American male is diagnosed with stage IVA mixed cellularity Hodgkin lymphoma after excisional biopsy is performed of a right inguinal mass. Bone marrow involvement is present at diagnosis and FDG avid lesions are seen in the liver. His International Prognostic Score is 5 with the following risk factors: low albumin, low lymphocyte count, low hemoglobin, stage IV, and male gender. There are no bulky sites of disease. He is treated with escalated BEACOPP for six cycles and achieves a complete remission by PET/CT post-therapy. His PET/CT after two cycles of escalated BEACOPP was negative as well. Five months later, he has biopsy proven relapsed Hodgkin lymphoma after left axillary lymph node enlargement prompts an excisional biopsy. His relapse stage is III, and GDP is administered for three cycles. He achieves a partial metabolic remission on PET/CT with a negative bone marrow biopsy. Organ function is preserved, and he receives a BEAM-conditioned autologous transplant. He suffers another biopsy-proven relapse with stage III disease seven months post autologous transplant. He is treated with IGEV salvage chemotherapy for three cycles, and achieves another partial metabolic response. Given that his organ function is preserved, he undergoes a reduced-intensity allogeneic hematopoietic stem cell transplant with Flu/Bu conditioning. He is alive three years post-allogeneic transplant with mild chronic graft versus host disease.

Case 2 Discussion. This young man was given an appropriate initial therapy, escalated BEACOPP, given his high risk disease. In fact, escalated BEACOPP is reasonable for any advanced Hodgkin lymphoma patient <60 years without pregnancy, HIV, or abnormal organ function regardless of IPS. He was given six cycles rather than the current standard of eight cycles established by the GHSG. Would he still have suffered a relapse if given eight cycles, is it appropriate to administer six cycles in this situation, and is it appropriate to obtain interim PET/CT scans outside the context of clinical trials? The answer to each of these questions is obviously controversial. The author believes that it is reasonable to perform interim PET/CT scans off study, and to make certain therapeutic decisions on the basis of those scans. Because the PET/CT was negative after two cycles, the author believes that it was a reasonable clinical decision to administer six rather than eight total cycles. Although impossible at present to know, the author believes that it is unlikely that two more cycles of escalated BEACOPP would have cured the case patient. Again, it is the author's strong preference to obtain further prospective data regarding interim PET/CT and therapy adjustment, which is why the optimal treatment for current patients with Hodgkin lymphoma is a clinical trial. The choice of GDP as salvage chemotherapy is very reasonable, as is the choice to take a patient in partial remission to a BEAM conditioned autologous transplant. Given at least three adverse prognostic factors associated with this relapse, which are: early relapse, relapse after high intensity initial chemotherapy, and partial rather than complete metabolic response pre-transplant, the author believes, even though randomized data are not available, that performing a tandem transplant as in the H96 study would have been reasonable in this patient. Once relapse after autologous transplant occurs, prognosis is poor and this case example illustrates that a reduced-intensity allogeneic hematopoietic stem cell transplant can be curative in this setting. In addition to the chronic adverse health effects associated with allogeneic transplant, Hodgkin lymphoma survivors do have persistent challenges in health related quality of life, particularly in regards to chronic fatigue (Baxi and Matasar 2010). This patient would likely benefit from multidisciplinary follow-up care including input from psychiatry and social work.

14. Conclusion

There are many unanswered questions the clinician faces in the care of the individual patient with advanced Hodgkin lymphoma throughout the course of the disease. Polychemotherapy with regimens such as ABVD or escalated BEACOPP for six to eight cycles are the standard of care for newly diagnosed patients, and the role of radiotherapy is uncertain. Refinement of morbidity and mortality related to chemotherapy and radiotherapy may be possible in the future with a sincere commitment of physicians to enroll patients on the current generation of clinical trials testing PET/CT directed strategies. Several newer agents are likely to be incorporated into polychemotherapy in the future based on promising results in the relapsed setting. The goal of therapy in the short term is a PET/CT without FDG avidity, or complete remission, and in the long term a cure. For most patients with relapsed or refractory Hodgkin lymphoma, polychemotherapy for approximately three cycles followed by autologous hematopoietic stem cell transplantation is the current standard of care. Radiotherapy should be considered in the relapsed setting to optimize curative potential of treatment in spite of the potential morbidity and lack of clear evidence base. Reduced intensity allogeneic hematopoietic stem cell transplantation should be considered as the primary curative treatment modality in those patients without significant comorbidity who relapse after autolgous transplantation.

15. Acknowledgments

I would like to acknowledge my family, who I love including my wife Ellen, sons Luke, Gabriel, and Michael, as well as my parents, Dennis and Patricia. Without these people in my life, this work would not be possible.

I would like to also acknowledge my mentors who give me daily guidance as physicians and friends, and were kind enough to review my work shortly before the deadline, Paul J. Petruska, M.D. and Friedrich G. Schuening, M.D.
I would like to also acknowledge my patients and their families. Hopefully I help you as much as you teach me.
I would also like to acknowledge Carol Murray and Kim Lipsey, who provided valuable assistance in referencing this chapter.

16. References

Aleman, B. M., J. M. Raemaekers, U. Tirelli, R. Bortolus, M. B. van 't Veer, M. L. Lybeert, J. J. Keuning, P. Carde, T. Girinsky, R. W. van der Maazen, R. Tomsic, M. Vovk, A. van Hoof, G. Demeestere, P. J. Lugtenburg, J. Thomas, W. Schroyens, K. De Boeck, J. W. Baars, J. C. Kluin-Nelemans, C. Carrie, M. Aoudjhane, D. Bron, H. Eghbali, W. G. Smit, J. H. Meerwaldt, A. Hagenbeek, A. Pinna, M. Henry-Amar, Research European Organization for, and Group Treatment of Cancer Lymphoma. 2003. Involved-field radiotherapy for advanced Hodgkin's lymphoma. *N Engl J Med* 348 (24):2396-406.

Andre, M., M. Henry-Amar, J. L. Pico, P. Brice, D. Blaise, M. Kuentz, B. Coiffier, P. Colombat, J. Y. Cahn, M. Attal, J. Fleury, N. Milpied, G. Nedellec, P. Biron, H. Tilly, J. P. Jouet, and C. Gisselbrecht. 1999. Comparison of high-dose therapy and autologous stem-cell transplantation with conventional therapy for Hodgkin's disease induction failure: a case-control study. Societe Francaise de Greffe de Moelle. *J Clin Oncol* 17 (1):222-9.

Aparicio, J., A. Segura, S. Garcera, A. Oltra, A. Santaballa, A. Yuste, and M. Pastor. 1999. ESHAP is an active regimen for relapsing Hodgkin's disease. *Ann Oncol* 10 (5):593-5.

Baetz, T., A. Belch, S. Couban, K. Imrie, J. Yau, R. Myers, K. Ding, N. Paul, L. Shepherd, J. Iglesias, R. Meyer, and M. Crump. 2003. Gemcitabine, dexamethasone and cisplatin is an active and non-toxic chemotherapy regimen in relapsed or refractory Hodgkin's disease: a phase II study by the National Cancer Institute of Canada Clinical Trials Group. *Ann Oncol* 14 (12):1762-7.

Bartlett, N. L., S. A. Rosenberg, R. T. Hoppe, S. L. Hancock, and S. J. Horning. 1995. Brief chemotherapy, Stanford V, and adjuvant radiotherapy for bulky or advanced-stage Hodgkin's disease: a preliminary report. *J Clin Oncol* 13 (5):1080-8.

Baxi, S. S., and M. J. Matasar. 2010. State-of-the-art issues in Hodgkin's lymphoma survivorship. *Curr Oncol Rep* 12 (6):366-73.

Boll, B., P. Borchmann, M. S. Topp, M. Hanel, K. S. Reiners, A. Engert, and R. Naumann. 2010. Lenalidomide in patients with refractory or multiple relapsed Hodgkin lymphoma. *Br J Haematol* 148 (3):480-2.

Bonadonna, G., P. Valagussa, and A. Santoro. 1986. Alternating non-cross-resistant combination chemotherapy or MOPP in stage IV Hodgkin's disease. A report of 8-year results. *Ann Intern Med* 104 (6):739-46.

Bonadonna, G., R. Zucali, S. Monfardini, M. De Lena, and C. Uslenghi. 1975. Combination chemotherapy of Hodgkin's disease with adriamycin, bleomycin, vinblastine, and imidazole carboxamide versus MOPP. *Cancer* 36 (1):252-9.

Cancer and Leukemia Group B. 2011. Chemotherapy Based on Positron Emission Tomography Scan in Treating Patients With Stage I or Stage II Hodgkin

Lymphoma. In *ClinicalTrials.gov [Internet]*. Bethesda (MD): National Library of Medicine (US). 2011- [cited 2011 Sept 15]. Available from: http://clinicaltrials.gov/show/NCT01132807.

Canellos, G. P., J. R. Anderson, K. J. Propert, N. Nissen, M. R. Cooper, E. S. Henderson, M. R. Green, A. Gottlieb, and B. A. Peterson. 1992. Chemotherapy of advanced Hodgkin's disease with MOPP, ABVD, or MOPP alternating with ABVD. *N Engl J Med* 327 (21):1478-84.

Chen, Robert, Ajay K. Gopal, Scott E. Smith, Stephen M. Ansell, Joseph D. Rosenblatt, Richard Klasa, Joseph M. Connors, Andreas Engert, Emily K. Larsen, Dana A. Kennedy, Eric L. Sievers, and Anas Younes. 2010. Results of a Pivotal Phase 2 Study of Brentuximab Vedotin (SGN-35) in Patients with Relapsed or Refractory Hodgkin Lymphoma. *ASH Annual Meeting Abstracts* 116 (21):283-.

Cheson, B. D., S. J. Horning, B. Coiffier, M. A. Shipp, R. I. Fisher, J. M. Connors, T. A. Lister, J. Vose, A. Grillo-Lopez, A. Hagenbeek, F. Cabanillas, D. Klippensten, W. Hiddemann, R. Castellino, N. L. Harris, J. O. Armitage, W. Carter, R. Hoppe, and G. P. Canellos. 1999. Report of an international workshop to standardize response criteria for non-Hodgkin's lymphomas. NCI Sponsored International Working Group. *J Clin Oncol* 17 (4):1244.

Connors, J. M. 2005. State-of-the-art therapeutics: Hodgkin's lymphoma. *J Clin Oncol* 23 (26):6400-8.

Connors, J. M., P. Klimo, G. Adams, B. F. Burns, I. Cooper, R. M. Meyer, S. E. O'Reilly, J. Pater, I. Quirt, A. Sadura, C. Shustik, J. Skillings, S. Sutcliffe, S. Verma, S. Yoshida, and B. Zee. 1997. Treatment of advanced Hodgkin's disease with chemotherapy--comparison of MOPP/ABV hybrid regimen with alternating courses of MOPP and ABVD: a report from the National Cancer Institute of Canada clinical trials group. *J Clin Oncol* 15 (4):1638-45.

Constans, Mireia, Anna Sureda, Reyes Arranz, Maria Dolores Caballero, Juan Jose Lahuerta, Juan Carlos Hernandez-Boluda, Maria Jesus Vidal, Jose Garcia-Larana, Jose Rifon, Josep Maria Ribera, Pascual Fernandez-Abellan, Jose Maria Moraleda, Maria Teresa Bernal, Maria Victoria Mateos, Maria Martin-Mateos, Rafael Cordoba, Javier Garcia-Conde, Jorge Sierra, Eulogio Conde, and for the Spanish Cooperative Group GEL/TAMO. 2004. Prognostic Factors and Long-Term Outcome for Patients with Hodgkin's Lymphoma Who Relapse after an Autologous Stem Cell Transplantation. *ASH Annual Meeting Abstracts* 104 (11):1649-.

Copeland, Amanda R, Yumei Cao, Michelle Fanale, Luis Fayad, Peter McLaughlin, Barbara Pro, Fredrick Hagemeister, Jorge Romaguera, Felipe Samaniego, Alma Rodriguez, and Anas Younes. 2009. Final Report of a Phase-II Study of Rituximab Plus ABVD for Patients with Newly Diagnosed Advanced Stage Classical Hodgkin Lymphoma.: Results of Long Follow up and Comparison to Institutional Historical Data. *ASH Annual Meeting Abstracts* 114 (22):1680-.

Crump, M. 2008. Management of Hodgkin lymphoma in relapse after autologous stem cell transplant. *Hematology Am Soc Hematol Educ Program*:326-33.

DeVita, V. T., Jr., B. J. Lewis, M. Rozencweig, and F. M. Muggia. 1978. The chemotherapy of Hodgkin's disease: past experiences and future directions. *Cancer* 42 (2 Suppl):979-90.

Devita, V. T., Jr., A. A. Serpick, and P. P. Carbone. 1970. Combination chemotherapy in the treatment of advanced Hodgkin's disease. *Ann Intern Med* 73 (6):881-95.

DeVita, Vincent T. Lawrence Theodore S. Rosenberg Steven A. 2008. *DeVita, Hellman, and Rosenberg's cancer : principles & practice of oncology*: Wolters Kluwer/Lippincott Williams & Wilkins.

Dickinson, M., D. Ritchie, D. J. DeAngelo, A. Spencer, O. G. Ottmann, T. Fischer, K. N. Bhalla, A. Liu, K. Parker, J. W. Scott, M. Bishton, and H. M. Prince. 2009. Preliminary evidence of disease response to the pan deacetylase inhibitor panobinostat (LBH589) in refractory Hodgkin Lymphoma. *Br J Haematol* 147 (1):97-101.

Diehl, V., J. Franklin, D. Hasenclever, H. Tesch, M. Pfreundschuh, B. Lathan, U. Paulus, M. Sieber, J. U. Rueffer, M. Sextro, A. Engert, J. Wolf, R. Hermann, L. Holmer, U. Stappert-Jahn, E. Winnerlein-Trump, G. Wulf, S. Krause, A. Glunz, K. von Kalle, H. Bischoff, C. Haedicke, E. Duehmke, A. Georgii, and M. Loeffler. 1998. BEACOPP, a new dose-escalated and accelerated regimen, is at least as effective as COPP/ABVD in patients with advanced-stage Hodgkin's lymphoma: interim report from a trial of the German Hodgkin's Lymphoma Study Group. *J Clin Oncol* 16 (12):3810-21.

Diehl, V., M. Loeffler, M. Pfreundschuh, U. Ruehl, D. Hasenclever, H. Nisters-Backes, M. Sieber, K. Smith, H. Tesch, W. Geilen, and et al. 1995. Further chemotherapy versus low-dose involved-field radiotherapy as consolidation of complete remission after six cycles of alternating chemotherapy in patients with advance Hodgkin's disease. German Hodgkins' Study Group (GHSG). *Ann Oncol* 6 (9):901-10.

Diehl, Volker, Heinz Haverkamp, Rolf Peter Mueller, Hans Theodor Eich, Hans Konrad Mueller-Hermelink, Thomas Cerny, Jana Markova, Anthony Ho, Lothar Kanz, Richard Greil, Wolfgang Hiddemann, and Andreas Engert. 2008. Eight Cycles of BEACOPP Escalated Compared with 4 Cycles of BEACOPP Escalated Followed by 4 Cycles of BEACOPP Baseline with Our without Radiotherapy in Patients in Advanced Stage Hodgkin Lymphoma (HL): Final Analysis of the Randomised HD12 Trial of the German Hodgkin Study Group (GHSG). *ASH Annual Meeting Abstracts* 112 (11):1558-.

Duggan, D. B., G. R. Petroni, J. L. Johnson, J. H. Glick, R. I. Fisher, J. M. Connors, G. P. Canellos, and B. A. Peterson. 2003. Randomized comparison of ABVD and MOPP/ABV hybrid for the treatment of advanced Hodgkin's disease: report of an intergroup trial. *J Clin Oncol* 21 (4):607-14.

Ekstrand, B. C., J. B. Lucas, S. M. Horwitz, Z. Fan, S. Breslin, R. T. Hoppe, Y. Natkunam, N. L. Bartlett, and S. J. Horning. 2003. Rituximab in lymphocyte-predominant Hodgkin disease: results of a phase 2 trial. *Blood* 101 (11):4285-9.

Engert, A., V. Diehl, J. Franklin, A. Lohri, B. Dorken, W. D. Ludwig, P. Koch, M. Hanel, M. Pfreundschuh, M. Wilhelm, L. Trumper, W. E. Aulitzky, M. Bentz, M. Rummel, O. Sezer, H. K. Muller-Hermelink, D. Hasenclever, and M. Loffler. 2009. Escalated-dose BEACOPP in the treatment of patients with advanced-stage Hodgkin's lymphoma: 10 years of follow-up of the GHSG HD9 study. *J Clin Oncol* 27 (27):4548-54.

European Organization for Research and Treatment of Cancer. 2002. Comparison of Two Combination Chemotherapy Regimens in Treating Patients With Stage III or Stage IV Hodgkin's Lymphoma. In *ClinicalTrials.gov [Internet]*. Bethesda (MD): National Library of Medicine (US). 2011- [cited 2011 Sept 15]. Available from: http://clinicaltrials.gov/show/NCT00049595.

Fabian, C. J., C. M. Mansfield, S. Dahlberg, S. E. Jones, T. P. Miller, E. Van Slyck, P. N. Grozea, F. S. Morrison, C. A. Coltman, Jr., and R. I. Fisher. 1994. Low-dose involved field radiation after chemotherapy in advanced Hodgkin disease. A Southwest Oncology Group randomized study. *Ann Intern Med* 120 (11):903-12.

Federico, M., M. Bellei, P. Brice, M. Brugiatelli, A. Nagler, C. Gisselbrecht, L. Moretti, P. Colombat, S. Luminari, F. Fabbiano, N. Di Renzo, A. Goldstone, A. M. Carella, and Ebmt Gisl Anzlg Sfgm Gela Intergroup HD01 Trial. 2003. High-dose therapy and autologous stem-cell transplantation versus conventional therapy for patients with advanced Hodgkin's lymphoma responding to front-line therapy. *J Clin Oncol* 21 (12):2320-5.

Federico, M., S. Luminari, E. Iannitto, G. Polimeno, L. Marcheselli, A. Montanini, A. La Sala, F. Merli, C. Stelitano, S. Pozzi, R. Scalone, N. Di Renzo, P. Musto, L. Baldini, G. Cervetti, F. Angrilli, P. Mazza, M. Brugiatelli, P. G. Gobbi, and H. D. Gruppo Italiano per lo Studio dei Linfomi Trial. 2009. ABVD compared with BEACOPP compared with CEC for the initial treatment of patients with advanced Hodgkin's lymphoma: results from the HD2000 Gruppo Italiano per lo Studio dei Linfomi Trial. *J Clin Oncol* 27 (5):805-11.

Fehniger, Todd A, Sarah Larson, Kathryn Trinkaus, Marilyn J Siegel, Amanda F Cashen, Kristie A Blum, Timothy S. Fenske, David D Hurd, Andre Goy, John F. DiPersio, and Nancy L Bartlett. 2009. A Phase II Multicenter Study of Lenalidomide in Relapsed or Refractory Classical Hodgkin Lymphoma. *ASH Annual Meeting Abstracts* 114 (22):3693-.

Ferme, C., C. Sebban, C. Hennequin, M. Divine, P. Lederlin, J. Gabarre, A. Ferrant, D. Caillot, D. Bordessoule, P. Brice, I. Moullet, F. Berger, and E. Lepage. 2000. Comparison of chemotherapy to radiotherapy as consolidation of complete or good partial response after six cycles of chemotherapy for patients with advanced Hodgkin's disease: results of the groupe d'etudes des lymphomes de l'Adulte H89 trial. *Blood* 95 (7):2246-52.

Fondazione Giovanni Pascale. 2011. A Phase 1/2 Study of Lenalidomide in Combination With Bendamustine in Relapsed and Primary Refractory Hodgkin Lymphoma (LEBEN). In *ClinicalTrials.gov [Internet].* Bethesda (MD): National Library of Medicine (US). 2011- [cited 2011 Sept 15]. Available from: http://clinicaltrials.gov/ct2/show/NCT01412307?term=NCT01412307&rank=1.

Gajewski, J. L., G. L. Phillips, K. A. Sobocinski, J. O. Armitage, R. P. Gale, R. E. Champlin, R. H. Herzig, D. D. Hurd, S. Jagannath, J. P. Klein, H. M. Lazarus, P. L. McCarthy, Jr., S. Pavlovsky, F. B. Peterson, P. A. Rowlings, J. A. Russell, S. M. Silver, J. M. Vose, P. H. Wiernik, M. M. Bortin, and M. M. Horowitz. 1996. Bone marrow transplants from HLA-identical siblings in advanced Hodgkin's disease. *J Clin Oncol* 14 (2):572-8.

Gallamini, A., M. Hutchings, L. Rigacci, L. Specht, F. Merli, M. Hansen, C. Patti, A. Loft, F. Di Raimondo, F. D'Amore, A. Biggi, U. Vitolo, C. Stelitano, R. Sancetta, L. Trentin, S. Luminari, E. Iannitto, S. Viviani, I. Pierri, and A. Levis. 2007. Early interim 2-[18F]fluoro-2-deoxy-D-glucose positron emission tomography is prognostically superior to international prognostic score in advanced-stage Hodgkin's lymphoma: a report from a joint Italian-Danish study. *J Clin Oncol* 25 (24):3746-52.

Gobbi, P. G., A. Levis, T. Chisesi, C. Broglia, U. Vitolo, C. Stelitano, V. Pavone, L. Cavanna, G. Santini, F. Merli, M. Liberati, L. Baldini, G. L. Deliliers, E. Angelucci, R.

Bordonaro, M. Federico, and Linfomi Intergruppo Italiano. 2005. ABVD versus modified stanford V versus MOPPEBVCAD with optional and limited radiotherapy in intermediate- and advanced-stage Hodgkin's lymphoma: final results of a multicenter randomized trial by the Intergruppo Italiano Linfomi. *J Clin Oncol* 23 (36):9198-207.

Goldie, J. H., and A. J. Coldman. 1979. A mathematic model for relating the drug sensitivity of tumors to their spontaneous mutation rate. *Cancer Treat Rep* 63 (11-12):1727-33.

Gordon, Leo I, Fanxing Hong, Richard I Fisher, Nancy L. Bartlett, Joseph M. Connors, Randy D. Gascoyne, Henry Wagner, Patrick J Stiff, Bruce D. Cheson, Mary Gospodarowicz, Ranjana Advani, Brad Kahl, Jonathan W. Friedberg, Kristie A. Blum, Thomas M. Habermann, Joseph Tuscano, Richard Hoppe, and Sandra J. Horning. 2010. A Randomized Phase III Trial of ABVD Vs. Stanford V +/- Radiation Therapy In Locally Extensive and Advanced Stage Hodgkin's Lymphoma: An Intergroup Study Coordinated by the Eastern Cooperatve Oncology Group (E2496). *ASH Annual Meeting Abstracts* 116 (21):415-.

Gutierrez-Delgado, F., L. Holmberg, H. Hooper, S. Petersdorf, O. Press, R. Maziarz, D. Maloney, T. Chauncey, F. Appelbaum, and W. Bensinger. 2003. Autologous stem cell transplantation for Hodgkin's disease: busulfan, melphalan and thiotepa compared to a radiation-based regimen. *Bone Marrow Transplant* 32 (3):279-85.

Hamblett, K. J., P. D. Senter, D. F. Chace, M. M. Sun, J. Lenox, C. G. Cerveny, K. M. Kissler, S. X. Bernhardt, A. K. Kopcha, R. F. Zabinski, D. L. Meyer, and J. A. Francisco. 2004. Effects of drug loading on the antitumor activity of a monoclonal antibody drug conjugate. *Clin Cancer Res* 10 (20):7063-70.

Hancock, B. W. 1986. Randomised study of MOPP (mustine, Oncovin, procarbazine, prednisone) against LOPP (Leukeran substituted for mustine) in advanced Hodgkin's disease. British National Lymphoma Investigation. *Radiother Oncol* 7 (3):215-21.

Hasenclever, D., and V. Diehl. 1998. A prognostic score for advanced Hodgkin's disease. International Prognostic Factors Project on Advanced Hodgkin's Disease. *N Engl J Med* 339 (21):1506-14.

Hasenclever, D., M. Loeffler, and V. Diehl. 1996. Rationale for dose escalation of first line conventional chemotherapy in advanced Hodgkin's disease. German Hodgkin's Lymphoma Study Group. *Ann Oncol* 7 Suppl 4:95-8.

Huguley, C. M., Jr., J. R. Durant, R. R. Moores, Y. K. Chan, R. F. Dorfman, and L. Johnson. 1975. A comparison of nitrogen mustard, vincristine, procarbazine, and prednisone (MOPP) vs. nitrogen mustard in advanced Hodgkin's disease. *Cancer* 36 (4):1227-40.

Jabbour, E., C. Hosing, G. Ayers, R. Nunez, P. Anderlini, B. Pro, I. Khouri, A. Younes, F. Hagemeister, L. Kwak, and L. Fayad. 2007. Pretransplant positive positron emission tomography/gallium scans predict poor outcome in patients with recurrent/refractory Hodgkin lymphoma. *Cancer* 109 (12):2481-9.

Johnson, P. W., J. A. Radford, M. H. Cullen, M. R. Sydes, J. Walewski, A. S. Jack, K. A. MacLennan, S. P. Stenning, S. Clawson, P. Smith, D. Ryder, B. W. Hancock, and L. Y. Trial United Kingdom Lymphoma Group. 2005. Comparison of ABVD and alternating or hybrid multidrug regimens for the treatment of advanced Hodgkin's lymphoma: results of the United Kingdom Lymphoma Group LY09 Trial (ISRCTN97144519). *J Clin Oncol* 23 (36):9208-18.

Josting, A., J. Franklin, M. May, P. Koch, M. K. Beykirch, J. Heinz, C. Rudolph, V. Diehl, and A. Engert. 2002. New prognostic score based on treatment outcome of patients with relapsed Hodgkin's lymphoma registered in the database of the German Hodgkin's lymphoma study group. *J Clin Oncol* 20 (1):221-30.

Josting, A., H. Muller, P. Borchmann, J. W. Baars, B. Metzner, H. Dohner, I. Aurer, L. Smardova, T. Fischer, D. Niederwieser, K. Schafer-Eckart, N. Schmitz, A. Sureda, J. Glossmann, V. Diehl, D. DeJong, M. L. Hansmann, J. Raemaekers, and A. Engert. 2010. Dose intensity of chemotherapy in patients with relapsed Hodgkin's lymphoma. *J Clin Oncol* 28 (34):5074-80.

Josting, A., L. Nogova, J. Franklin, J. P. Glossmann, H. T. Eich, M. Sieber, T. Schober, H. D. Boettcher, U. Schulz, R. P. Muller, V. Diehl, and A. Engert. 2005. Salvage radiotherapy in patients with relapsed and refractory Hodgkin's lymphoma: a retrospective analysis from the German Hodgkin Lymphoma Study Group. *J Clin Oncol* 23 (7):1522-9.

Josting, A., C. Rudolph, M. Reiser, M. Mapara, M. Sieber, H. H. Kirchner, B. Dorken, D. K. Hossfeld, V. Diehl, A. Engert, and Centers Participating. 2002. Time-intensified dexamethasone/cisplatin/cytarabine: an effective salvage therapy with low toxicity in patients with relapsed and refractory Hodgkin's disease. *Ann Oncol* 13 (10):1628-35.

Josting, A., U. Rueffer, J. Franklin, M. Sieber, V. Diehl, and A. Engert. 2000. Prognostic factors and treatment outcome in primary progressive Hodgkin lymphoma: a report from the German Hodgkin Lymphoma Study Group. *Blood* 96 (4):1280-6.

Kobe, C., M. Dietlein, J. Franklin, J. Markova, A. Lohri, H. Amthauer, S. Klutmann, W. H. Knapp, J. M. Zijlstra, A. Bockisch, M. Weckesser, R. Lorenz, M. Schreckenberger, R. Bares, H. T. Eich, R. P. Mueller, M. Fuchs, P. Borchmann, H. Schicha, V. Diehl, and A. Engert. 2008. Positron emission tomography has a high negative predictive value for progression or early relapse for patients with residual disease after first-line chemotherapy in advanced-stage Hodgkin lymphoma. *Blood* 112 (10):3989-94.

Kuruvilla, J., T. Nagy, M. Pintilie, R. Tsang, A. Keating, and M. Crump. 2006. Similar response rates and superior early progression-free survival with gemcitabine, dexamethasone, and cisplatin salvage therapy compared with carmustine, etoposide, cytarabine, and melphalan salvage therapy prior to autologous stem cell transplantation for recurrent or refractory Hodgkin lymphoma. *Cancer* 106 (2):353-60.

Kuruvilla, John, Diane Taylor, Lisa Wang, Chantale Blattler, Armand Keating, and Michael Crump. 2008. Phase II Trial of Lenalidomide in Patients with Relapsed or Refractory Hodgkin Lymphoma. *ASH Annual Meeting Abstracts* 112 (11):3052-.

Lazarus, H. M., P. A. Rowlings, M. J. Zhang, J. M. Vose, J. O. Armitage, P. J. Bierman, J. L. Gajewski, R. P. Gale, A. Keating, J. P. Klein, C. B. Miller, G. L. Phillips, D. E. Reece, K. A. Sobocinski, K. van Besien, and M. M. Horowitz. 1999. Autotransplants for Hodgkin's disease in patients never achieving remission: a report from the Autologous Blood and Marrow Transplant Registry. *J Clin Oncol* 17 (2):534-45.

Linch, D. C., D. Winfield, A. H. Goldstone, D. Moir, B. Hancock, A. McMillan, R. Chopra, D. Milligan, and G. V. Hudson. 1993. Dose intensification with autologous bone-marrow transplantation in relapsed and resistant Hodgkin's disease: results of a BNLI randomised trial. *Lancet* 341 (8852):1051-4.

Longo, D. L., P. L. Duffey, V. T. DeVita, Jr., P. H. Wiernik, S. M. Hubbard, J. C. Phares, A. W. Bastian, E. S. Jaffe, and R. C. Young. 1991. Treatment of advanced-stage Hodgkin's disease: alternating noncrossresistant MOPP/CABS is not superior to MOPP. *J Clin Oncol* 9 (8):1409-20.

M.D. Anderson Cancer Center. 2011. Panobinostat Plus Ifosfamide, Carboplatin, and Etoposide (ICE) Compared With ICE For Relapsed Hodgkin Lymphoma. In *ClinicalTrials.gov [Internet]*. Bethesda (MD): National Library of Medicine (US). 2011- [cited 2011 Sept 15]. Available from: http://clinicaltrials.gov/ct2/show/NCT01169636?term=NCT01169636&rank=1.

Repeated Author. 2011. Phase II R-ABVD Versus ABVD for Advanced Stage Classical Hodgkin Lymphoma. In *ClinicalTrials.gov [Internet]*. Bethesda (MD): National Library of Medicine (US). 2011- [cited 2011 Sept 15]. Available from: http://clinicaltrials.gov/ct2/show/NCT00654732?term=pHASE+II+R-ABVD+VERSUS+ABVD&rank=1.

Martin, A., M. C. Fernandez-Jimenez, M. D. Caballero, M. A. Canales, J. A. Perez-Simon, J. Garcia de Bustos, L. Vazquez, F. Hernandez-Navarro, and J. F. San Miguel. 2001. Long-term follow-up in patients treated with Mini-BEAM as salvage therapy for relapsed or refractory Hodgkin's disease. *Br J Haematol* 113 (1):161-71.

Milpied, N., A. K. Fielding, R. M. Pearce, P. Ernst, and A. H. Goldstone. 1996. Allogeneic bone marrow transplant is not better than autologous transplant for patients with relapsed Hodgkin's disease. European Group for Blood and Bone Marrow Transplantation. *J Clin Oncol* 14 (4):1291-6.

Morschhauser, F., P. Brice, C. Ferme, M. Divine, G. Salles, R. Bouabdallah, C. Sebban, L. Voillat, O. Casasnovas, A. Stamatoullas, K. Bouabdallah, M. Andre, J. P. Jais, D. Cazals-Hatem, C. Gisselbrecht, and Gela Sfgm Study Group. 2008. Risk-adapted salvage treatment with single or tandem autologous stem-cell transplantation for first relapse/refractory Hodgkin's lymphoma: results of the prospective multicenter H96 trial by the GELA/SFGM study group. *J Clin Oncol* 26 (36):5980-7.

Moskowitz, A. J., M. A. Perales, T. Kewalramani, J. Yahalom, H. Castro-Malaspina, Z. Zhang, J. Vanak, A. D. Zelenetz, and C. H. Moskowitz. 2009. Outcomes for patients who fail high dose chemoradiotherapy and autologous stem cell rescue for relapsed and primary refractory Hodgkin lymphoma. *Br J Haematol* 146 (2):158-63.

Moskowitz, C. H., S. D. Nimer, A. D. Zelenetz, T. Trippett, E. E. Hedrick, D. A. Filippa, D. Louie, M. Gonzales, J. Walits, N. Coady-Lyons, J. Qin, R. Frank, J. R. Bertino, A. Goy, A. Noy, J. P. O'Brien, D. Straus, C. S. Portlock, and J. Yahalom. 2001. A 2-step comprehensive high-dose chemoradiotherapy second-line program for relapsed and refractory Hodgkin disease: analysis by intent to treat and development of a prognostic model. *Blood* 97 (3):616-23.

Nissen, N. I., T. F. Pajak, O. Glidewell, J. Pedersen-Bjergaard, L. Stutzman, G. Falkson, J. Cuttner, J. Blom, L. Leone, A. Sawitsky, M. Coleman, F. Haurani, C. L. Spurr, J. B. Harley, B. Seligman, C. Cornell, Jr., P. Henry, H. J. Senn, K. Brunner, G. Martz, P. Maurice, A. Bank, L. Shapiro, G. W. James, and J. F. Holland. 1979. A comparative study of a BCNU containing 4-drug program versus MOPP versus 3-drug combinations in advanced Hodgkin's disease: a cooperative study by the Cancer and Leukemia Group B. *Cancer* 43 (1):31-40.

Novartis Pharmaceuticals. 2011. A Phase III Randomized, Double Blind, Placebo Controlled Multi-center Study of Panobinostat for Maintenance of Response in Patients With

Hodgkin's Lymphoma, edited by C. g. [Internet]. Bethesda (MD): National Library of Medicine (US). 2011- [cited 2011 Sept 15]. Available from: http://clinicaltrials.gov/ct2/show/NCT01034163?term=NCT01034163&rank=1.

O'Reilly, S. E., P. Hoskins, P. Klimo, and J. M. Connors. 1991. MACOP-B and VACOP-B in diffuse large cell lymphomas and MOPP/ABV in Hodgkin's disease. *Annals of Oncology* 2 (SUPPL. 1):17-23.

Peggs, K. S., A. Hunter, R. Chopra, A. Parker, P. Mahendra, D. Milligan, C. Craddock, R. Pettengell, A. Dogan, K. J. Thomson, E. C. Morris, G. Hale, H. Waldmann, A. H. Goldstone, D. C. Linch, and S. Mackinnon. 2005. Clinical evidence of a graft-versus-Hodgkin's-lymphoma effect after reduced-intensity allogeneic transplantation. *Lancet* 365 (9475):1934-41.

Peniket, A. J., M. C. Ruiz de Elvira, G. Taghipour, C. Cordonnier, E. Gluckman, T. de Witte, G. Santini, D. Blaise, H. Greinix, A. Ferrant, J. Cornelissen, N. Schmitz, A. H. Goldstone, and Registry European Bone Marrow Transplantation Lymphoma. 2003. An EBMT registry matched study of allogeneic stem cell transplants for lymphoma: allogeneic transplantation is associated with a lower relapse rate but a higher procedure-related mortality rate than autologous transplantation. *Bone Marrow Transplant* 31 (8):667-78.

Proctor, S. J., M. Mackie, A. Dawson, J. White, R. J. Prescott, H. L. Lucraft, B. Angus, G. H. Jackson, A. L. Lennard, A. Hepplestone, and P. R. Taylor. 2002. A population-based study of intensive multi-agent chemotherapy with or without autotransplant for the highest risk Hodgkin's disease patients identified by the Scotland and Newcastle Lymphoma Group (SNLG) prognostic index. A Scotland and Newcastle Lymphoma Group study (SNLG HD III). *Eur J Cancer* 38 (6):795-806.

Radford, J. A., A. Z. S. Rohatiner, D. J. Dunlop, A. Rossi, W. D. J. Ryder, D. P. Deakin, and et al. 1997. Preliminary results of a four-centre randomised trial comparing weekly VAPEC-B chemptherapy with the CHLVPP/EVA hybrid regimen in previously regimen in previously untreated Hodgkin's disease. Paper read at Program/Proceedings, American Society of Clinical Oncology : thirty-third annual meeting, May 17-20, 1997, Denver, CO.

Santoro, A., G. Bonadonna, P. Valagussa, R. Zucali, S. Viviani, F. Villani, A. M. Pagnoni, V. Bonfante, R. Musumeci, F. Crippa, and et al. 1987. Long-term results of combined chemotherapy-radiotherapy approach in Hodgkin's disease: superiority of ABVD plus radiotherapy versus MOPP plus radiotherapy. *J Clin Oncol* 5 (1):27-37.

Schmid, C., L. Pan, T. Diss, and P. G. Isaacson. 1991. Expression of B-cell antigens by Hodgkin's and Reed-Sternberg cells. *Am J Pathol* 139 (4):701-7.

Schmitz, N., B. Pfistner, M. Sextro, M. Sieber, A. M. Carella, M. Haenel, F. Boissevain, R. Zschaber, P. Muller, H. Kirchner, A. Lohri, S. Decker, B. Koch, D. Hasenclever, A. H. Goldstone, V. Diehl, Group German Hodgkin's Lymphoma Study, Blood Lymphoma Working Party of the European Group for, and Transplantation Marrow. 2002. Aggressive conventional chemotherapy compared with high-dose chemotherapy with autologous haemopoietic stem-cell transplantation for relapsed chemosensitive Hodgkin's disease: a randomised trial. *Lancet* 359 (9323):2065-71.

Schulz, H., U. Rehwald, F. Morschhauser, T. Elter, C. Driessen, T. Rudiger, P. Borchmann, R. Schnell, V. Diehl, A. Engert, and M. Reiser. 2008. Rituximab in relapsed lymphocyte-predominant Hodgkin lymphoma: long-term results of a phase 2 trial by the German Hodgkin Lymphoma Study Group (GHSG). *Blood* 111 (1):109-11.

Seattle Genetics, Inc. 2011. A Phase 1 Study of Brentuximab Vedotin Combined With Multi-Agent Chemotherapy for Hodgkin Lymphoma. In *ClinicalTrials.gov [Internet]*. Bethesda (MD): National Library of Medicine (US). 2011- [cited 2011 Sept 15]. Available from: http://clinicaltrials.gov/ct2/show/NCT01060904?term=NCT01060904&rank=1.

Repeated Author. 2011. A Phase 3 Study of Brentuximab Vedotin (SGN-35) in Patients at High Risk of Residual Hodgkin Lymphoma Following Stem Cell Transplant (The AETHERA Trial). In *ClinicalTrials.gov [Internet]*. Bethesda (MD): National Library of Medicine (US). 2011- [cited 2011 Sept 15]. Available from: http://clinicaltrials.gov/ct2/show/NCT01100502?term=NCT01100502&rank=1.

Sieber, M., H. Tesch, B. Pfistner, U. Rueffer, B. Lathan, O. Brosteanu, U. Paulus, T. Koch, M. Pfreundschuh, M. Loeffler, A. Engert, A. Josting, J. Wolf, D. Hasenclever, J. Franklin, E. Duehmke, A. Georgii, K. P. Schalk, H. Kirchner, G. Doelken, R. Munker, P. Koch, R. Herrmann, R. Greil, A. P. Anselmo, and V. Diehl. 2002. Rapidly alternating COPP/ABV/IMEP is not superior to conventional alternating COPP/ABVD in combination with extended-field radiotherapy in intermediate-stage Hodgkin's lymphoma: final results of the German Hodgkin's Lymphoma Study Group Trial HD5. *J Clin Oncol* 20 (2):476-84.

Sirohi, B., D. Cunningham, R. Powles, F. Murphy, T. Arkenau, A. Norman, J. Oates, A. Wotherspoon, and A. Horwich. 2008. Long-term outcome of autologous stem-cell transplantation in relapsed or refractory Hodgkin's lymphoma. *Ann Oncol* 19 (7):1312-9.

Southwest Oncology Group. 2011. A Phase II Trial of Response-Adapted Therapy of Stage III-IV Hodgkin Lymphoma Using Early Interim FDG-PET Imaging. In *ClinicalTrials.gov [Internet]*. Bethesda (MD): National Library of Medicine (US). 2011- [cited 2011 Sept 15]. Available from: http://clinicaltrials.gov/archive/NCT00822120/2011_09_06.

Sureda, A., R. Arranz, A. Iriondo, E. Carreras, J. J. Lahuerta, J. Garcia-Conde, I. Jarque, M. D. Caballero, C. Ferra, A. Lopez, J. Garcia-Larana, R. Cabrera, D. Carrera, M. D. Ruiz-Romero, A. Leon, J. Rifon, J. Diaz-Mediavilla, R. Mataix, M. Morey, J. M. Moraleda, A. Altes, A. Lopez-Guillermo, J. de la Serna, J. M. Fernandez-Ranada, J. Sierra, E. Conde, and Group Grupo Espanol de Linformas/Transplante Autologo de Medula Osea Spanish Cooperative. 2001. Autologous stem-cell transplantation for Hodgkin's disease: results and prognostic factors in 494 patients from the Grupo Espanol de Linfomas/Transplante Autologo de Medula Osea Spanish Cooperative Group. *J Clin Oncol* 19 (5):1395-404.

Sureda, A., S. Robinson, C. Canals, A. M. Carella, M. A. Boogaerts, D. Caballero, A. E. Hunter, L. Kanz, S. Slavin, J. J. Cornelissen, M. Gramatzki, D. Niederwieser, N. H. Russell, and N. Schmitz. 2008. Reduced-intensity conditioning compared with conventional allogeneic stem-cell transplantation in relapsed or refractory Hodgkin's lymphoma: an analysis from the Lymphoma Working Party of the European Group for Blood and Marrow Transplantation. *J Clin Oncol* 26 (3):455-62.

Sureda, Anna, Anas Younes, Dina Ben-Yehuda, Tee-Chuan Ong, Jonathan L. Kaufman, Christophe Le Corre, Jennifer Gallagher, Angela Shen, and Andreas Engert. 2010. Final Analysis: Phase II Study of Oral Panobinostat In Relapsed/Refractory Hodgkin Lymphoma Patients Following Autologous Hematopoietic Stem Cell Transplant. *ASH Annual Meeting Abstracts* 116 (21):419-.

Svoboda, J., C. Andreadis, R. Elstrom, E. A. Chong, L. H. Downs, A. Berkowitz, S. M. Luger, D. L. Porter, S. Nasta, D. Tsai, A. W. Loren, D. L. Siegel, E. Glatstein, A. Alavi, E. A. Stadtmauer, and S. J. Schuster. 2006. Prognostic value of FDG-PET scan imaging in lymphoma patients undergoing autologous stem cell transplantation. *Bone Marrow Transplant* 38 (3):211-6.

Tesch, H., V. Diehl, B. Lathan, D. Hasenclever, M. Sieber, U. Ruffer, A. Engert, J. Franklin, M. Pfreundschuh, K. P. Schalk, G. Schwieder, G. Wulf, G. Dolken, P. Worst, P. Koch, N. Schmitz, U. Bruntsch, C. Tirier, U. Muller, and M. Loeffler. 1998. Moderate dose escalation for advanced stage Hodgkin's disease using the bleomycin, etoposide, adriamycin, cyclophosphamide, vincristine, procarbazine, and prednisone scheme and adjuvant radiotherapy: a study of the German Hodgkin's Lymphoma Study Group. *Blood* 92 (12):4560-7.

Tsang, R. W., M. K. Gospodarowicz, S. B. Sutcliffe, M. Crump, and A. Keating. 1999. Thoracic radiation therapy before autologous bone marrow transplantation in relapsed or refractory Hodgkin's disease. PMH Lymphoma Group, and the Toronto Autologous BMT Group. *Eur J Cancer* 35 (1):73-8.

University of Cologne 2011. AVD-Rev in Elderly Hodgkin Lymphoma Patients. In *ClinicalTrials.gov [Internet]*. Bethesda (MD): National Library of Medicine (US). 2011- [cited 2011 Sept 15]. Available from: http://clinicaltrials.gov/ct2/show/NCT01056679?term=NCT01056679&rank=1.

University of Cologne. 2011. HD18 for Advanced Stages in Hodgkins Lymphoma. In *ClinicalTrials.gov [Internet]*. Bethesda (MD): National Library of Medicine (US). 2011- [cited 2011 Sept 15]. Available from: http://clinicaltrials.gov/ct2/show/NCT00515554?term=NCT00515554&rank=1.

Varterasian, M., V. Ratanatharathorn, J. P. Uberti, C. Karanes, E. Abella, F. Momin, C. Kasten-Sportes, A. Al-Katib, L. Lum, L. K. Heilbrun, and et al. 1995. Clinical course and outcome of patients with Hodgkin's disease who progress after autologous transplantation. *Leuk Lymphoma* 20 (1-2):59-65.

Viviani, S., G. Bonadonna, A. Santoro, V. Bonfante, M. Zanini, L. Devizzi, F. Soncini, and P. Valagussa. 1996. Alternating versus hybrid MOPP and ABVD combinations in advanced Hodgkin's disease: ten-year results. *J Clin Oncol* 14 (5):1421-30.

Viviani, S., P. L. Zinzani, A. Rambaldi, E. Brusamolino, A. Levis, V. Bonfante, U. Vitolo, A. Pulsoni, A. M. Liberati, G. Specchia, P. Valagussa, A. Rossi, F. Zaja, E. M. Pogliani, P. Pregno, M. Gotti, A. Gallamini, D. Rota Scalabrini, G. Bonadonna, A. M. Gianni, Foundation Michelangelo, Linfomi Gruppo Italiano di Terapie Innovative nei, and Linfomi Intergruppo Italiano. 2011. ABVD versus BEACOPP for Hodgkin's lymphoma when high-dose salvage is planned. *N Engl J Med* 365 (3):203-12.

Washington University School of Medicine. 2011. Lenalidomide Maintenance Therapy Post Autologous Transplant for Hodgkins Lymphoma. In *ClinicalTrials.gov [Internet]*. Bethesda (MD): National Library of Medicine (US). 2011- [cited 2011 Sept 15] Available from: http://clinicaltrials.gov/ct2/show/NCT01207921.

Younes, A., J. Romaguera, F. Hagemeister, P. McLaughlin, M. A. Rodriguez, P. Fiumara, A Goy, S. Jeha, J. T. Manning, Jr., D. Jones, L. V. Abruzzo, and L. J. Medeiros. 2003. A pilot study of rituximab in patients with recurrent, classic Hodgkin disease. *Cancer* 98 (2):310-4.

Part 7

Evolving Therapies in Relapsed and Refractory Hodgkin's Lymphoma

7

Evolving Therapies in Relapsed and Refractory Hodgkin Lymphoma

Sulada Pukiat and Francisco J. Hernandez-Ilizaliturri*
Departments of Medical Oncology and Immunology,
Roswell Park Cancer Institute,
Buffalo, NY,
USA

1. Introduction

Approximately 20% of Hodgkin Lymphoma (HL) patients do not achieve a durable remission or fail to respond to front-line chemotherapy. Despite the attempt to improve clinical outcomes by using the risk adaptive therapy, a significant number of patients die as a results of relapsed/refractory (rel/ref) disease.[1] Advances in understanding the etiology and molecular biology of HL are leading the development of novel therapeutic strategies that could be applied to improve clinical outcome of rel/ref HL patients. The pathologic features of HL reflect a defect in immune responses resulting from various cytokines and chemokines secreted partially by Hodgkin Reed-Sternberg (HRS) cells. HRS cells are unique in the way that they lost typical B cell gene expression pattern but retain the expression of surface molecules involving in antigen presentation (tumor necrosis factor receptor (CD30, CD40), CD80, MHC class II, and CD86). Aberration of Notch signaling pathway may contribute to their reprogramming.[2,3] Multiple genetic lesions, deregulated signaling pathway and transcription factors play important role in pathogenesis of HL including constitutive activation of nuclear factor kappa B (NFκB) and the Janus kinase-signal transducer and activator of transcription (JAK-STAT) signaling pathway.[4-6] Moreover, the role of the microenvironment in HL has been increasingly recognized. The majority of the cell population in HL-affected tissue is composition of the inflammatory cellular infiltrate, not the HRS cells that represents only small population (<1%). Understanding the complex relationship between the HRS cells and the microenvironment and chemokines milieu involved in its formation is crucial for the development of new therapeutic strategies.

In addition, Epstein Barr Virus (EBV) infection may plays a role in the pathogenesis of HL since it can influence the expression of certain chemokines (i.e. CXCL9, CXCL10, CCL3, and CCL5) that are highly expressed in HRS cells and the EBV gene encoding the latent membrane protein 1 (LMP1) can mimic constitutively active TNF receptor (via a CD40/CD40L interaction) and promote IκB turnover leading to activation of NFκB and downstream signaling events.[7] Ongoing efforts are focused in developing adaptive or adoptive immune therapies targeting EVB related proteins in rel/ref HL patients.

* Corresponding Author

This chapter will provide an overview of the emerging therapeutic strategies for patients with relapsed and refractory HL (rel/ref HL) that had failed standard front line therapy, salvage chemotherapy and high-dose chemotherapy and autologous stem cell support (HDC-ASCS).

2. Systemic chemotherapy

Salvage systemic chemotherapy is often used in patients with rel/ref HL failing HDC-ASCS. Response rates are modest and response duration is usually short. Participation in clinical trials evaluating novel therapeutic approaches is strongly recommended. On the other hand, two chemotherapy agents had proven anti-tumor activity in highly refractory HL patients: gemcitabine and bendamustine.

Gemcitabine had been studied in the rel/ref HL either as single agent or combination therapy (i.e. with Vinorelbine).[8,9] Favorable toxicity profile and significant clinical anti-tumor activity were observed in heavily pre-treated HL patients, with overall response rates (ORR) up to 70% when used in combination regimens.[10,11] On the other hand, the duration of response is limited stressing the need to develop novel therapeutic strategies or to use this agent as a bridge rel/ref HL patient into more definitive treatments (i.e. allogeneic bone marrow transplant or other cellular-based therapies).

Bendamustine hydrochloride is a bifunctional mechlorethamine derivative with alkylating and antimetabolite properties. The exact antitumor mechanism is unknown though it appears to crosslink macromolecules resulting in DNA damage and subsequently apoptosis. It may also inhibit mitotic checkpoints and induce mitotic catastrophe. Bendamustine showed marked antiproliferative and proapoptotic effects on HL cell lines.[12] Moskowitz et al reported the activity of single agent bendamustine in rel/ref HL that previously failed HDC-ASCT, allogeneic stem cell transplantation (AlloSCT) or ineligible for transplant.[13] In this phase II clinical trial, bendamustine was administered at a dose of 120 mg/m^2 for two consecutive days, every 28 days, for up to maximum of 6 cycles. Of evaluable 16 patients, there were 6 complete responses (CRs) (38%) and 6 partial responses (PRs) (38%) for an ORR of 75%. Further studies of both single agent bendamustine and in combination with other chemotherapy are warranted in rel/ref HL patients.

3. Passive immunotherapy targeting the tumor microenvironment and/or HRS cells (Table 1)

3.1 CD80 (B7-1)

Immunohistochemical analysis has shown strong expression of CD80 on HRS cells, antigen presenting cells (APCs), T-cells and activated B-cells but not on resting B-cells and plasma cells and is absolutely absent on CD34+ cells, making CD80 an excellent target in HL. Preclinical data demonstrated that an anti-B7-1 immunotoxin had significant anti-tumor activity in HL-cell lines and minimal toxicity to CD34+ hematopoietic stem cell.[14,15] Galiximab is a primatized IgG1 monoclonal antibody, which binds to CD80 with high affinity and induces cell death via antibody-dependent cell-mediated cytotoxicity (ADCC). Smith et al studied the clinical activity of single agent Galiximab in patients with rel/ref HL not eligible for or had failed HDC-ASCT/AlloSCT.[16] Galiximab was administered at a dose of 500 mg/m^2 weekly for 4 weeks followed by 500 mg/m^2 every 4 weeks until disease

Author	Agent	Study Design (Phase)	Patient population	Clinical Activity	Median Duration of Response	Adverse Reaction
Smith et al[10]	Galiximab	II	Rel/ref HL (N=30)	ORR 6.9%; 1 CR, 1 PR	2 responders progressed after 7.5 and 3 mo.	Gr 3-4 hypo-phosphatemia, elevated SGOT/ SGPT, infection
Freedman et al[20]	Lucatumumab	Ia/II	Rel/ref HL (N=28) or NHL (N=31)	Ia N=10: ORR 10%; 1 PR II N=18: ORR 17%; 3 PR	NR	Gr 3-4 asymptomatic/ reversible elevated amylase/lipase, SGOT/SGPT
Younes et al[23]	Rituximab	N/A	Rel/ref HL (N=22)	ORR 22%; 1 CR, 4 PR	DOR 8.7 mo. (3.3⁺-14.9 mo.)	NR
Corazzelli et al[26]	Rituximab + Gemcitabine, Ifosfamide, Oxaliplatin (R+GIFOX)	N/A	Rel/ref HL (N=21)	ORR 86%; 16 CR, 2 PR	NR	Gr 4 TCP, infection
Oki et al[27]	Rituximab + Gemcitabine	II	Rel/ref HL (N=33)	ORR 48%; 5 CR, 11 PR	FFS 2.7 mo.	Gr 3-4 neutropenia, TCP
Ekstrand et al[29]	Rituximab	II	CD20+ newly diagnosed and rel/ref NLPHL (N=22)	ORR 100%; 10 CR, 12 PR	FFP 10.2 mo.	Infusion related reaction, Gr 1 hematologic toxicities, No Gr 3-4 toxicity
Rehwald et al[30]	Rituximab	II	NLPHL or CD20+ relapsed cHL (N=14)	ORR 86%; 8 CR, 4 PR	Not reach at 20^+ mo.	Infusion related reaction, Gr 1-2 chill, fever, rhinitis, nausea, pruritus, leucopenia, dizziness
Eichenauer et al[31]	Rituximab	II	Newly diagnosed stage IA NLPHL (N=28)	ORR 100%; 24 CR, 4 PR	NR	No Gr 3-4 toxicity
Schulz et al[32]	Rituximab	II	Rel/ref NLPHL (N=15); cHL (N=4)	NLPHL: ORR 94%; 8 CR, 6 PR HL: 3 CR	TTP 33 mo. OS not reached	NR

HL = Hodgkin Lymphoma; Rel/ref = relapsed/refractory; ORR = overall response rate; CR = complete response; PR = partial response; Gr = grade; NLPHL = Nodular lymphocyte predominant Hodgkin lymphoma; TTP = time to progression; FFP = freedom from progression; OS = overall survival; NR = Not reported; TCP = thrombocytopenia

Table 1. Monoclonal antibodies targeting HRS cells or accessory cells in relapsed/refractory Hodgkin Lymphoma.

progression or unacceptable toxicity. The results were disappointing with ORR of only 6.9% and very short median time to progression (TTP) of 1.6 month. The authors concluded that single agent galiximab seems to have minimal activity in heavily pretreated rel/ref HL.

3.2 CD40

CD40 is a member of TNFR family (TNFRSF5) that is constantly expressed in HRS cells. In addition, CD40+ HRS cells are surrounded by CD40L-expressing T-cell lymphocytes. The CD40/CD40L interaction contributes to the pathobiology of HL possibly by NFκB activation and increased autocrine growth factor CCL5 resulting in inhibition of apoptosis, increased proliferation and microenvironment formation.[17-19]

Lucatumumab is a monoclonal antibody targeting the transmembrane receptor CD40. The safety and clinical activity of lucatumumab (HCD122) was evaluated in both NHL and HL patients who have progressed after at least two previous therapies [NCT00670592].[20] Patients received lucatumumab at a dose of 3 or 4 or 6 mg/kg intravenous weekly for 4 weeks followed by a 4-weeks rest period. The maximum tolerated dose (MTD) and dose limiting toxicity (DLT) were 4 mg/kg and 6 mg/kg, respectively. DLTs were consisted of clinically asymptomatic and reversible grade 3-4 elevation of amylase/lipase or transminase enzymes. For rel/ref HL patients, three of eighteen (17%) patients in phase II study component achieved a PR.

3.3 CD52

CD52 is highly expressed in surrounding reactive B-cells, T-cells and monocytes, although not on HRS cells itself. Depleting CD52+ accessory cells, which appear to provide survival signals to HRS cells, may have therapeutic value. Alemtuzumab is a humanized monoclonal antibody directed against CD52 resulting in cell lysis via antibody dependent cellular-mediated cytotoxicity. A phase II study addressing the clinical efficacy of alemtuzumab in rel/ref HL was unfortunately terminated due to slow accrual [NCT00129753].[21] Another phase II study focusing on the clinical outcome in rel/ref DLBCL and HL treated with alemtuzumab in combination with dose-adjusted EPOCH-Rituximab is currently enrolling patients [NCT01030900].[22]

3.4 CD20

A pilot study evaluating rituximab monotherapy in rel/ref HL has shown that depletion of B lymphocytes may has therapeutic potential.[23] The rationale of using rituximab in classical HL (cHL) is based on several laboratory and clinical observations: HRS stem cells express CD20 even though HRS cells infrequently express CD20, elimination of CD20+ B lymphocytes supporting HRS cells may deprive survival signals and improve immune response against HRS cell.[24,25] Studies of evaluating the addition of rituximab to conventional chemotherapy in patients with rel/ref cHL demonstrated promising results.[26,27] Copeland et al showed significant improvement of 5-year event free survival (EFS) in patients with newly diagnosed advanced stage cHL treated rituximab plus ABVD compared to historical data of patients treated with ABVD from the same institute.[28]

Targeting CD20 in patients with lymphocyte predominant HL (LPHL, had show to be an effective therapeutic strategy in contrast to other subtypes of HL. The efficacy of rituximab in LPHL was documented in several phase II studies with an ORR up to 100% in both relapsed and newly diagnosed patients.[29-32] Zojer et al and Schnell et al reported 2 cases of rel/ref HL patients treated with radiolabeled anti-CD20 monoclonal antibody, Yttrium-90 ibritumomab tiuxetan.[33,34] One patient had LPHL and another patient had cHL (lymphocyte rich) both achieved a complete remission following radioimmunotherapy (RIT). A Phase I/II study of safety and efficacy of I^{131} tositumomab rel/ref CD20+ cHL is currently enrolling patients [NCT00484874].[35]

4. Signaling pathway targets on HRS cells

4.1 CD30 signaling (Table 2)

CD30, a member of tumor necrosis factor receptor family (TNFR super family 8) involved in the activation of the canonical NFκB pathway and provides tumor cell survival signaling. CD30 is express in almost 100% of the HRS cells and serve as an attractive target of immunotherapy for cHL.[36,37] Borchmann et al had summarized the upsides and downsides of immunotherapy in HL.[38] Immunotoxins (ITs) containing ricin A, a ribosome inactivating protein, linked with surface marker CD30 as well as other ITs had shown disappointing clinical results with regard to response and toxicity in HL. Bi-specific constructs of monoclonal antibodies or molecules (BSMs) targeting CD30 and CD16 (NK cells) or CD64 (monocytes) were though well tolerated and showed some objective responses, production of BSMs is very expensive and time consuming. Low dose radioimmunotherapy (RIT), I-131 labeled anti-CD30 antibofy (131I-Ki-4) used in phase I trial in patients with relapsed HL showed some clinical activity with limitation to hematotoxicity particularly thrombocytopenia.[39] Better choice of radionuclides and the carriers would be necessary to

Author	Agent	Study Design (Phase)	Patient population	Clinical Activity	Median Duration of Response	Adverse Reaction
Ansell et al[41]	Iratumumab MDX-060	Phase I/II	Rel/ref HL (N=63)	4 responses; 2 CR, 2 PR	DOR 4 mo.	Gr 3 elevation of transaminase enzyme, epitaxis, anemia; gr3-4 dyspnea, cardiac temponade, ARDS
Younes et al[43]	Brentuximab vedotin	I	Rel CD30+ lymphomas (N=45; HL=43)	ORR 40%; CR 27%, PR 13% (for HL)	DOR 9.7+ mo. PFS 5.9 mo.	Peripheral neuropathy
Chen et al[44]	Brentuximab vedotin	II	Rel/ref HL (N=102)	ORR 75%; CR 34%	DOR not reach (for CR pts)	Peripheral neuropathy, neutropenia, TCP, anemia

HL = Hodgkin Lymphoma; Rel/ref = relapsed/refractory; ORR = overall response rate; CR = complete response; PR = partial response; Gr = grade; NLPHL = Nodular lymphocyte predominant Hodgkin lymphoma; DOR = duration of response; PFS = progression free survival

Table 2. Selected Clinical studies targeting CD30 in relapsed/refractory Hodgkin Lymphoma.

further development of this approach. Preclinical study targeting CD30 demonstrated significant anti-tumor activity.[40] Initial clinical studies evaluated naked antibodies targeting CD30 (MDX-030 and SGN-30) in patients with rel/ref HL. Both antibodies failed to demonstrate anti-tumor activity and in some cases accelerated tumor growth was observed upon CD30 binding by MDX-060.[41]

Previously unknown factors influenced the negative results observed in such trials such as 1) the agonist effects of the antibodies initially tested, 2) the modulation of CD30 in HRS cells (i.e. antigen shedding and/or internalization), and/or 3) impaired immune effector function in heavily pre-treated patients with HL. Two therapeutic approaches (i.e. development of drug conjugates or antibody re-engineering) had been explored clinically with significant improvement in clinical activity.

SGN-35 (brentuximab vedotin) is a drug conjugated designed to improve the clinical activity of SGN-30 in lymphomas. Brentuximab vedotin (SGN-35) is a antibody-drug conjugate containing the anti-tubulin agent, monomethylauristatin E (MMAE) linked to antiCD30 monoclonal antibody to enhance antitumor activity.[42]

Younes et al reported encouraging results in a phase I study of brentuximab vedotin in patients with relapsed CD30+ lymphomas.[43] Most of patients in the study had rel/ref HL (42/45), were heavily pre-treated (median number of previous regimens was 3), and almost 75% had previous HDC-ASCT. Seventeen patients had objective response including 11 CRs. Fifty percent (6/12) of patients who received maximum tolerating dose (MTD) (1.8mg/kg/dose) had objective responses.

Subsequently, a pivotal phase II of brentuximab vedotin in patients with rel/ref HL reported similar results.[44] All patients had failed HDC-ASCT and had median of 3.5 prior treatments. The ORR was 75% (76/102) with 34% of the patients achieving a CR (35/102). Currently, a randomized, double blind, placebo-controlled phase III study is evaluating SGN-35 versus placebo in patients at high-risk for residual disease after HDC-ASCT is ongoing [NCT01100502].[45] Brentuximab vedotin in combination with standard chemotherapy (ABVD) was now being evaluated in patients with newly diagnosed Hodgkin lymphoma stage IIA-IV [NCT01060904].[46] SGN-35 received fast track designation from the U.S. Food and Drug Administration (FDA) for the treatment of HL in 2009.

5. Downstream signaling targets (Table 3)

5.1 NFκB activity

As previously noted, constitutive activation of NFκB is one of the most important events in pathogenesis of HL and the result of multiple mechanisms. Downstream signaling of TNF receptors, expression of the EBV LMP1, and/or mutation of IκB gene have been described as the cause of constitutive NFκB activation. Inhibition of NFκB has been an area of drug development for the treatment of multiple hematological malignancies including HL. Pre-clinical data demonstrated that the proteasome inhibitor, PS-341 (Bortezomib) affects tumor cell proliferation and survival via inhibiting NFkB pathway, which is constitutively activated in HRS cells. As a result, bortezomib was evaluated in patients with rel/ref HL. The Cancer and Leukemia Group B (CALGB) conducted a phase II clinical trials (CALGB 50206) evaluating bortezomib monotherapy in rel/ref HL. Disappointingly, no clinical activity was observed in treated patients.[47] The lack of anti-tumor activity of bortezomib in rel/ref HL was confirmed by two subsequent studies reported by Younes et al and Trelle et al.[48,49] More recent studies that evaluated bortezomib in combination with conventional chemotherapy showed mix results.[50,51]

Author	Agent	Study Design (Phase)	Patient population	Clinical Activity	Median Duration of Response	Adverse Reaction
Blum et al[47]	Bortezomib	II	Rel/ref HL (N=30)	9 SD	PFS 1.4 mo. OS 14.8 mo.	Gr 3-4 TCP
Youne et al[48]	Bortezomib	N/A	Rel/ref HL (N=14)	1 PR	NR	Gr 3 TCP, dyspnea and neutropenic fever
Trelle et al[49]	Bortezomib + Dexamethasone	II	Rel HL (N=12)	No response	NR	TCP
Mendler et al[50]	Bortezomib + Gemcitabine	N/A	Rel HL (N=18)	ORR 22%	NR	Gr 3 elevation of transaminase enzyme
Fanale et al[51]	Bortezomib + ICE	I	Rel/ref HL (N=13)	CR 33%; 9 Response (8/9 underwent HDC-ASCS)	NR	Gr 4 TCP 35%, Gr 4 neutropenia 18%
Kirschbaum et al[54]	Vorinostat	II	Rel/ref HL (N=25)	ORR 4%; 1 PR	PFS 4.8 mo.	Gr 4 anemia, lymphopenia, and Gr 3 TCP
Younes et al[57]	Mocetinostat	II	Rel/ref HL, (N=51)	110 mg: ORR 35%; 2 CR, 6 PR 85 mg: ORR 21%; 6 PR	NR	Gr 3 TCP, fatigue, neutropenia, non-fatal pericardial effusion
Dickinson et al[56]	Panobinostat	IA/II	Hematologic malignancies (N=128; HL=23 with 13 evaluable pts)	PR by CT 38%; PR by PET 58%	NR	TCP, neutropenia, febrile neutropenia, fatigue, anemia
Sureda et al[63]	Panobinostat	II	Rel/ref HL after ASCT (N=129)	ORR 27%; 5 CR, 30 PR	PFS 6.1 mo.	Gr 1-2 anemia, N/V/D, gr 3-4 TCP, aneima, neutropenia
Younes et al[68]	Entinostat	II	Rel/ref HL (N=23)	Disease control rate (CR+PR+SD) 65%	NR	Gr 1-2 GI causalities, fatique, pyrexia,; gr 3-4 TCP, anemia, neutropenia

Author	Agent	Study Design (Phase)	Patient population	Clinical Activity	Median Duration of Response	Adverse Reaction
Viviani et al[70]	Givinostat	II	Rel/ref HL (N=15; 13 evaluable pts)	7 SD (54%)	N	Gr 1 leukopenia, 1 diarrhea/ abdominal pain; Gr 2 TCP; 20% had QTc prolongation
Carlo-Stella et al[71]	Givinostat + Meclorethamine	II	Rel/ref HL (N= 35)	ORR 38%; CR 15%. PR 23%	OS 28 mo. TTP 3 mo.	Gr 1-2 nausea and fatigue; gr 3-4 TCP, anemia neutropenia
Johnston et al[75]	Everolimus	II	Rel/ref HL (N=19)	ORR 47%; 1 CR, 8 PR	TTP 7.2 mo.	Gr ≥3 pulmonary toxicity (4 pts)

HL = Hodgkin Lymphoma; Rel/ref = relapsed/refractory; ORR = overall response rate; CR = complete response; PR = partial response; Gr = grade; TCP = thrombocytopenia; TTP= time to progression; PFS = progression free survival; OS = overall survival; HDC-ASCS = high dose chemotherapy and autologous stem cell support; NR = Not reported

Table 3. Selected clinical studies evaluating target specific agents in relapsed/refractory Hodgkin lymphoma.

More potent and/or irreversible proteasome inhibitors (i.e. carfilzomib, MLN2238) had demonstrated high efficacy in rel/ref multiple myeloma and now are being evaluated in other hematologic malignancies.[52] However, their clinical activity in HL remains unknown.

5.2 Deacetylation of histone and other cellular proteins in HL biology: The therapeutic role of deacetylase inhibitors (DACi)

Gene expression profiling studies had demonstrated that HL is characterized by the silencing of key regulatory genes involved in B-cell maturation (i.e. CD79a, CD19, CD20, etc). In general gene expression is a tightly regulated process that is influenced by the 1) DNA/mRNA sequence, 2) expression/activity of transcription factors, 3) epigenetics (including the DNA, chromatin, and histone modifications); and 4) messenger RNA stability.

Post-transcriptional histone modification plays an important role in regulating gene transcription and is mediated by two groups of enzymes: histone acetyltransferase (HATs) and histone deacetylase (HDACs). The balance between HATs and HDACs is crucial in regulating the expression/function of several proteins involved in cell proliferation, cell cycle, apoptosis, angiogenesis, and immune regulation. Altering balance between HATs and HDACs had been found to be associated with various malignancies including HL.

To date, 18 HDACs have been identified in humans. HDACs are grouped in two major categories and four classes; zinc-dependent HDACs (Class I, II and IV) and NAD-dependent HDACs (Class III). Class I includes HDAC 1, 2, 3, 8, and 11; Class II includes HDAC 4, 5, 6, 7, 9, and 10; Class III includes homologues of yeast SIRT 1–7, and Class IV, which includes only HDAC 11. As a group, HDAC are known to regulate several key cellular functions such cell proliferation, cell cycle, apoptosis, angiogenesis, migration, antigen presentation, and/or immune regulation. The activity spectrum of each HDAC is yet to be defined and there is overlap between the function of different HDAC regardless of their group or class.

HATs and HDACs interact also with non-histone proteins such as transcription factors (i.e. p53, STAT3, MYC , E2F, NFκB, etc.), α-tubulin, and chaperons (heat shock protein-90 [HSP90]), adding complexity to their cellular functions in normal and malignant cells. Given their influence in multiple regulatory pathways, HDACs became an attractive strategy to develop novel pharmacologic inhibitors for the treatment of cancer. Several pan- or selective-HDAC inhibitors (class I and IV) had been developed. Pre-clinical studies demonstrated significant anti-tumor activity in various cancer models including non-Hodgkin lymphoma and HL. Laboratory experiments suggest that HDAC inhibitors can induce cell cycle arrest, apoptosis or autophagy in cancer cell lines and can potentiate the anti-tumor activity of chemotherapy agents including proteasome inhibitors. Two HDAC inhibitors had been approved for the management of relapsed/refractory cutaneous T-cell lymphoma (vorisnostat and romidepsin). A second generation of more potent and selective (i.e. less toxic) of HDAC inhibitors (entinostat, panobinostat and MGCD103) had entered into clinical studies for patients with relapsed/refractory HL.

Vorinostat (SAHA), the first FDA approved HDAC inhibitor, is a potent inhibitor of class I and II HDAC and was the first of its class agent evaluated in patients with rel/ref HL. At the pre-clinical level, vorinostat has anti-proliferative and pro-apoptotic effects on HL cell lines by inducing p21 expression and down regulation of Bcl-xL respectively.[53] Kirschbaum et al presented on behalf of the South Western Oncology Group (SWOG), the results of a phase II clinical trial evaluating the safety and efficacy of Vorinostat in refractory/relapsed HL.[54] A total of 25 patients were treated with vorinostat at 200 mg given orally twice per day for 14 days every 21-day cycle. The activity of vorinostat was modest and only one patient achieved a partial remission (PR). Adverse events reported were similarly to those reported in vorinostat clinical trials in patients with cutaneous T-cell lymphoma (CTCL).

Preclinical data by Hartlapp et al demonstrated the activity of depsipeptide (**romidepsin**) in cHL cell lines *in vitro*.[55] In addition, the investigators demonstrated that romidepsin several cellular events leading to cell cycle arrest and apoptosis in HL cell lines such as and increased DNA binding capacity of RelA/p65, PARP-cleavage, decreased transcription of anti-apoptotic proteins (eg. XIAP, Bcl-xL), and down-regulation of STAT6. Romidepsin has not been formally evaluated in rel/ref HL patients.

An isotype-selective histone deacetylase inhibitor, **mocetinostat (MGCD-0103)**, inhibits class I and class IV and minimal class II HDAC inhibition. A phase II trial of 2 different doses (85 mg and 110 mg thrice weekly every 28 days) of mocetinostat in rel/ref HL had shown promising results with ORR of 38%.[56] The updated results from the same group demonstrated activity of single agent mocetinostat in heavily pretreated rel/ref HL with clinical responses observed in approximately 35% of patients with slightly better responses with 110 mg cohort.[57] Of 51 patients, 2 patients (110 mg cohort) achieved complete responses and 6 patients each from both cohort achieved partial response. Over eighty percent of patients in the study had previously failed HDC-ASCS and more than half of patients received four or more previous treatments. Serum thymus and activation-regulated chemokine (TARC) or CCL17 which is highly expressed in HRS cells, decreased in patients treated with mocetinostat.[58] This findings were similar what had been previously observed following in vitro exposure of HL cell lines to vorinostat.[53] Together these findings, suggests that a decline in serum TARC may be a biomarker to predict clinical response to DAC inhibition therapy. Buglio et al found that MGCD0103 induced apoptosis in HL cell lines via the induction of TNFα expression and that inhibition of NF-κB activation with bortezomib resulted in synergistic anti-tumor activity.[59]

Bhalla et al observed similar findings with **PCI-24781**, a phenyl hydroxamic acid-based broad spectrum HDAC inhibitor.[60] PCI-24781 combined with bortezomib enhances apoptosis via reactive oxygen species (ROS), caspase activation (increased cleavage of caspase 8 and caspase 9), PARP activation, cell cycle arrest (G0/G1), and upregulation of p21 in HL cell lines and several non-Hodgkin lymphoma (Burkitt's lymphoma, follicular lymphoma, and large B-cell lymphoma) cell lines. While the biological interaction between bortezomib and multiple DAC inhibitors had been demonstrated in pre-clinical models and is been pursued in several clinical studies in multiple myeloma and mantle cell lymphoma patients, the limited activity of bortezomib as a single agent had damped the interest for pursuing this combination strategy in rel/ref HL patients.

Panobinostat (LBH-589) is a potent pan-HDAC inhibitor with anti-tumor activity observed in pre-clinical studies at nanomolar concentrations. Moreover, pre-clinical studies suggest that panobinostat is more potent than vorinostat in lymphoma pre-clinical models. Panobinostat was evaluated in phase IA/II study in 128 patients with advanced hematologic malignancies including rel/ref HL.[56] Patients received 2 schedules of oral administration (MWF every week at a dose of 20, 30, 40, 60, 80 mg/dose or MWF every other week at a dose of 30, 45, 60, 80 mg/dose). Out of 23 patients with rel/ref HL, 13 patients were evaluable for response. Five out of thirteen (38%) patients had PR by CT and 7/12 patients (58%) had metabolic PR by PET. The maximum tolerated dose (MTD) was 40 mg/dose every week schedule and the principal dose-limiting toxicity (DTL) was thrombocytopenia.

Younes et al confirmed efficacy of panobinostat in phase II study in patients with rel/ref HL.[61] Panobinostat was administered at a dose of 40 mg thrice weekly in 21-day cycle until disease progression. The update results showed encouraging clinical activity of panobinostat with 1 patient achieved CR and 10 pateints achieved PR.[62] Moreover, disease control rate (CR+PR+SD) was 79%. Panobinostat was well tolerated and reversible thrombocytopenia was managed by dose delay or dose reduction. The interim results for this phase II study continues to demonstrate encouraging activity of panobinostat.[63] The final results are currently not available. As previously demonstrated with other DAC inhibitors, a decrease in serum TARC levels was observed in panobinostat treated patients achieving an objective response (i.e. PR or CR).[64]

The safety and efficacy of the oral agent **belinostat (PXD-101)** was evaluated in patients with rel/ref NHL or cHL by Zain et al.[65] Tumor size reduction found in 1/3 of patients with HL using the recommended dose-schedule for patients with solid tumors (750 mg daily, D1-14 every 21days).

Entinostat (SNDX-275) is a class I isotype-selective HDAC inhibitor with longer half-life. Pre-clinical data from Khaskhely et al demonstrated *in vitro* activity in HL-derived cell lines.[66] Entinostat induced cell death with an IC50 of 0.4 μM. At the molecular level, entinostat up-regulates p21 expression, increased H3 acetylation and down-regulates the anti-apoptotic X-linked inhibitor of apoptosis (XIAP) resulting in apoptosis. Moreover, the combination entinostat with gemcitabine or bortezomib has shown synergistic effects. Jóna et al found that entinostat down-regulates anti-apotoptic Bcl-2 and Bcl-xL expression without altering Mcl-1 or Bax levels and its effect was enhanced by two Bcl-2 inhibitors (ABT-737 and obatoclax).[67]

Younes et al recently presented an update of a phase II clinical study evaluating the safety and efficacy of entinostat as a single agent in relapsed/refractory HL.[68] Interim results from a phase II open-label multicenter study of entinostat (ENGAGE-501) administered in an alternate dosing schedule (the first stage: 10 mg every 14 days, 28-day cycle; the second stage: 15mg every 14 days beginning C1d15) showed that of 23 patients with rel/ref HL, 65% have disease control (CR+PR+SD). Entinostat was well tolerable with minimal AEs consisting of grade 1/2 fatigue, fever and GI symptoms. Serious grade 3/4 AEs were primarily hematological and consisted of thrombocytopenia (59.4%) and neutropenia (28.1%). Accrual into the study continues and the final results of this clinical trial are eagerly anticipated. Given the safety profile of and the long half-life of this promising agent, combination studies with chemotherapeutic agents based in pre-clinical studies are warranted to further define the role of entinostat in the management of HL.

Givinostat (ITF-2357) is a hydroxamate pan-HDAC inhibitor with anti-inflammatory properties. Furlan et al reported a phase I safety and pharmacokinetics study in healthy males.[69] They found no serious side effects and no organ toxicity. Several phase II studies of givinostat are in process to evaluate the safety and efficacy in rel/ref HL. A phase II open label non-randomized study by Viviani et al enrolled 15 patients with rel/ref disease, 13 patients had failed HDC-ASCT, and 4 of those patients had also failed an alloSCT.[70] Givinostat was administered at a dose of 100 mg orally daily in three 4-week cycles. Seven of 13 patients (54%) whom completed at least one cycle of therapy were evaluable for response, SD was observed in 46% of the patients. Toxicity includes grade 1-2 thrombocytopenia, leukopenia, diarrhea and/or abdominal pain; nonetheless, twenty percent of patients had transient drug discontinuation due to prolonged QTc. Another phase II study evaluated the safety and clinical activity of givinostat in combination with meclorethamine in patients with rel/ref HL.[71] Anti-tumor activity was observed and correlated with a reduction in serum TARC levels.

5.3 Targeting the PI3K/AKT/mTOR pathway in HL

Everolimus (RAD001) binds to FK506-binding protein 12 (FKBP12) forming a complex that has mTOR kinase inhibition activity, inhibit tumor cell proliferation and angiogenesis by decreasing hypoxia-inducible factor 1a (HIF1a) expression.[72,73] Everolimus demonstrated anti-proliferative effect in several solid tumor and hematologic malignancies including HL. Jundt et al showed that everolimus markedly suppress tumor cell proliferation of HL *in vivo* and down-regulates constitutively activated NFκB activity in HL cell lines.[74] A phase II trial evaluated the clinical activity and toxicity of everolimus in patients with heavily pretreated rel/ref HL (median of 6 prior therapies and 84% had prior HDC-ASCS).[75] Of 19 patients, one patient achieved CR, 8 patients achieved PR resulting in ORR of 47%, although median time to response was only 7.2 months.

Preclinical data from Georgakis et al showed **temsirolimus** (CCI-779) induced cell cycle arrest at G0/G1 phase and autophagy in HL-derived cell lines suggesting that this particular mTOR inhibitor may have therapeutic value in patients with HL.[76] Several phase I/II trials studying the safety and efficacy of single agent various mTOR inhibitors (i.e. temsirolimus or everolimus) monotherapy, or combination with lenalidomide or sorafinib are being conducted to test the concept of mTOR inhibition in treatment rel/ref HL.

5.4 Heat Shock Protein (HSP)

Heat shock protein acting as chaperones are essential in promoting cell survival by maintaining the structure and function of key regulatory proteins involved in cell cycle, proliferation and apoptosis. HSP over-expression had been demonstrated in several malignancies including HL. Inhibition of HSP is another attractive target in cancer therapeutics. Boll et al demonstrated the biological effects of a HSP90 inhibitor, **BIIB021** on HL-derived cell lines.[77] The investigators demonstrated that, BIIB021 inhibited the constitutive activity of NFκB independent of IκB mutation status and increased susceptibility of HL cells for NK cell-mediated killing via inducing the expression of activating NK-cell ligands. Schoof et al showed that inhibition of HSP90 by either geldanamycin derivative 17-AAG or RNA interference in HL cells led to decrease cell proliferation and inhibition of STAT1, STAT3, STAT5, and STAT6 tyrosine phosphorylation possible secondary to reduced protein expression of Janus kinase (Jaks).[78] HSP90 may be a promising target in patients with rel/ref cHL.

6. Immune therapy for rel/ref HL

6.1 Lenalidomide

Lenalidomide, a novel IMiDs® immunomodulatory drug is emerging as an attractive therapeutic option for patients with B-cell lymphoproliferative neoplasms, including HL. Studies in lymphoma and multiple myeloma (MM) models have demonstrated that lenalidomide exerts higher anti-tumor activity than thalidomide, has a unique capacity to enhance the innate immune system, enhance the anti-tumor activity of rituximab, and inhibit angiogenesis.[79,80] Abnormal immune response, increased angiogenesis, and apoptosis resistance, which contribute to the development of HL, support the scientific standpoint of evaluating lenalidomide in rel/ref HL.[81-83]

Lenalidomide was evaluated in patients with relapsed/refractory HL in three phase II clinical trials (Table 4). A phase II study presented by Böll et al and subsequently validated by Kuruvilla et al suggested lenalidomide had anti-tumor activity in rel/ref HL patients achieved a clinical response (CR or PR).[84,85] More importantly, lenalidomide monotherapy was well tolerated and toxicities were manageable. Fehniger et al reported similar anti-neoplastic activity in rel/ref HL patients.[86] Recently and as had been observed in other lenalidomide treated patients, tumor flare reaction (TFR) syndrome with sudden onset painful re-enlargement of tumor following early tumor shrinkage was reported in 3 cases of relapsed HL after hematopoietic stem cell transplantation which mimic tumor progression but manageable with anti-inflammatory/analgesic upon continuation of lenalidomide.[87]

Author	Agent	Study Design (Phase)	Patient population	Clinical Activity	Median Duration of Response	Adverse Reaction
Böll et al[84]	Lenalidomide	N/A	Rel/ref HL (N=42; 24 evaluable pts)	ORR 50%; 1CR, 11 PR	NR	Diarrhea, constipation, neuropathy, and mild dyspnea
Kuruvilla et al[85]	Lenalidomide	II	Rel/ref HL (N=15; 14 evaluable pts)	ORR 14%; 2 PR	TTP 3.2 mo. OS 9.1 mo	Gr 3-4 neutropenia, TCP, anemia; Gr 2 rash
Fehniger et al[86]	Lenalidomide	II	Rel/ref HL (N=38; 36 evaluable pts)	ORR 19%; 1 CR, 6 PR	NR	Gr 3-4 neutropenia, anemia, TCP, (4 discontinued d/t rash, elevated billirubin)

HL = Hodgkin Lymphoma; Rel/ref = relapsed/refractory; ORR = overall response rate; CR = complete response; PR = partial response; Gr = grade; TCP = thrombocytopenia; TTP= time to progression; NR = Not reported

Table 4. Clinical trials evaluating lenalidomide monotherapy in relapsed/refractory Hodgkin lymphoma patients.

6.2 EBV specific CTL therapy

In general, while chemotherapy agents, small molecule inhibitors, drug immunoconjugates or immunodulatory drugs exhibit promising anti-tumor activity in patients with rel/ref HL, the duration of response to each agent when reported by investigators is rather short. Giving the median age of patients with rel/ref HL the incorporation of therapeutic strategies with durable remissions is necessary. Two therapeutic approaches are been actively evaluated with promising results: 1) Autologous or allogeneic LMP2-specific cytotoxic T-cell lymphocytes (CTL) and 2) allogeneic bone marrow transplantation.

Approximately 30-40% of HL cases are associated with EBV infection of the HRS cells as proven by the expression of viral latent membrane protein (LMP).[88,89] EBV is known to induce the surface expression of three latent antigens in EBV-infected HRS cells: LMP1, LMP2 and Epstein Barr nuclear antigen 1 (EBNA1). Immunotherapy targeting EBV related proteins in HRS cells is an area of active translational research. The generation and ex vivo expansion of cytotoxic T-cell lymphocytes (CTLs) specific for one or more EBV antigens had been studied in patients with hematological malignancies such as post-transplant lymphorpoliferative disorders and rel/ref HL. In general two EBV-related immunotherapy approached had been studied: 1) adoptive immunotherapy (administration of autologous or allogeneic EBV specific CTLs) and 2) vaccination of relevant epitopes from one of the EBV antigens to boost the patients' own immune response.[90,91]

Lucas et al demonstrated the clinical efficacy of allogeneic EBV-specific CTLs in EBV-positive rel/ref HL who had previously failed HDC-ASCT.[92] Significant clinical activity was observed following allogenic CTLs infusion despite a lack to detect donor chimerism. In addition, in the limited number of patients evaluated the administration of fludarabine prior to CTLs infusion enhanced the clinical responses observed. While clinical effects had been observed in HL patients treated with EBV-specific CTLs, the anti-tumor effects are not as robust as what has been observed in patients with PTLDs. Several observations can account for such differences, EBV infected HRS usually express less immunogenic EBV proteins in contrast to PTLD patients (LMP2). In addition, HRS cell have mechanisms to evade immune response to EBV infection including down-regulation of the immunogenicity of latent EBV antigen (i.e. LMP2) and secretion of the immunosuppressive cytokines such as IL10, IL-13, TARC, TRAFs (tumor necrosis factor receptor-associated factors) and TGFβ which may suppress the efficacy of EBV specific CTL.[93-95] Using the strategies to enhance Th1 CTLs development and decrease Th2 cytokine production may overcome the defective immune recognition of HRS cells and improve the efficacy of the EBV specific CTL therapy in rel/ref HL (Table 5).

Clinical trial	Agent	Study design	Patient population	Clinical outcome	N	Location
NCT00058617	Autologous EBV Specific CTLs	Phase I	EBV positive HL, NHL, Plasma cell neoplasm	Safety, immunological efficacy and anti-tumor effects	N=18	Baylor College of Medicine
NCT01192464	Autologous Chimeric Receptors CD30 (CARCD30) + EBV Specific CTLs	Phase I	Rel CD30+ HL, NHL or newly diagnosed but unable to receive standard therapy CD30+ HL or CD30 + NHL with plan for high dose therapy and ASCT	Safety and anti-tumor effects of CARCD30 EBV Specific CTLs	N=18	Baylor College of Medicine
NCT00082225	Autologous/synergeic/allogeneic LMP2a Specific CTLs following anti-CD45 antibody	Phase I	Rel EBV positive HL or NHL	Safety and anti-tumor effects	N=4	Baylor College of Medicine
NCT00062868	Autologous/allogeneic LMP Specific CTLs	Phase I	Rel EBV positive HL or NHL	Safety and anti-tumor effects	N=108	Baylor College of Medicine
NCT00368082	Autologous/syngeneic/ allogeneic TGFβ resistant LMP Specific CTLs	Phase I	Rel EBV positive lymphomas	Safety and anti-tumor effects	N=20	Baylor College of Medicine
NCT00608478	Autologous LMP1 and LMP2 Specific CTLs plus antiCD45 antibody	Phase I	Rel EBV positive lymphomas	Safety and anti-tumor effects	N=24	Baylor College of Medicine

N= number of patients; HL = Hodgkin Lymphoma; NHL = Non-Hodgkin lymphoma; Rel/ref = relapsed/refractory; EBV = Epstein Barr Virus; CTL = cytotoxic T-cell lymphocytes; LMP = Latent membrane protein; LMP2a = Latent membrane protein 2a.

Table 5. Ongoing trials of EBV-Specific CTLs for patients with relapsed/refractory Hodgkin lymphoma.

6.3 Allogeneic bone marrow transplant (AlloSCT)

Approximately 50% of patients with relapsed Hodgkin lymphoma who undergo HDC-ASCT relapse as a consequence of refractory disease, usually within the first year post-transplant.[96,97] Relapsed HL patients after HDC-ASCT have a poor clinical outcome and represent a therapeutic challenge for the practicing oncologist. There are several proposed risk factors to identify patients at high risk to develop disease progression following HDC-ASCT such as chemotherapy resistant disease prior to HDC-ASCT, B symptoms at the time of relapse, residual disease at the time of transplantation by functional imaging, extra-nodal disease at the time of relapse, and bulky disease.[98,99] Patients with any of these high risk factors may be suited for alternative therapeutic strategies such as tandem transplant, allogeneic bone marrow transplant, and/or post-HDC-ASCT maintenance therapy in the context of a clinical trial.

A second HDC-ASCT could be considered for patients with a long period of remission following the initial transplant (>3 years) or those whom alloSCT is not feasible.[100]

AlloSCT has been used in patients with rel/ref HL with controversial results. Often the high incidence of transplant related mortality (TRM) offsets the potential clinical benefit.[101] While the incorporation of reduced intensity conditioning regimens has been associated with lower TRM rates, the long-term PFS rates rarely exceed 20-25% questioning the validity of this approach. Patients who have chemotherapy sensitive disease, non-bulky disease, and have greater than 1 year of remission after the first HDC-ASCT seem to have most benefited with this approach.[102]

Despite early good responses, the results of RIC-AlloSCT demonstrate a disappointing clinical outcome and lack of long term disease control with 2 year OS of 29-66% and 2 year PFS of 20-39% regardless of conditioning regimens or donor types.[103-105] Peggs et al reported durable response to donor lymphocyte infusion (DLI) in patients with relapsed HL post alloSCT that incorporated *in vivo* T-cell depletion.[106] DLI was administered to 46 patients for mixed chimerism (n=22) and relapsed disease post-alloSCT (n=24). Eighty-six percent of patients with mixed chimerism converted to full donor status and had a 4-year relapse incidence of 5%. More importantly, CR and PR were noted in 58.3% and 20.8% of 24 patients with relapsed disease respectively, suggesting the existence of graft vs. HL effects. Ongoing clinical studies are investigating the role of alloSCT in relapsed HL patients with poor-risk features who are at high risk to relapse after HDC-ASCT.

In summary, promising therapies are emerging for the treatment of rel/ref HL. Substantial and occasionally durable remissions have been observed with some therapeutic interventions, such as HDACi, drug immunoconjugates, and cellular therapy. Ongoing studies will hopefully guide the integration of these therapies in the current treatment of high-risk HL in an attempt to improve cure rates. In addition, ongoing scientific and translational research and the importance of the development of novel therapeutics for patients with ref/rel HL should not be underemphasized.

7. References

[1] Kuruvilla J. Standard therapy for advanced Hodgkin lymphoma. Hematology Am Soc Hematol Educ Program 2009:497-506 2009.

[2] Jundt F, Anagnostopoulos I, Forster R, Mathas S, Stein H, Dorken B. Activated Notch1 signaling promotes tumor cell proliferation and survival in Hodgkin and anaplastic large cell lymphoma. Blood 2002;99:3398-403.
[3] Jundt F, Acikgoz O, Kwon SH, et al. Aberrant expression of Notch1 interferes with the B-lymphoid phenotype of neoplastic B cells in classical Hodgkin lymphoma. Leukemia 2008;22:1587-94.
[4] Skinnider BF, Elia AJ, Gascoyne RD, et al. Signal transducer and activator of transcription 6 is frequently activated in Hodgkin and Reed-Sternberg cells of Hodgkin lymphoma. Blood 2002;99:618-26.
[5] Holtick U, Vockerodt M, Pinkert D, et al. STAT3 is essential for Hodgkin lymphoma cell proliferation and is a target of tyrphostin AG17 which confers sensitization for apoptosis. Leukemia 2005;19:936-44.
[6] Bargou RC, Emmerich F, Krappmann D, et al. Constitutive nuclear factor-kappaB-RelA activation is required for proliferation and survival of Hodgkin's disease tumor cells. J Clin Invest 1997;100:2961-9.
[7] Teruya-Feldstein J, Tosato G, Jaffe ES. The role of chemokines in Hodgkin's disease. Leuk Lymphoma 2000;38:363-71.
[8] Venkatesh H, Di Bella N, Flynn TP, Vellek MJ, Boehm KA, Asmar L. Results of a phase II multicenter trial of single-agent gemcitabine in patients with relapsed or chemotherapy-refractory Hodgkin's lymphoma. Clin Lymphoma 2004;5:110-5.
[9] Aurer I, Radman I, Nemet D, et al. Gemcitabine in the treatment of relapsed and refractory Hodgkin's disease. Onkologie 2005;28:567-71.
[10] Suyani E, Sucak GT, Aki SZ, Yegin ZA, Ozkurt ZN, Yagci M. Gemcitabine and vinorelbine combination is effective in both as a salvage and mobilization regimen in relapsed or refractory Hodgkin lymphoma prior to ASCT. Ann Hematol 2011;90:685-91.
[11] Cole PD, Schwartz CL, Drachtman RA, de Alarcon PA, Chen L, Trippett TM. Phase II study of weekly gemcitabine and vinorelbine for children with recurrent or refractory Hodgkin's disease: a children's oncology group report. J Clin Oncol 2009;27:1456-61.
[12] De Filippi R, Aldinucci, D., Galati, D., Esposito, A, Borghese, C., Crisci, S., Abagnale, G., Morelli, E., Frigeri, F., Corazzelli, G., Pinto, A.,. Effects of bendamustine on apoptosis and colony-initiating precursors in Hodgkin lymphoma cells [abstract]. ASCO Annual Meeting 2011;29 Suppl abstr e18559.
[13] Moskowitz AJ, Hamin, P.A., Gerecitano, J., Horwitz, S.M., Matasar, M., Melkie, J., Noy, A., Lia Palomba, M., Portlock, C.S., Straus, D.J., Vanak, J.M., Zelenetz, A.D., Moskowitz, C.G. . Bendamustine Is Highly Active in Heavily Pre-Treated Relapsed and Refractory Hodgkin Lymphoma and Serves as a Bridge to Allogeneic Stem Cell Transplant [abstract]. ASH Annual Meeting 114:720 2009.
[14] Vooijs WC, Otten HG, van Vliet M, et al. B7-1 (CD80) as target for immunotoxin therapy for Hodgkin's disease. Br J Cancer 1997;76:1163-9.
[15] Bolognesi A, Polito L, Tazzari PL, et al. In vitro anti-tumour activity of anti-CD80 and anti-CD86 immunotoxins containing type 1 ribosome-inactivating proteins. Br J Haematol 2000;110:351-61.
[16] Smith SM. Galiximab in relapsed hodgkin lymphoma. Clin Adv Hematol Oncol 2010;8:669-70.

[17] Gruss HJ, Hirschstein D, Wright B, et al. Expression and function of CD40 on Hodgkin and Reed-Sternberg cells and the possible relevance for Hodgkin's disease. Blood 1994;84:2305-14.
[18] Aldinucci D, Gloghini A, Pinto A, Colombatti A, Carbone A. The role of CD40/CD40L and interferon regulatory factor 4 in Hodgkin lymphoma microenvironment. Leuk Lymphoma 2011.
[19] Aldinucci D, Celegato M, Borghese C, Colombatti A, Carbone A. IRF4 silencing inhibits Hodgkin lymphoma cell proliferation, survival and CCL5 secretion. Br J Haematol 2011;152:182-90.
[20] Freedman A, Kuruvilla, J., Assouline, S.E., Engert, A., Heo, D., Solal-Celigny, P., Corradini, P., Verhoef, G., Fanale, M.A., Bendiske, J., Ewald, B., Dey, J., Baeck, J., Younes, A. Clinical Activity of Lucatumumab (HCD122) In Patients (pts) with Relapsed/Refractory Hodgkin or non-Hodgkin Lymphoma Treated In a Phase Ia/II Clinical Trial (NCT00670592) [abstract].. ASH Annual Meeting Abstracts 2010 116:284 2010.
[21] http://clinicaltrials.gov/ct2/search. NCT00129753. Last access January 23, 2012.
[22] http://clinicaltrials.gov/ct2/search. NCT01030900. Last access January 23, 2012.
[23] Younes A, Romaguera J, Hagemeister F, et al. A pilot study of rituximab in patients with recurrent, classic Hodgkin disease. Cancer 2003;98:310-4.
[24] Jones RJ, Gocke CD, Kasamon YL, et al. Circulating clonotypic B cells in classic Hodgkin lymphoma. Blood 2009;113:5920-6.
[25] Inoue S, Leitner WW, Golding B, Scott D. Inhibitory effects of B cells on antitumor immunity. Cancer Res 2006;66:7741-7.
[26] Corazzelli G, Frigeri, F., Marcacci, G., Capobianco, G., Arcamone, M., Becchimanzi, C., Russo, F., Pinto, A. Rituximab plus gemcitabine, ifosfamide, oxaliplatin (R-GIFOX) as salvage therapy for recurrent Hodgkin lymphoma [abstract]. ASCO Annual Meeting 2009;27:Suppl abstr 8579.
[27] Oki Y, Pro B, Fayad LE, et al. Phase 2 study of gemcitabine in combination with rituximab in patients with recurrent or refractory Hodgkin lymphoma. Cancer 2008;112:831-6.
[28] Copeland A, Cao, Y., Fanale, M., Fayad, L., McLaughlin, P., Pro, B., Hagemeister, F., Romaguera, J., Samaniego, F., Rodriguez, A., Younes, A. Final Report of a Phase-II Study of Rituximab Plus ABVD for Patients with Newly Diagnosed Advanced Stage Classical Hodgkin Lymphoma : Results of Long Follow up and Comparison to Institutional Historical Data [abstract]. ASH Annual Meeting Abstracts 2009 114:1680 2009.
[29] Ekstrand BC, Lucas JB, Horwitz SM, et al. Rituximab in lymphocyte-predominant Hodgkin disease: results of a phase 2 trial. Blood 2003;101:4285-9.
[30] Rehwald U, Schulz H, Reiser M, et al. Treatment of relapsed CD20+ Hodgkin lymphoma with the monoclonal antibody rituximab is effective and well tolerated: results of a phase 2 trial of the German Hodgkin Lymphoma Study Group. Blood 2003;101:420-4.
[31] Eichenauer DA, Fuchs M, Pluetschow A, et al. Phase 2 study of rituximab in newly diagnosed stage IA nodular lymphocyte-predominant Hodgkin lymphoma: a report from the German Hodgkin Study Group. Blood 2011;118:4363-5.

[32] Schulz H, Rehwald U, Morschhauser F, et al. Rituximab in relapsed lymphocyte-predominant Hodgkin lymphoma: long-term results of a phase 2 trial by the German Hodgkin Lymphoma Study Group (GHSG). Blood 2008;111:109-11.
[33] Zojer N, Mirzaei S, Ludwig H. Successful treatment of a patient with lymphocyte-predominant Hodgkin's lymphoma with yttrium-90-ibritumomab tiuxetan. Eur J Haematol 2008;81:322-4.
[34] Schnell R, Dietlein M, Schomacker K, et al. Yttrium-90 ibritumomab tiuxetan-induced complete remission in a patient with classical lymphocyte-rich Hodgkin's Lymphoma. Onkologie 2008;31:49-51.
[35] http://clinicaltrials.gov/ct2/search. NCT00484874. Last access January 23, 2012.
[36] Gruss HJ, Pinto A, Gloghini A, et al. CD30 ligand expression in nonmalignant and Hodgkin's disease-involved lymphoid tissues. Am J Pathol 1996;149:469-81.
[37] Pinto A, Aldinucci D, Gloghini A, et al. Human eosinophils express functional CD30 ligand and stimulate proliferation of a Hodgkin's disease cell line. Blood 1996;88:3299-305.
[38] Borchmann P, Schnell R, Engert A. Immunotherapy of Hodgkin's lymphoma. Eur J Haematol Suppl 2005:159-65.
[39] Schnell R, Dietlein M, Staak JO, et al. Treatment of refractory Hodgkin's lymphoma patients with an iodine-131-labeled murine anti-CD30 monoclonal antibody. J Clin Oncol 2005;23:4669-78.
[40] Borchmann P, Treml JF, Hansen H, et al. The human anti-CD30 antibody 5F11 shows in vitro and in vivo activity against malignant lymphoma. Blood 2003;102:3737-42.
[41] Ansell SM, Horwitz SM, Engert A, et al. Phase I/II study of an anti-CD30 monoclonal antibody (MDX-060) in Hodgkin's lymphoma and anaplastic large-cell lymphoma. J Clin Oncol 2007;25:2764-9.
[42] Okeley NM, Miyamoto JB, Zhang X, et al. Intracellular activation of SGN-35, a potent anti-CD30 antibody-drug conjugate. Clin Cancer Res 2010;16:888-97.
[43] Younes A, Bartlett NL, Leonard JP, et al. Brentuximab vedotin (SGN-35) for relapsed CD30-positive lymphomas. N Engl J Med 2010;363:1812-21.
[44] Chen R, Gopal, AK., Smith, SE., Ansell, SM., Rosenblatt, JD., Savage KJ., Connors, JM., Engert, A., Larsen, EK., Kennedy, DA., Sievers, EL., Younes, A. Results from a pivotal phase II study of brentuximab vedotin (SGN-35) in patients with relapsed or refractory hodgkin lymphoma (HL) [abstract]. ASCO Annual Meeting 2011;29 Suppl abstr 8031.
[45] http://clinicaltrials.gov/ct2/search. NCT01100502. Last access January 23, 2012.
[46] http://clinicaltrials.gov/ct2/search. NCT01060904. Last access January 23, 2012.
[47] Blum KA, Johnson JL, Niedzwiecki D, Canellos GP, Cheson BD, Bartlett NL. Single agent bortezomib in the treatment of relapsed and refractory Hodgkin lymphoma: cancer and leukemia Group B protocol 50206. Leuk Lymphoma 2007;48:1313-9.
[48] Younes A, Pro B, Fayad L. Experience with bortezomib for the treatment of patients with relapsed classical Hodgkin lymphoma. Blood 2006;107:1731-2.
[49] Trelle S, Sezer O, Naumann R, et al. Bortezomib in combination with dexamethasone for patients with relapsed Hodgkin's lymphoma: results of a prematurely closed phase II study (NCT00148018). Haematologica 2007;92:568-9.
[50] Mendler JH, Kelly J, Voci S, et al. Bortezomib and gemcitabine in relapsed or refractory Hodgkin's lymphoma. Ann Oncol 2008;19:1759-64.

[51] Fanale M, Fayad L, Pro B, et al. Phase I study of bortezomib plus ICE (BICE) for the treatment of relapsed/refractory Hodgkin lymphoma. Br J Haematol 2011;154:284-6.
[52] Jain S, Diefenbach C, Zain J, O'Connor OA. Emerging role of carfilzomib in treatment of relapsed and refractory lymphoid neoplasms and multiple myeloma. Core Evid 2011;6:43-57.
[53] Buglio D, Georgakis GV, Hanabuchi S, et al. Vorinostat inhibits STAT6-mediated TH2 cytokine and TARC production and induces cell death in Hodgkin lymphoma cell lines. Blood 2008;112:1424-33.
[54] Kirschbaum MH, Goldman BH, Zain JM, et al. A phase 2 study of vorinostat for treatment of relapsed or refractory Hodgkin lymphoma: Southwest Oncology Group Study S0517. Leuk Lymphoma 2011.
[55] Hartlapp I, Pallasch C, Weibert G, Kemkers A, Hummel M, Re D. Depsipeptide induces cell death in Hodgkin lymphoma-derived cell lines. Leuk Res 2009;33:929-36.
[56] Dickinson M, Ritchie D, DeAngelo DJ, et al. Preliminary evidence of disease response to the pan deacetylase inhibitor panobinostat (LBH589) in refractory Hodgkin Lymphoma. Br J Haematol 2009;147:97-101.
[57] Younes A, Oki Y, Bociek RG, et al. Mocetinostat for relapsed classical Hodgkin's lymphoma: an open-label, single-arm, phase 2 trial. Lancet Oncol 2011;12:1222-8.
[58] Younes A PB, Fanale M, McLaughlin P, Neelapu S, Fayad L, Wedgwood A, Buglio D, Patterson T, Dubay M, Li Z, Martell RE, Ward R, Bociek RG. Isotype-Selective HDAC inhibitor MGCD0103 Decreases Serum TARC Concentrations and produces Clinical Response in Heavily Pretreated Patients with Relapsed Classical Hodgkin Lymphoma (HL) [abstract]. ASH Annual Meeting Abstracts 2007 110:2566 2007.
[59] Buglio D, Mamidipudi V, Khaskhely NM, et al. The class-I HDAC inhibitor MGCD0103 induces apoptosis in Hodgkin lymphoma cell lines and synergizes with proteasome inhibitors by an HDAC6-independent mechanism. Br J Haematol 2010;151:387-96.
[60] Bhalla S, Balasubramanian S, David K, et al. PCI-24781 induces caspase and reactive oxygen species-dependent apoptosis through NF-kappaB mechanisms and is synergistic with bortezomib in lymphoma cells. Clin Cancer Res 2009;15:3354-65.
[61] Younes A SA, Ben-Yehuda D, Ong TC, Tan D, Engert A, Le Corre C, Gallagher J, Hirawat S, Prince M. Phase II Study of Oral Panobinostat in Patients with Relapsed/refractory Hodgkin Lymphoma after High-dose Chemotherapy with Autologous Stem Cell Transplant [abstract]. Haematologica 2009;94:34 abs. 0088.
[62] Younes A OT, Ribrag V, Engert a, Ben-Yehuda D, McCabe R, Shen A, Le Corre C, Hirawat S, Sureda A. Efficacy of Panobinostat in Phase II study in Patients with Relapsed/Refractory Hodgkin Lymphoma (HL) After High-DOse Chemotherapy with Autologous Stem Cell Transplant [abstract]. ASH Annual Meeting Abstracts 2009 114:923 2009.
[63] Sureda A EA, Browett PJ, Radford JA, Verhoef GE, Ramchandren R, Myke N, Shen A, Le Corre C, Younes A. Interim results for the phase II study of panobinostat (LBH589) inpatients (Pts) with relapsed/refractory Hodgkin's lymphoma (HL) after autologous hematopoietic stem cell transplant (AHSCT) [abstract]. ASCO Annual Meeting 2010;28.
[64] HarrisonSJ HA, Meeson PJ, Younes A, Sureda A, Engert A, Li M, Savage P, Bugarini R, Le Corre C, Williams DE, Gllagher JD, Shen A, Ritchie D Biomarker analysis of

pivotal phase II study of oral panobinostat (PAN) in relapsed/refractory Hodgkin lymphoma (HL) patients following autologous stem cell transplant (ASCT) [abstract]. ASCO Annual Meeting 2011;29.
[65] Zain JM FF, Kelly WK, DeBono J, Petrylak D, Narwal A, Neylon E, Blumenschein G, Lassen U, O'Connor OA. Final results of a phase I study of oral belinostat (PXD101) in patients with lymphoma [abstract]. ASCO Annual Meeting 2009;27.
[66] Khaskhely NM, Buglio, D., Shafer, J., Younes, A. The Histone Deacetylase (HDAC) Inhibitor Entinostat (SNDX-275) Targets Hodgkin lymphoma through a Dual Mechnism of Immune Modulation and Apoptosis Induction [abstract]. ASH Annual Meeting Abstracts 2009 114:1562 2009.
[67] Jona A, Khaskhely N, Buglio D, et al. The histone deacetylase inhibitor entinostat (SNDX-275) induces apoptosis in Hodgkin lymphoma cells and synergizes with Bcl-2 family inhibitors. Exp Hematol 2011;39:1007-17 e1.
[68] Younes A, Hernandez-Ilizaliturri, F.J., Bociek, R.G., Kasamon, Y.L., Lee, P., Gore, L., Buglio, D., Copeland, A. . ENGAGE-501:Phase 2 Study Investigating the Role of Epigenetic Therapy with Entinostat (SNDX-275) In Relapsed and Refractory Hodgkin's Lymphoma (HL), Interim Results [abstract]. ASH Annual Meeting Abstracts 2010 116:3959 2010.
[69] Furlan A, Monzani V, Reznikov LL, et al. Pharmacokinetics, safety and inducible cytokine responses during a phase 1 trial of the oral histone deacetylase inhibitor ITF2357 (givinostat). Mol Med 2011;17:353-62.
[70] Viviani S, Bonfante, V., Fasola, C., Valagussa, A., Gianni, M. Phase II study of the histone-deacetylase inhibitor ITF2357 in relapsed/refractory Hodgkin's lymphoma patients [abstract]. ASCO Annual Meeting 2008;26 Suppl abs 8532.
[71] Carlo-Stella C, Guidetti, A., Viviani, S., Bonfante, V., Marchiano, A., Gatti, B., D'Urzo, C., Di Nicola, M., Corradini, P., Giannai, AM. Safety and clinical activity of the histone deacetylase inhibitor givinostat in combination with meclorethamine in relapsed/refractory Hodgkin lymphoma (HL) [abstract]. ASCO Annual Meeting 2010;28 15 Suppl:3069.
[72] Faivre S, Kroemer G, Raymond E. Current development of mTOR inhibitors as anticancer agents. Nat Rev Drug Discov 2006;5:671-88.
[73] Lane HA, Wood JM, McSheehy PM, et al. mTOR inhibitor RAD001 (everolimus) has antiangiogenic/vascular properties distinct from a VEGFR tyrosine kinase inhibitor. Clin Cancer Res 2009;15:1612-22.
[74] Jundt F, Raetzel N, Muller C, et al. A rapamycin derivative (everolimus) controls proliferation through down-regulation of truncated CCAAT enhancer binding protein {beta} and NF-{kappa}B activity in Hodgkin and anaplastic large cell lymphomas. Blood 2005;106:1801-7.
[75] Johnston PB, Inwards DJ, Colgan JP, et al. A Phase II trial of the oral mTOR inhibitor everolimus in relapsed Hodgkin lymphoma. Am J Hematol 2010;85:320-4.
[76] Georgakis G, Yazbeck, VY., Li, Y., Younes, A. Preclinical rationale for therapeutic targeting of mTOR by CC-I779 and rapamycin in hodgkin lymphoma [abstract]. ASCO Annual Meeting Suppl 24:10070 2006.
[77] Boll B, Eltaib F, Reiners KS, et al. Heat shock protein 90 inhibitor BIIB021 (CNF2024) depletes NF-kappaB and sensitizes Hodgkin's lymphoma cells for natural killer cell-mediated cytotoxicity. Clin Cancer Res 2009;15:5108-16.

[78] Schoof N, von Bonin F, Trumper L, Kube D. HSP90 is essential for Jak-STAT signaling in classical Hodgkin lymphoma cells. Cell Commun Signal 2009;7:17.
[79] Chang DH, Liu N, Klimek V, et al. Enhancement of ligand-dependent activation of human natural killer T cells by lenalidomide: therapeutic implications. Blood 2006;108:618-21.
[80] Dredge K, Marriott JB, Macdonald CD, et al. Novel thalidomide analogues display anti-angiogenic activity independently of immunomodulatory effects. Br J Cancer 2002;87:1166-72.
[81] Enblad G, Molin D, Glimelius I, Fischer M, Nilsson G. The potential role of innate immunity in the pathogenesis of Hodgkin's lymphoma. Hematol Oncol Clin North Am 2007;21:805-23.
[82] Re D, Kuppers R, Diehl V. Molecular pathogenesis of Hodgkin's lymphoma. J Clin Oncol 2005;23:6379-86.
[83] Steidl C, Connors JM, Gascoyne RD. Molecular pathogenesis of Hodgkin's lymphoma: increasing evidence of the importance of the microenvironment. J Clin Oncol 2011;29:1812-26.
[84] Boll B, Fuchs, M., Reiners, KS., Engert, A., Borchmann, P. Lenalidomide In Patients with Relapsed or Refractory Hodgkin Lymphoma [abstract]. ASH Annual Meeting Abstracts 2010 116:2828 2010.
[85] Kuruvilla J, Taylor, D., Wang, L., Blattler, C., Keating, A., Crump, M. Phase II Trials of Lenalidomide in Patients with Relapsed or Refractory Hodgkin Lymphoma [abstract]. ASH Annual Meeting Abstracts 2008 112:3052 2008.
[86] Fehniger TA, Larson S, Trinkaus K, et al. A phase 2 multicenter study of lenalidomide in relapsed or refractory classical Hodgkin lymphoma. Blood 2011;118:5119-25.
[87] Corazzelli G, De Filippi R, Capobianco G, et al. Tumor flare reactions and response to lenalidomide in patients with refractory classic Hodgkin lymphoma. Am J Hematol 2010;85:87-90.
[88] Glaser SL, Lin RJ, Stewart SL, et al. Epstein-Barr virus-associated Hodgkin's disease: epidemiologic characteristics in international data. Int J Cancer 1997;70:375-82.
[89] Herbst H, Dallenbach F, Hummel M, et al. Epstein-Barr virus latent membrane protein expression in Hodgkin and Reed-Sternberg cells. Proc Natl Acad Sci U S A 1991;88:4766-70.
[90] Deacon EM, Pallesen G, Niedobitek G, et al. Epstein-Barr virus and Hodgkin's disease: transcriptional analysis of virus latency in the malignant cells. J Exp Med 1993;177:339-49.
[91] Grasser FA, Murray PG, Kremmer E, et al. Monoclonal antibodies directed against the Epstein-Barr virus-encoded nuclear antigen 1 (EBNA1): immunohistologic detection of EBNA1 in the malignant cells of Hodgkin's disease. Blood 1994;84:3792-8.
[92] Lucas KG, Salzman D, Garcia A, Sun Q. Adoptive immunotherapy with allogeneic Epstein-Barr virus (EBV)-specific cytotoxic T-lymphocytes for recurrent, EBV-positive Hodgkin disease. Cancer 2004;100:1892-901.
[93] Newcom SR, Gu L. Transforming growth factor beta 1 messenger RNA in Reed-Sternberg cells in nodular sclerosing Hodgkin's disease. J Clin Pathol 1995;48:160-3.

[94] Skinnider BF, Elia AJ, Gascoyne RD, et al. Interleukin 13 and interleukin 13 receptor are frequently expressed by Hodgkin and Reed-Sternberg cells of Hodgkin lymphoma. Blood 2001;97:250-5.

[95] Peh SC, Kim LH, Poppema S. TARC, a CC chemokine, is frequently expressed in classic Hodgkin's lymphoma but not in NLP Hodgkin's lymphoma, T-cell-rich B-cell lymphoma, and most cases of anaplastic large cell lymphoma. Am J Surg Pathol 2001;25:925-9.

[96] Varterasian M, Ratanatharathorn V, Uberti JP, et al. Clinical course and outcome of patients with Hodgkin's disease who progress after autologous transplantation. Leuk Lymphoma 1995;20:59-65.

[97] Martinez C, Canals, C., Alessandrino, E., Karakasis, D., Leone, G., Trneny, M., Snowden, J., Apperley, J., Milpied, N., Sureda, A. Relapse of Hodgkin's lymphoma (HL) after autologous stem cell transplantation (ASCT): Prognostic factors in 462 patients registered in the database of the EBMT. ASCO Annual Meeting 2010;15s Suppl abstr 8060.

[98] Majhail NS, Weisdorf DJ, Defor TE, et al. Long-term results of autologous stem cell transplantation for primary refractory or relapsed Hodgkin's lymphoma. Biol Blood Marrow Transplant 2006;12:1065-72.

[99] Smith SD, Moskowitz CH, Dean R, et al. Autologous stem cell transplant for early relapsed/refractory Hodgkin lymphoma: results from two transplant centres. Br J Haematol 2011;153:358-63.

[100] Smith SM, van Besien K, Carreras J, et al. Second autologous stem cell transplantation for relapsed lymphoma after a prior autologous transplant. Biol Blood Marrow Transplant 2008;14:904-12.

[101] Gajewski JL, Phillips GL, Sobocinski KA, et al. Bone marrow transplants from HLA-identical siblings in advanced Hodgkin's disease. J Clin Oncol 1996;14:572-8.

[102] Thomson KJ, Peggs KS, Blundell E, Goldstone AH, Linch DC. A second autologous transplant may be efficacious in selected patients with Hodgkin's lymphoma relapsing after a previous autograft. Leuk Lymphoma 2007;48:881-4.

[103] Robinson SP, Sureda A, Canals C, et al. Reduced intensity conditioning allogeneic stem cell transplantation for Hodgkin's lymphoma: identification of prognostic factors predicting outcome. Haematologica 2009;94:230-8.

[104] Sarina B, Castagna L, Farina L, et al. Allogeneic transplantation improves the overall and progression-free survival of Hodgkin lymphoma patients relapsing after autologous transplantation: a retrospective study based on the time of HLA typing and donor availability. Blood 2010;115:3671-7.

[105] Devetten MP, Hari PN, Carreras J, et al. Unrelated donor reduced-intensity allogeneic hematopoietic stem cell transplantation for relapsed and refractory Hodgkin lymphoma. Biol Blood Marrow Transplant 2009;15:109-17.

[106] Peggs KS, Kayani I, Edwards N, et al. Donor lymphocyte infusions modulate relapse risk in mixed chimeras and induce durable salvage in relapsed patients after T-cell-depleted allogeneic transplantation for Hodgkin's lymphoma. J Clin Oncol 2011;29:971-8.

Part 8

Therapy for Relapsed and Refractory Pediatric Hodgkin's Lymphoma

8

Therapy for Relapsed and Refractory Pediatric Hodgkin Lymphoma

Karen S. Fernández and Pedro A. de Alarcón
University of Illinois, College of Medicine at Peoria
Children's Hospital of Illinois,
USA

1. Introduction

The treatment of Hodgkin lymphoma (HL) has improved dramatically over the past two decades. The reported five-year event free survival ranges between 80 – 90% with combined modality chemotherapy and radiotherapy. However, 10 - 15% of patients with localized disease and 25% of patients with advanced classical Hodgkin Lymphoma (cHL) have recurrent disease after first line treatment. (Lohri, Barnett et al. 1991; Longo, Duffey et al. 1992; Ferme, Mounier et al. 2002). Refractory patients are also problematic occurring in 2 - 5% of patient with low stage (I/II) and 5 – 10% of high stage (III/IV) cHL (Diehl, Franklin et al. 2003). Retrieval of patients with relapsed and refractory Hodgkin Lymphoma (RR-HL) can be achieved with the use of salvage chemotherapy that includes front-line chemotherapy agents and high dose therapy (HDT) followed by autologous stem cell transplantation (ASCT) (Andre, Henry-Amar et al. 1999; Lazarus, Rowlings et al. 1999). This chapter will discuss the various second line therapeutic approaches for retrieval of patients with RR-HL.

2. Prognostic factors and risk stratification at the time of relapse

Several adverse risk factors have been identified to have prognostic significance in patients with RR-HL. In adults as in the pediatric population, time to initial treatment failure is a strong predictor of survival for patients receiving salvage therapy regardless of high dose chemotherapy and ASCT. (Josting, Rueffer et al. 2000; Schellong, Dorffel et al. 2005). Chemosensitivity to induction or salvage therapy prior to HDT and ASCT is also a strong predictor of outcome (Chopra, McMillan et al. 1993), and in fact helps to define subsequent treatment plan. Patients with induction failure at the time of relapse have the worse outcome (Moskowitz, Kewalramani et al. 2004).

Over the past 15 years, two retrospective studies demonstrated that time to relapse, site of relapse, clinical stage at relapse, and the presence of anemia at the time of relapse were significant predictors of outcome (Brice, Bouabdallah et al. 1997; Josting, Engert et al. 2002).

The scoring system developed by Justing et al, demonstrated that time to relapse (<12months vs. > 12 months), clinical stage at relapse (Stage III/IV) and the presence of anemia (< 10.5 g/dL in females, < 12 g/L in males) at the time of relapse were independent predictors of outcome with a freedom from second failure of 45%, 32% and 18% for patients with 0, 1, 2, or 3 of the above mentioned risk factors, respectively (Josting, Engert et al. 2002).

Another prospective study by Moskowitz et al, indentified the presence of B symptoms, extranodal disease, and less than 12 months to relapse as adverse prognostic factors. They estimated a EFS of 83% for patients with 0-1 adverse prognostic factors, 27% for patients with 2 factors and 10% for patients with 3 factors (Moskowitz, Nimer et al. 2001).

In the pediatric population significant predictors of poor OS and EFS are extranodal disease, mediastinal mass at relapse, stage IV at relapse and primary refractory disease (Lieskovsky, Donaldson et al. 2004; Schellong, Dorffel et al. 2005). In adolescents the presence of B symptoms at the time of relapse confers an 11-year OS of 27% after HDT and ASCT (Akhtar, El Weshi et al. 2010).

The recognition of adverse risk factors at the time of relapse in cHL defines risk group and allows assignment of treatment according to risk stratification. For instance, using time to relapse (> 12 months) and extranodal disease as predictors of outcome, Brice proposes that adult patients with no adverse prognostic factors (favorable risk), should not be exposed to HDT and ASCT to prevent long term toxicity, but instead be treated with conventional chemotherapy such as BEACOPP or MOPP/ABV. Patients with one risk factor (intermediate risk), may benefit from HDT and ASCT +/- Radiation depending on the site of relapse. Finally, patients with two risk factors (high risk for relapse), or those with induction failure or refractory disease, stage IIIB or with anemia required salvage therapy prior to HDT and ASCT (Brice 2008).

In Pediatrics, the identification of prognostic factors is used by individual groups to select therapy, however, there is no agreement across the international groups among a model for risk stratification and treatment assignment according to the prognostic parameters. The EuroNet-PHL-C1 protocol is using this concept and is stratifying patients, depending on time of relapse. Late relapse (< 12 months after primary therapy) is considered low risk, primary progression is high risk and intermediate risk are all other relapses (Daw, Wynn et al. 2011).

Patients with RR-HL regardless of their prognostic factors at the time of relapse/recurrence have several therapeutic options. The role of salvage chemotherapy, high dose therapy followed by ASCT, allogeneic stem cell transplantation (Allo SCT), and other alternatives are discussed below.

3. Salvage chemotherapy regimens (Re-induction chemotherapy)

There is no consensus on the gold-standard second-line chemotherapy for retrieval of RR-HL. Several regimens have been used over the past decades, as summarized in Table 1. This regimes could be classified into:

3.1 Intensive conventional regimens

Mini BEAM (carmustine, etoposide, cytarabine and melphalan); **Dexa - BEAM** (dexamethasone, carmustine, etoposide, cytarabine and melphalan).

3.2 Platinum based regimens

ESHAP (etoposide, methylprednisolone, high dose cytarabine and cisplatin); **DHAP** (dexamethasone, high-dose cytarabine, cisplatin); **APE** (cytarabine, cisplatin, etoposide)

3.3 Ifosfamide-Etoposide based regimens

ICE (ifosfamide, carboplatin, etoposide); **MINE** (mitoxantrone, ifosfamide, vinorelbine and etoposide); **EPIC** (etoposide, prednisolone, ifosfamide, and cisplatin); **OIE** (oxaliplatin, ifosfamide, etoposide); **IEP-ABVD** (ifosfamide, etoposide, prednisolone, adriamycin, bleomycin, vinblastine and dacarbazine).

3.4 Other novel combinations

IGEV (ifosfamide, gemcitabine and vinorelbine), with reported response rates of 65- 85%in RR-HL. **GV** (gemcitabine, vinorelbine).

Selection of the salvage regimen should take into consideration the primary therapy. The ideal regimen would include non-cross-resistant chemotherapy, produce high response rate with acceptable toxicity and allow peripheral stem cell mobilization (Kuruvilla, Keating et al. 2011). The number of chemotherapy cycles prior to ASCT is not known, however most authors advocate for two to four cycles. The goal of salvage chemotherapy is to assess cytoreduction and chemo sensitivity, as those factors are predictors of outcome and define the need of subsequent HDT followed by ASCT. Therefore, salvage chemotherapy should facilitate stem cell harvesting and enable patients to proceed to ASCT.

Disease status before HDT and ASCT is the most important prognostic factor for success as reported by multiple authors (Bierman, Bagin et al. 1993; Andre, Henry-Amar et al. 1999; Popat, Hosing et al. 2004) and discussed previously in this chapter. Response to salvage therapy or response to re-induction chemotherapy prior to high dose chemotherapy is a significant predictor of overall survival (OS) (Yuen, Rosenberg et al. 1997). Sirohi et al reported that patients with complete response prior to transplant, had a 5-year progression-free survival (PFS) rate of 79% compared to 59% for those with partial response and 17% for those with resistant disease (Sirohi, Cunningham et al. 2008).

In the pediatric population several strategies of combined chemotherapeutic regimens have been used in RR-HL. These include the use of ifosfamide, carboplatin and etoposide (ICE) pioneered by Memorial Sloan Kettering Cancer Center (MSKCC), reporting an 88% response rate in a combined trial with adult and pediatric patients with RR-HL. (Moskowitz, Nimer et al. 2001). In Europe the current standard approach for pediatric RR-HL retrieval is alternating IEP-ABVD. Furthermore, this regimen is using response to therapy by using functional imaging with FDG-PET prior to the use of HDT (Daw, Wynn et al. 2011).

In the United States, ICE is the most widely used re-induction treatment option in children and adolescents. Although, the use of ICE can put patients in second remission, it is not optimal, since it is associated to an increased risk of treatment-related secondary malignant neoplasm associated with the use of alkylating agents and epipodophyllotoxins. For this reason the Children's Oncology Group (COG) considering this risk of treatment-related second malignant neoplasms explored other retrieval regimens, such as the combination of ifosfamide with vinorelbine (IV) on their AHOD00P1 protocol. On AHOD00P1, each chemotherapy cycle consisted of Ifosfamide 3000 mg/m2/day during 4 consecutive days and vinorelbine 25 mg/m2 dose on days 1 and 5. Sixty one of 66 patients (92%) had a response after 2 cycles, and 44 (72%) achieved at least a partial response. More than 90% of the patients completed induction without disease progression. This study showed Ifosfamide/Vinorelbine (IV) regimen to be a safe and effective for reinduction therapy. The toxicity profile was acceptable, with primarily hematologic toxicity (Trippet 2004).

Regimen	Drugs Involved	Response	Reference
Dexa-BEAM	Dexamethasone BCNU Etoposide Cytarabine Melphalan	CR 27% PR 54% ORR 81%	(Schmitz, Pfistner et al. 2002)
Mini-BEAM	BCNU Etoposide Cytarabine Melphalan	CR 49% PR 33% ORR 82%	(Martin, Fernandez-Jimenez et al. 2001)
ICE	Ifosfamide Carboplatin Etoposide	CR 26% PR 59% ORR 85%	(Moskowitz, Nimer et al. 2001)
DHAP Q2 weeks	Dexamethasone High-dose Cytarabine Cisplatin	CR 21% PR 68% ORR 89%	(Josting, Rudolph et al. 2005)
GVD	Gemcitabine Vinorelbine Doxil	CR 19% PR 51% ORR 70%	(Bartlett, Niedzwiecki et al. 2007)
GV	Gemcitabine Vinorelbine	ORR 76%	(Cole, Schwartz et al. 2009)
IEP-ABVD	Ifosfamide Etoposide Prednisolone Adriamycin Bleomycin Vinblastine Dacarbazine	ORR 85%	(Schellong, Dorffel et al. 2005)
IV	Ifosfamide Vinorelbine	ORR 83%	(Bonfante, Santoro et al. 1997)
MINE	Mitoguazone Ifosfamide Vinorelbine Etoposide	ORR 75%	(Ferme, Mounier et al. 2002)

RR-HL: recurrent / relapsed Hodgkin Lymphoma; BCNU: Carmustine; CR: complete remission; PR: partial response; ORR: overall response rate

Table 1. Salvage Chemotherapy Regimens for Patients with RR – HL.

Another alternative regimen tested by the COG as a salvage regimen in pediatric patients with RR-HL is Gemcitabine in combination with Vinorelbine (**GV**). This combination was used by the Memorial Sloan-Kettering Cancer Center (MSKCC) in 13 adults with second relapse after HDT and ASCT. The doses used by MSKCC were Gemcitabine 1275 mg/m2 and 30 mg/m2 of vinorelbine every 21 days. The overall response rate was 62% (6 PR and 2 CR) (Hamlin PA 2002). Ozkaynak also reported a small limited experience in a pediatric series (Ozkaynak and Jayabose 2004). The Children's Oncology Group in the AHOD0321 protocol evaluated the Children's Oncology Group in the AHOD0321 protocol, that looked at the efficacy and toxicity of the combination of gemcitabine/vinorelbine in pediatric cHL patients in in second or greater recurrence. The doses used in the COG study were Gemcitabine 1000 mg/m2/dose on day 1 - 8 and Vinorelbine 25 mg/m2 on day 1 and 8. The study accrued 26 evaluable patients. Of those, 19 were responders (CR or PR). The 2-year EFS and OS were 60% and 87% respectively. The regimen proved to be effective and well tolerated (Cole, Trippett et al. 2007; Cole, Schwartz et al. 2009).

Both of these regimens substantiated the use of these novel approaches as acceptable salvage or re-induction regimen for pediatric patients with RR-HL. These regimens, VI or GV, were very well tolerated with a very acceptable toxicity profile and have the advantage of eliminating the use of etoposide and reducing the increased incidence of treatment-related secondary myelodysplasia and acute myelocytic leukemia associated with this medication.

More recently, COG completed another phase II pilot study (AHOD0521) for RR-HL pediatric patients. The study evaluated the addition of bortezomib, a proteasome inhibitor, to ifosfamide / vinorelbine (IV). The study was designed to test the efficacy and safety of bortezomib as a chemo-sensitizing agent in primary RR-HL in first relapse by comparing the results to the historical data of AHOD00P1 with IV regimen alone. The study accrued 23 evaluable patients with RR-HL in first relapse; 48% (11/23patients) had negative FGD-PET scans after 2 cycles. The overall response after 4 cycles of chemotherapy was 89%. Fourteen patients (74%) achieved complete response, and 3 (16%) had a partial response. Four patients had progressive disease and went off protocol. The 2-year EFS and overall survival were 69 and 87%, respectively, demonstrated better results than with ifosfamide/vinorelbine alone (Horton 2010).

Another single-institution pediatric trial has used a combination of Methotrexate, Ifosfamide, etoposide and dexamethasone for children with RR-HL, with an overall response of 84% (Sandlund, Pui et al. 2011).

Table 2. demonstrates the most recent salvage chemotherapy regimens introduced by COG, and provides detail of their schema, chemotherapy doses and timing of administration.

Although all of the salvage regimens produce remission rates in the range of 50 - 65% for RR-HL, they are not curative and the disease free survival (DFS) remains low for this group of patients. Addition of more intensive chemotherapy regimens followed by stem cell rescue has shown to improve DFS compared to salvage chemotherapy alone (Linch, Winfield et al. 1993; Schmitz, Pfistner et al. 2002).

4. High Dose Therapy (HDT) as conditioning regime for ASCT

The current standard therapy for RR-HL, after re-induction or salvage chemotherapy, is high dose therapy (HDT) followed by autologous stem cell transplantation (ASCT). The two landmark studies that proved that high dose chemotherapy followed by ASCT improved survival were conducted by the British National Lymphoma Investigation Group lead by Linch in 1993. This small randomized clinical trial for patients with RR-HL compared BEAM (carmustine, etoposide, cytarabine and melphalan) followed by ASCT vs. mini-BEAM alone.

The 3-year event free survival (EFS) was 53% in the first group and 10% in the second group. (Linch, Winfield et al. 1993).

Later in 2002, the German Hodgkin Lymphoma Study Group performed a larger randomized study that included 161 patients. All patients received Dexa-BEAM (dexamethasone, carmustine, etoposide, cytarabine and melphalan) for 2 cycles. Patients with complete or partial response where randomized to receive two additional cycles of Dexa-BEAM vs. high dose BEAM followed by ASCT. The 3-year failure free survival (FFS) was 55% in the transplant group compared to 34% in the Dexa-BEAM group (Schmitz, Pfistner et al. 2002).

Josting et al compared intensification of the pre ASCT conditioning regimen, by using two cycles of DHAP (dexamethasone, high-dose cytarabine, cisplatin) followed by ASCT vs. DHAP plus cyclophosphamide, high dose MTX, vincristine and etoposide. The 30 months freedom from treatment failure (FFTF) was 69% with no difference in the two arms (Josting, Rudolph et al. 2005).

AHOD00P1 - Phase II Study of Ifosfamide /Vinorelbine (VI)

	Course 1			Course 2		
Days	1	5 6	21/1	5 6		21
Drugs	IV	V	IV	V		IV
	Mesna		Mesna			
		GCSF			**GCSF**	

Vinorelbine (V) 25 mg /m²/dose IV over 6 - 10 minutes on days 1 and 5
Ifosfamide (I) 3000 mgm²/day IV continuous infusion on days 1- 4
MESNA 3000 mg/m²/ day IV continuous infusion on days 1- 4
GCSF (Filgastrim) cycle 1: 5 mcg/kg/dose SQ/IV daily from day 6 until ANC > 1000 or 3 consecutive days or > 10,000 for 1 day; Cycle 2: Dose increased 10 mcg/kg/dose SQ/IV

AHOD0321 - Phase II Study of Gemcitabine / Vinorelbine (GV)

	Course 1			Course 2		
Days	1	8 9	21/1	8 9		21
	G	G	G	G		
	V	V	V	V		
		GCSF			**GCSF**	

Vinorelbine (V) 25 mg /m²/dose IV over 6 - 10 minutes on days 1 and 8
Gemcitabine (G) 1000 mg/m²/day IV continuous infusion on days 1- 8
GCSF (Filgastrim) 5 mcg/kg/dose SQ daily from day 9 until ANC > 1000 or 3 consecutive days or > 10,000 for 1 day for > 7 days until ANC > 1500

AHOD0521-A Phase II Study of Bortezomib in Combination with Ifosfamide/Vinorelbine (IVB)

	Cycle 1				Cycle 2		
Days	1	4 5 6 8		21/1	4 5 6 8		21
Drugs	IV	V		IV	V		IV
	Mesna	**GCSF**		Mesna	**GCSF**		
	B	B	B	B	B	B	

Vinorelbine (V), Ifosfamide (I), MESNA, GCSF as in AHOD00P1(above)
Bortezomib (B) 1200 mg /m²/ dose on day 1, 4, and 8
Give 2 - 4 cycles depending on response
If after 2 cycles there is no evidence of malignancy, patient proceed for stem cell harvesting

Table 2. Pediatric Salvage Chemotherapy Regimen for Relapsed / Recurrent Hodgkin Lymphoma.

Although the outcome with HDT followed by ASCT has proven superior to salvage chemotherapy alone, nospecific regimen has shown to be superior. Comparing toxicity and efficacy of the various conditioning regimen using HDT prior to ASCT is somewhat difficult, because the doses used in each of the trials are different. For comparison, Table 3 contrasts the specific chemotherapy doses.

Group	Regimen Name	Regimen Drugs +and Doses	Outcome	Reference
British National Lymphoma Investigation Group1993	BEAM + ASCT	Carmustine: 300 mg/m^2 x1 Etoposide: 800 mg/m^2 x1 Cytarabine: 1600 mg/m^2 x1 Melphalan: 140 mg/m^2 x1	3-year-EFS 53%	(Linch, Winfield et al. 1993)
	Mini-BEAM	BCNU /Carmustine:60 mg/m^2 Etoposide: 300 mg/m^2 Cytarabine: 800 mg/m^2 Melphalan: 30 mg/m2	3-year-EFS 10%	
German Hodgkin Lymphoma Study Group 2002	Dexa-BEAM	Dexamethasone 24 mg x 10 Carmustine 60 mg/m^2 x Etoposide 250 mg/m^2 x 4 Cytarabine 200 mg/m^2 IV x 4 Melphalan 20 mg/m^2 x 1	3-year –FF2F 34%	(Schmitz, Pfistner et al. 2002)
	BEAM + ASCT	Carmustine 300 mg/m^2 x 1 Etoposide 300 mg/m^2 x 4 Cytarabine 400 mg/m^2 x 4 Melphalan 140 mg/m^2 x1	3-year-FF2F 54%	
German Hodgkin Lymphoma Study Group 2005	DHAP + ASCT	Dexamethasone 40 mg/m^2 x 4 HD-Cytarabine 4000mg/m^2 x 2 Cisplatin 100 mg/m^2 x 1	Median Follow up 30 months FFTF 59% OS 78%	(Josting, Rudolph et al. 2005)
	DHAP x 2 + CPM, HD-MTX, VCR ETO	Dexamethasone 40 mg/m^2 x 4 HD-Cytarabine 4000mg/m^2 x 2 Cisplatin 100 mg/m^2 x 1 Cyclophosphamide 4 g/m^2 High dose MTX 8 g/m^2 Vincristine 1.4 g/m^2 Etoposide 2500 mg/m^2		
	BEAM + ASCT	Bendamustine 200 mg /m^2 Etoposide 800 mg/m^2 Cytarabine 1600 mg/m^2 Melphalan 140 mg/m^2	Median DFS 19 months	(Visani, Malerba et al. 2011)

EFS: event free survival; FF2F: freedom from second failure; FFTF: freedom from treatment failure; DFS: disease free survival ; ASCT autologous stem cell transplantation

Table 3. High Dose Therapy as Conditioning Regimen Prior to ASCT Comparative Doses.

It is important to recognized that although carmustine (BCNU)-containing regimens are the most widely used as conditioning regimen for the treatment of RR-HL, there are some major pitfalls such as a high incidence of interstitial pneumonitis or idiopathic pneumonia (2- 23%), a still high incidence of relapse, and the risk of non-relapse related death (Seiden, Elias et al. 1992; Reece, Nevill et al. 1999; Alessandrino, Bernasconi et al. 2000). In addition, the increase of secondary malignancies after treatment with alkylating agents and epidophylotoxins is of great concern, particularly in children and adolescents and young adults (AYA). For these reasons the search for new and optimal conditioning regimens continues.

In search for this optimal conditional regimen, Visai et al. recently presented the results of a phase I / II trial using BeEAM (bendamustine, etoposide, cytarabine and melphalan) as a conditioning regimen for ASCT in patients with lymphomas. The phase I study used escalating doses of bendamustine (160 mg/m^2, 180 mg/m^2 and 200 mg/m^2). This study included 15 HL patients out of the 43. None of the 43 patients had dose limiting toxicities. The regimen was well tolerated with minimal treatment related mortality. Although the regimen seemed to have worked better for non-Hodgkin lymphoma (NHL) patients, the median DFS for HL patients was 19 months after ASCT. The major limitations of this study is the small number of patients with HL, and therefore this regimen warrants further studies to confirm the efficacy of this novel regimen in the treatment of RR-HL (Visani, Malerba et al. 2011).

Even with the use of HDT and ASCT approximately 50% of patients continue to have refractory disease or recur after ASCT (Chopra, McMillan et al. 1993) so that more effective therapy is still needed.

In Pediatrics, the use of HDT and ASCT is reserved for patients with high risk for relapse or those with primary progressive disease. There is very little evidence to support the use of this approach in first relapse for children and adolescents. The implementation of this approach in the pediatric population has been adapted from the adult experience described above.

5. Tandem autologous transplantation

The use of tandem autologous transplants seem to have a role for a subset of patients with RR-HL and certain risk factors at the time of initial salvage therapy.

Brice et al used two different conditioning regimen CBV (cyclophosphamide, carmustine, etoposide) vs. CBV (cyclophosphamide, carmustine, etoposide) plus mitoxantrone (30 mg/m^2) for the first ASCT and a second conditioning regimen with total body irradiation (TBI) of 12 Gy or busulfan (12 mg/kg) followed by high dose cytarabine (6 g/m^2) and melphalan (140 mg/m^2). The two-year survival rate from the date of progression were respectively at 65% and at 74%.(Brice, Divine et al. 1999)

A US group lead by Fung used a preparative regimen of melphalan (150 mg/m^2) and a second preparative regimen with fractionated TBI (1200cGy) or carmustine (450 mg/m^2) plus etoposide (60mg/kg) and cyclophosphamide (100mg/kg). This US group reported a 5-year FF2F of 55% and a OS of 54% suggesting that in patients with primary progressive or poor risk recurrent HL, tandem ASCT is well tolerated and compares favorably with the conventional single transplant. (Fung, Stiff et al. 2007).

Castagna et al investigated the feasibility and toxicity of ifosfamide, gemcitabine and vinorelbine (IGEV) as salvage therapy followed by two tandem ASCT using melphalan

($200mg/m^2$) alone as the first conditioning regimen and BEAM as the second conditioning regimen. The response rate increased with each step, from 47% after salvage chemotherapy, to 65% after first ASCT to 75% after second transplant. The 3-year FFP was 63% and the OS was 72% (Castagna, Magagnoli et al. 2007).

The Group d'Etude des Lymphomes de L'adulte (GELA) tested the feasibility of tandem ASCT vs. single ASCT in patients with primary refractory disease or high risk for relapse as defined by the presence of at least two of the following three adverse risk factors: 1) relapse in a previous radiation field, 2) stage III/IV at the time of relapse or 3) time to relapse < 12 months; or intermediate-risk patients those with one risk factor. Intermediate risk patients received single ASCT showing a FF2F and OS of 73% and 85%, respectively. High risk patients received tandem ASCT with a FF2F and OS of 46% and 57% respectively, which was comparable to previous reports. The results of this study suggest that single ASCT is appropriate for intermediate-risk patients, and that high risk patients with RR-HL may benefit of tandem ASCT (Morschhauser, Brice et al. 2008). In spite of these encouraging results the use of tandem ASCT for RR-HL is still considered experimental.

6. Second autologous transplants

For patients who relapse after a previous ASCT a second auto graft is a viable option, although very limited data exist to support this strategy (Smith, van Besien et al. 2008). This option can be considered as a treatment alternative in patient with a time to relapse > 1 year after the initial transplant. Allografting after ASCT in general is not recommended (Kuruvilla, Keating et al. 2011). Nonetheless, it can still be used in certain circumstances as described below.

7. Allogeneic stem cell transplantation

In the past, allogeneic stem cell transplant (Allo-SCT) offered a chance for a better disease free survival (DFS) but the procedure associated mortality has negated this advantage yielding a worse event free survival. ASCT substituted allo-SCT due to this high treatment-related mortality and the non-infrequent incidence of relapse. However, the introduction of reduced-intensity chemotherapy (RIC) as the preparative regimen for allogeneic transplantation has improved the safety of the procedure. RIC allo-SCT is now being considered an effective approach for selected patients, including those who have failed HDT with ASCT, or for patients with bone marrow involvement at relapse or insufficient stem-cell collection for a second HDT (Brice 2008; Salit, Bishop et al. 2010). Although, the feasibility of RIC allo-SCT has improved, there is still a lack of durable response (Peggs, Sureda et al. 2007; Devetten, Hari et al. 2009). The use of a RIC allo-SCT strategy is best used within the context of prospective clinical trials, as its use remain highly controversial.

8. Standard-dose chemotherapy

A non-ASCT-based strategy has a role in some patients with late relapse (>1 year after completion of induction chemotherapy) and chemo sensitive disease. The Italian group lead by Bonfante found an 8-year freedom from second progression (FF2P) and OS of 53% and 62% respectively in patients treated with mechlorethamine, vincristine, procarbazine, prednisone (MOPP) and Adriamycin, bleomycin, vinblastine, and dacarbazine (ABVD) (Bonfante, Santoro et al. 1997). The German group demonstrated good results for patient with the above mentioned characteristics treated with IEP-ABVD regimen followed by radiation therapy to nodal regions involved at the time of relapse and original regions had they not been irradiate. A 10-year DFS and OS was 57% and 75% respectively was reported (Schellong, Dorffel et al. 2005).

9. Role of radiotherapy for RR-HL

Radiotherapy alone can achieve long-term remission, but only in a small proportion of patients. Radiotherapy (RT) is used less as a first line therapy in RR-HL due to its limited efficacy in patients with advanced disease. In some ongoing pediatric clinical trials the use of RT has been omitted from the upfront therapy for patients with good response to initial chemotherapy. Therefore, some patients may be radiation naïve at the time of relapse or have received only limited RT. This fact, makes the use of RT at the time of relapse an attractive alternative for certain relapsed patients, particularly the ones with limited stage disease and relapse at the site of original disease only.

Josting et al reported a 5-year freedom from treatment failure (FFTF) and OS of 29% and 51% respectively for RR-HL treated with radiotherapy alone. The presence of B symptoms, advanced stage (III/IV) at relapse, Karnofsky of < 90% were identified as poor prognostic factors for those patients (Josting, Nogova et al. 2005).

10. Role of chemotherapy plus radiation without ASCT

Combined modality therapy with multi-agent chemotherapy followed by radiotherapy is the standard treatment for limited-stage HL (Press, LeBlanc et al. 2001; Engert, Franklin et al. 2007; Ferme, Eghbali et al. 2007). This modality is particularly attractive for patients who have not received radiotherapy with prior treatment or have relapsed with disease in sites that have not previously been radiated (Press, LeBlanc et al. 2001; Kuruvilla, Keating et al. 2011). Radiotherapy can also be given to patients with RR-HL and bulky disease after standard HDT therapy and ASCT.

Kurovilla et al suggested the use of standard dose chemotherapy plus radiotherapy as a salvage therapy for patients with very late relapse (>5 years) after primary therapy who suffer localized relapse without B symptoms (Kuruvilla, Keating et al. 2011)

11. Salvage therapies following ASCT

More than 50% of patients with RR-HL will not be cured, either because their tumors are not chemotherapy sensitive to proceed with ASCT or because they do not achieve a durable response after ASCT. For those patients, single or combined conventional therapies that can provide disease control such as Gemcitabine / Vinorelbine or Vinorelbine / Ifosfamide plus bortezomib are possible re-induction regimens. As previously mentioned an allo-RIC SCT is also an alternative and should always be considered when in the context of a prospective clinical trial.

The Children's Oncology Group, in the US is performing a trial to evaluate immunomodulation after HDT and ASCT. The study had two parts. The first one is to determine toxicity and feasibility of administering cyclosporine, interferon-γ, and interleukin-2 following BEAM chemotherapy with ASCT. The second part aims to assess whether greater levels of autologous GVHD and/or autoreactive cytolytic lymphocytes are associated with improved survival, whether expression of the target molecule of autologous GVHD is associated with improved survival, and whether immunotherapy can produce better outcomes in patients identified as having high risk disease on the basis of high serum levels of interleukin-10 or soluble interleukin-2 receptor. The results of this trial have not been reported yet.

12. New agents

The development of novel drugs for the treatment of cHL has been slow partially due to the high success rate of the treatment of the disease. However, the better understanding of the pathology, biology and immunology has allow the introduction of several therapeutic targets. This new drug development not only is aiming for better survival but also to decrease toxic effects.

12.1 Antibody/receptor therapy

One of the defining features of cHL is CD30 expression by Reed-Stenberg cells. The use of an anti-CD30 molecule has been an attractive target in the treatment for HL (Forero-Torres, Leonard et al. 2009). Several anti CD30 antibodies have been engineered: MDX-060 (Medarex) a fully humanized antibody to CD30 (SGN-30), a chimeric monoclonal anti-CD30 antibody, both have shown to inhibit cell proliferation and to induce cell death in CD30 positive lymphomas. However, when used alone they were not effective as single agents, showing response rates much lower than traditional cytotoxic chemotherapy.

Newer generation of anti-CD30 antibodies with enhanced Fc receptor-antibody activity (Medarex, MDX-1401) and with antibody-drug conjugates are currently under study (Foyil and Bartlett 2010).

The recent introduction of a conjugated anti-CD30 antibody conjugated to the antitubuline agent, Brentuximab Vedotin, (SGN-35) has shown excellent results in CD30 positive lymphomas. In a phase I, open label, multicenter dose-escalation study published in the New England Journal of Medicine, 42 evaluable patients with refractory CD30 lymphomas demonstrated tumor regression of 86%. (Younes, Bartlett et al. 2010). An additional phase II clinical trials using Brentuximab Vedotin intravenously at a dose of 1.8 mg/kg every 3 weeks was reported at ASCO in 2011. The study found a response of 75% (76 out of 102) in patient with HL, with a complete remission in 34% of them. The average duration of response was 6.7 months. The excellent results of these studies resulted in the recent FDA approval of Brentuximab Vedotin for the treatment of patients with HL whose disease has progressed after autologous stem cell transplant, or after two prior multiagent chemotherapy treatments among patients ineligible to receive a transplant. Prospective studies in the pediatric population are warranted.

The use of the anti-CD20 antibody, Rituximab, has demonstrated excellent activity against nodular lymphocyte predominant HL (NLPHL) with overall response rates of 94% (Ekstrand, Lucas et al. 2003; Rehwald, Schulz et al. 2003). Rituximab is currently being studied in cHL (Younes, Romaguera et al. 2003).

12.2 Radioimmunotherapy (RIT)

Radioimmunotherapy uses the concept of targeted antibodies, typically antiferritin and anti-CD30 to deliver radiation with Yttrium-90 or iodine-131 to the tumor cells (Klimm, Schnell et al. 2005). The use of polyclonal antibodies, Ytrium 90-labelled antiferritin, In-labeled antiferritin antibody recently became available. They have been well tolerated and have shown activity in RR-HL with a response of approximately 8 months. Other attempts to increase the efficacy of antiCD30 monoclonal antibody include conjugation with Iodine-131 (Schnell, Dietlein et al. 2005).

The German group has developed an antiCD25 also known as anti IL-2 receptor (Daclizumab) and anti-CD25 linked to Ytrium-90. CD25 is found in a large proportion of Hodgkin Reed Stenberg cells and in the surrounding tumor-associated T-cell and therefore represents an attractive target therapy. Some preliminary studies using Y-90-CD25 (90Y-daclizumab) every 6 - 10 weeks yielded an overall response of 70% (O'Mahony D. Janik JE 2007).

12.3 Antiapoptotic molecules

Other novel pharmacological approaches include inhibition of NF-kB pathway. NF-kB is a transcription factor that is constitutively activated in HL, and that is thought to be responsible for cell proliferation and antiapoptosis in HL (Pajonk, Pajonk et al. 2000).

Bortezomib (Velcade) is a proteasome inhibitor that also inhibits NF-kB pathway. Bortezomib has shown some limited efficacy when used as a single agent or in combination with dexamethasone (Younes, Pro et al. 2006; Trelle, Sezer et al. 2007). However, NF-kB inhibition is postulated to sensitize malignant cells to chemotherapy, including Gemcitabine (Moskowitz, Nimer et al. 2001), TNF-related apoptosis-inducing ligand (TRAIL) (Zheng, Georgakis et al. 2004), dexamethasone and vinorelbine (Hinz, Lemke et al. 2002). Inhibition of the antiapoptotic molecule XIAP has shown some encouraging results in preclinical studies (LaCasse, Cherton-Horvat et al. 2006). As mentioned above the Children's Oncology Group recently completed a study that assess the safety of bortezomib in addition to ifosfamide / vinorelbine, the preliminary data suggest that bortezomib may have added additional efficacy to the backbone regimen of ifosfamide and vinorelbine .

12.4 Transcriptional pathways

The use of other molecules that are mediators of apoptosis, such as the histone deacetylase (HDAC) inhibitors in HL is currently under investigation. Some of these are Panobinostat, Vorinostat, Entinosat. A phase II study demonstrated 40% response in patients with RR-HL (Younes 2007; Jona and Younes 2010).

M-TOR inhibitors, particularly everolimus, have also shown some promising results with up to 42% overall response rate in patients with RR-HL (Johnston PB 2007) . The small molecule Nutlin 3A, stabilizes p53 protein via MDM2 binding, allowing to activate apoptotic pathways in Hodgkin Reed Stenberg cells (Drakos, Thomaides et al. 2007). This three novel molecules may have an interesting potential therapeutic intervention in cHL.

12.5 EBV-directed therapy

Nearly 50% of cHL patients are known to be EBV positive, making the use of EBV-targeted therapy very attractive. EBV specific cytotoxic T lymphocytes (CTL) can be generated in vitro and then given to the patients with the intent of targeting specific EBV-infected cancer cells. Portis et al demonstrated that by using this technology 30% of treated patients achieved a complete remission (Portis and Longnecker 2004).

13. Conclusions

The treatment of RR-HL has improved over the years. The use of HDT followed by ASCT has allow 50% of patients to have durable remission. However, the management of the patient with refractory disease is a real challenge. Treatment intensification with traditional chemotherapy agents is not sufficient and new approaches are needed. As the armamentarium for the treatment of patients that have failed initial therapy continuous to expand, we are foreseeing novel treatment modalities. Some of such agents, particularly the biologically target agents, have the potential to be incorporated into front line therapy of cHL as they may have a better therapeutic profile than our current cytotoxic chemotherapy agents. The use of novel biological and targeted therapies is very attractive for the retrieval of patients with RR-HL. As we develop a better understanding of the biology of cHL, we are likely to see more effective treatment strategies that will overcome resistance, and reduced short and long term toxicity for patients with primary and refractory cHL.

14. References

Akhtar, S., A. El Weshi, et al. (2010). "High-dose chemotherapy and autologous stem cell transplant in adolescent patients with relapsed or refractory Hodgkin's lymphoma." *Bone Marrow Transplant* 45(3): 476-482.

Alessandrino, E. P., P. Bernasconi, et al. (2000). "Pulmonary toxicity following carmustine-based preparative regimens and autologous peripheral blood progenitor cell transplantation in hematological malignancies." *Bone Marrow Transplant* 25(3): 309-313.

Andre, M., M. Henry-Amar, et al. (1999). "Comparison of high-dose therapy and autologous stem-cell transplantation with conventional therapy for Hodgkin's disease induction failure: a case-control study. Societe Francaise de Greffe de Moelle." *J Clin Oncol* 17(1): 222-229.

Bartlett, N. L., D. Niedzwiecki, et al. (2007). "Gemcitabine, vinorelbine, and pegylated liposomal doxorubicin (GVD), a salvage regimen in relapsed Hodgkin's lymphoma: CALGB 59804." *Ann Oncol* 18(6): 1071-1079.

Bierman, P. J., R. G. Bagin, et al. (1993). "High dose chemotherapy followed by autologous hematopoietic rescue in Hodgkin's disease: long-term follow-up in 128 patients." *Ann Oncol* 4(9): 767-773.

Bonfante, V., A. Santoro, et al. (1997). "Outcome of patients with Hodgkin's disease failing after primary MOPP-ABVD." *J Clin Oncol* 15(2): 528-534.

Brice, P. (2008). "Managing relapsed and refractory Hodgkin lymphoma." *Br J Haematol* 141(1): 3-13.

Brice, P., R. Bouabdallah, et al. (1997). "Prognostic factors for survival after high-dose therapy and autologous stem cell transplantation for patients with relapsing Hodgkin's disease: analysis of 280 patients from the French registry. Societe Francaise de Greffe de Moelle." *Bone Marrow Transplant* 20(1): 21-26.

Brice, P., M. Divine, et al. (1999). "Feasibility of tandem autologous stem-cell transplantation (ASCT) in induction failure or very unfavorable (UF) relapse from Hodgkin's disease (HD). SFGM/GELA Study Group." *Ann Oncol* 10(12): 1485-1488.

Castagna, L., M. Magagnoli, et al. (2007). "Tandem high-dose chemotherapy and autologous stem cell transplantation in refractory/relapsed Hodgkin's lymphoma: a monocenter prospective study." *Am J Hematol* 82(2): 122-127.

Chopra, R., A. K. McMillan, et al. (1993). "The place of high-dose BEAM therapy and autologous bone marrow transplantation in poor-risk Hodgkin's disease. A single-center eight-year study of 155 patients." *Blood* 81(5): 1137-1145.

Cole, P. D., C. L. Schwartz, et al. (2009). "Phase II Study of Weekly Gemcitabine and Vinorelbine for Children With Recurrent or Refractory Hodgkin's Disease: A Children's Oncology Group Report." *Journal of Clinical Oncology* 27(9): 1456-1461.

Cole, P. D., T. M. Trippett, et al. (2007). "AHOD0321: A cog phase II study of weekly gemcitabine and vinorelbine in children with recurrent or refractory Hodgkin disease." *Haematologica-the Hematology Journal* 92: 58-58.

Daw, S., R. Wynn, et al. (2011). "Management of relapsed and refractory classical Hodgkin lymphoma in children and adolescents." *Br J Haematol* 152(3): 249-260.

Devetten, M. P., P. N. Hari, et al. (2009). "Unrelated donor reduced-intensity allogeneic hematopoietic stem cell transplantation for relapsed and refractory Hodgkin lymphoma." *Biol Blood Marrow Transplant* 15(1): 109-117.

Diehl, V., J. Franklin, et al. (2003). "Standard and increased-dose BEACOPP chemotherapy compared with COPP-ABVD for advanced Hodgkin's disease." *N Engl J Med* 348(24): 2386-2395.

Drakos, E., A. Thomaides, et al. (2007). "Inhibition of p53-murine double minute 2 interaction by nutlin-3A stabilizes p53 and induces cell cycle arrest and apoptosis in Hodgkin lymphoma." *Clin Cancer Res* 13(11): 3380-3387.

Ekstrand, B. C., J. B. Lucas, et al. (2003). "Rituximab in lymphocyte-predominant Hodgkin disease: results of a phase 2 trial." *Blood* 101(11): 4285-4289.

Engert, A., J. Franklin, et al. (2007). "Two cycles of doxorubicin, bleomycin, vinblastine, and dacarbazine plus extended-field radiotherapy is superior to radiotherapy alone in early favorable Hodgkin's lymphoma: final results of the GHSG HD7 trial." *J Clin Oncol* 25(23): 3495-3502.

Ferme, C., H. Eghbali, et al. (2007). "Chemotherapy plus involved-field radiation in early-stage Hodgkin's disease." *N Engl J Med* 357(19): 1916-1927.

Ferme, C., N. Mounier, et al. (2002). "Intensive salvage therapy with high-dose chemotherapy for patients with advanced Hodgkin's disease in relapse or failure after initial chemotherapy: results of the Groupe d'Etudes des Lymphomes de l'Adulte H89 Trial." *J Clin Oncol* 20(2): 467-475.

Forero-Torres, A., J. P. Leonard, et al. (2009). "A Phase II study of SGN-30 (anti-CD30 mAb) in Hodgkin lymphoma or systemic anaplastic large cell lymphoma." *Br J Haematol* 146(2): 171-179.

Foyil, K. V. and N. L. Bartlett (2010). "Anti-CD30 Antibodies for Hodgkin lymphoma." *Curr Hematol Malig Rep* 5(3): 140-147.

Fung, H. C., P. Stiff, et al. (2007). "Tandem autologous stem cell transplantation for patients with primary refractory or poor risk recurrent Hodgkin lymphoma." *Biol Blood Marrow Transplant* 13(5): 594-600.

Hamlin PA, K. T., Schaindlin P, Moskowitz CH (2002). "Gemcitabine / Vinorelbine: A well tolerated and effective regimen for patetients with relapsed/refractory Hodgkin's Disease (HD) who fail autologus stem cell transplantation (ACST)." *Proc Am Soc Hem*(100): 634a.

Hinz, M., P. Lemke, et al. (2002). "Nuclear factor kappaB-dependent gene expression profiling of Hodgkin's disease tumor cells, pathogenetic significance, and link to constitutive signal transducer and activator of transcription 5a activity." *J Exp Med* 196(5): 605-617.

Horton, T. (2010). "A Phase II Study of Bortezomib in Combination with Ifosfamide/Vinorelbine in Pediatric Patients and Young Adults with Refractory/Recurrent Hodgkin Disease, Children's Oncology Group " *Annual American Society of Clinical Oncology (ASCO) meeting on June 6, 2010.*

Johnston PB, A. S., Colgan JP et al (2007). "Promising results for patients with relapsed or refractry Hodgkin lymphoma related with the oral MTOR inhibitor everolimus (RAD001)." *Presented at the Seventh International Symposium on Hodgking Lymphoma, Cologne* Abstract 099

Jona, A. and A. Younes (2010). "Novel treatment strategies for patients with relapsed classical Hodgkin lymphoma." *Blood Rev* 24(6): 233-238.

Josting, A., A. Engert, et al. (2002). "Prognostic factors and treatment outcome in patients with primary progressive and relapsed Hodgkin's disease." *Ann Oncol* 13 Suppl 1: 112-116.

Josting, A., L. Nogova, et al. (2005). "Salvage radiotherapy in patients with relapsed and refractory Hodgkin's lymphoma: a retrospective analysis from the German Hodgkin Lymphoma Study Group." *J Clin Oncol* 23(7): 1522-1529.

Josting, A., C. Rudolph, et al. (2005). "Cologne high-dose sequential chemotherapy in relapsed and refractory Hodgkin lymphoma: results of a large multicenter study of the German Hodgkin Lymphoma Study Group (GHSG)." *Ann Oncol* 16(1): 116-123.

Josting, A., U. Rueffer, et al. (2000). "Prognostic factors and treatment outcome in primary progressive Hodgkin lymphoma: a report from the German Hodgkin Lymphoma Study Group." *Blood* 96(4): 1280-1286.

Klimm, B., R. Schnell, et al. (2005). "Current treatment and immunotherapy of Hodgkin's lymphoma." *Haematologica* 90(12): 1680-1692.

Kuruvilla, J., A. Keating, et al. (2011). "How I treat relapsed and refractory Hodgkin lymphoma." *Blood* 117(16): 4208-4217.

LaCasse, E. C., G. G. Cherton-Horvat, et al. (2006). "Preclinical characterization of AEG35156/GEM 640, a second-generation antisense oligonucleotide targeting X-linked inhibitor of apoptosis." *Clin Cancer Res* 12(17): 5231-5241.

Lazarus, H. M., P. A. Rowlings, et al. (1999). "Autotransplants for Hodgkin's disease in patients never achieving remission: a report from the Autologous Blood and Marrow Transplant Registry." *J Clin Oncol* 17(2): 534-545.

Lieskovsky, Y. E., S. S. Donaldson, et al. (2004). "High-dose therapy and autologous hematopoietic stem-cell transplantation for recurrent or refractory pediatric Hodgkin's disease: results and prognostic indices." *J Clin Oncol* 22(22): 4532-4540.

Linch, D. C., D. Winfield, et al. (1993). "Dose intensification with autologous bone-marrow transplantation in relapsed and resistant Hodgkin's disease: results of a BNLI randomised trial." *Lancet* 341(8852): 1051-1054.

Lohri, A., M. Barnett, et al. (1991). "Outcome of treatment of first relapse of Hodgkin's disease after primary chemotherapy: identification of risk factors from the British Columbia experience 1970 to 1988." *Blood* 77(10): 2292-2298.

Longo, D. L., P. L. Duffey, et al. (1992). "Conventional-dose salvage combination chemotherapy in patients relapsing with Hodgkin's disease after combination chemotherapy: the low probability for cure." *J Clin Oncol* 10(2): 210-218.

Martin, A., M. C. Fernandez-Jimenez, et al. (2001). "Long-term follow-up in patients treated with Mini-BEAM as salvage therapy for relapsed or refractory Hodgkin's disease." *Br J Haematol* 113(1): 161-171.

Morschhauser, F., P. Brice, et al. (2008). "Risk-adapted salvage treatment with single or tandem autologous stem-cell transplantation for first relapse/refractory Hodgkin's lymphoma: results of the prospective multicenter H96 trial by the GELA/SFGM study group." *J Clin Oncol* 26(36): 5980-5987.

Moskowitz, C. H., T. Kewalramani, et al. (2004). "Effectiveness of high dose chemoradiotherapy and autologous stem cell transplantation for patients with biopsy-proven primary refractory Hodgkin's disease." *Br J Haematol* 124(5): 645-652.

Moskowitz, C. H., S. D. Nimer, et al. (2001). "A 2-step comprehensive high-dose chemoradiotherapy second-line program for relapsed and refractory Hodgkin disease: analysis by intent to treat and development of a prognostic model." *Blood* 97(3): 616-623.

O'Mahony D. Janik JE, C. J., et al (2007). "Yttrium-90 radiolabeled humanized anti-CD25 monoclonal antibody, daclizumab, provides effective therapy for refractory an relapased Hodking's Lymphoma " *Presented at the Seventh International Symposium on Hodgking Lymphoma, Cologne* Abstract 1069

Ozkaynak, M. F. and S. Jayabose (2004). "Gemcitabine and vinorelbine as a salvage regimen for relapse in Hodgkin lymphoma after autologous hematopoietic stem cell transplantation." *Pediatric Hematology and Oncology* 21(2): 107-113.

Pajonk, F., K. Pajonk, et al. (2000). "Apoptosis and radiosensitization of hodgkin cells by proteasome inhibition." *Int J Radiat Oncol Biol Phys* 47(4): 1025-1032.

Peggs, K. S., A. Sureda, et al. (2007). "Reduced-intensity conditioning for allogeneic haematopoietic stem cell transplantation in relapsed and refractory Hodgkin lymphoma: impact of alemtuzumab and donor lymphocyte infusions on long-term outcomes." *Br J Haematol* 139(1): 70-80.

Popat, U., C. Hosing, et al. (2004). "Prognostic factors for disease progression after high-dose chemotherapy and autologous hematopoietic stem cell transplantation for recurrent or refractory Hodgkin's lymphoma." *Bone Marrow Transplant* 33(10): 1015-1023.

Portis, T. and R. Longnecker (2004). "Epstein-Barr virus (EBV) LMP2A mediates B-lymphocyte survival through constitutive activation of the Ras/PI3K/Akt pathway." *Oncogene* 23(53): 8619-8628.

Press, O. W., M. LeBlanc, et al. (2001). "Phase III randomized intergroup trial of subtotal lymphoid irradiation versus doxorubicin, vinblastine, and subtotal lymphoid irradiation for stage IA to IIA Hodgkin's disease." *J Clin Oncol* 19(22): 4238-4244.

Reece, D. E., T. J. Nevill, et al. (1999). "Regimen-related toxicity and non-relapse mortality with high-dose cyclophosphamide, carmustine (BCNU) and etoposide (VP16-213) (CBV) and CBV plus cisplatin (CBVP) followed by autologous stem cell transplantation in patients with Hodgkin's disease." *Bone Marrow Transplant* 23(11): 1131-1138.

Rehwald, U., H. Schulz, et al. (2003). "Treatment of relapsed CD20+ Hodgkin lymphoma with the monoclonal antibody rituximab is effective and well tolerated: results of a phase 2 trial of the German Hodgkin Lymphoma Study Group." *Blood* 101(2): 420-424.

Salit, R. B., M. R. Bishop, et al. (2010). "Allogeneic hematopoietic stem cell transplantation: does it have a place in treating Hodgkin lymphoma?" *Curr Hematol Malig Rep* 5(4): 229-238.

Sandlund, J. T., C. H. Pui, et al. (2011). "Efficacy of high-dose methotrexate, ifosfamide, etoposide and dexamethasone salvage therapy for recurrent or refractory childhood malignant lymphoma." *Ann Oncol* 22(2): 468-471.

Schellong, G., W. Dorffel, et al. (2005). "Salvage therapy of progressive and recurrent Hodgkin's disease: results from a multicenter study of the pediatric DAL/GPOH-HD study group." *J Clin Oncol* 23(25): 6181-6189.

Schmitz, N., B. Pfistner, et al. (2002). "Aggressive conventional chemotherapy compared with high-dose chemotherapy with autologous haemopoietic stem-cell transplantation for relapsed chemosensitive Hodgkin's disease: a randomised trial." *Lancet* 359(9323): 2065-2071.

Schnell, R., M. Dietlein, et al. (2005). "Treatment of refractory Hodgkin's lymphoma patients with an iodine-131-labeled murine anti-CD30 monoclonal antibody." *J Clin Oncol* 23(21): 4669-4678.

Seiden, M. V., A. Elias, et al. (1992). "Pulmonary toxicity associated with high dose chemotherapy in the treatment of solid tumors with autologous marrow transplant: an analysis of four chemotherapy regimens." *Bone Marrow Transplant* 10(1): 57-63.

Sirohi, B., D. Cunningham, et al. (2008). "Long-term outcome of autologous stem-cell transplantation in relapsed or refractory Hodgkin's lymphoma." *Ann Oncol* 19(7): 1312-1319.

Smith, S. M., K. van Besien, et al. (2008). "Second autologous stem cell transplantation for relapsed lymphoma after a prior autologous transplant." *Biol Blood Marrow Transplant* 14(8): 904-912.

Trelle, S., O. Sezer, et al. (2007). "Bortezomib in combination with dexamethasone for patients with relapsed Hodgkin's lymphoma: results of a prematurely closed phase II study (NCT00148018)." *Haematologica* 92(4): 568-569.

Trippet, T. D. P., London W. (2004). "AHOD001, a pilot study of re-induction chemotherapy with ifosfamide and vinorelbine (IV) in children with refractory/relapsed Hodking Disease." *Proc Am Soc Hem.*

Visani, G., L. Malerba, et al. (2011). "BeEAM (bendamustine, etoposide, cytarabine, melphalan) before autologous stem cell transplantation is safe and effective for resistant/relapsed lymphoma patients." *Blood* 118(12): 3419-3425.

Younes, A., N. L. Bartlett, et al. (2010). "Brentuximab vedotin (SGN-35) for relapsed CD30-positive lymphomas." *N Engl J Med* 363(19): 1812-1821.

Younes, A., B. Pro, et al. (2006). "Experience with bortezomib for the treatment of patients with relapsed classical Hodgkin lymphoma." *Blood* 107(4): 1731-1732.

Younes, A., J. Romaguera, et al. (2003). "A pilot study of rituximab in patients with recurrent, classic Hodgkin disease." *Cancer* 98(2): 310-314.

Younes, A. F. M., Pro B. et al (2007). "A phase II study of a novel oral isotype-selective histone deacetylase (HDAC) inhibitor in patients with relapsed or refractory Hodgkin lymphoma." *J Clin Oncol*(25): 8000.

Yuen, A. R., S. A. Rosenberg, et al. (1997). "Comparison between conventional salvage therapy and high-dose therapy with autografting for recurrent or refractory Hodgkin's disease." *Blood* 89(3): 814-822.

Zheng, B., G. V. Georgakis, et al. (2004). "Induction of cell cycle arrest and apoptosis by the proteasome inhibitor PS-341 in Hodgkin disease cell lines is independent of inhibitor of nuclear factor-kappaB mutations or activation of the CD30, CD40, and RANK receptors." *Clin Cancer Res* 10(9): 3207-3215.

Part 9

Mucosa-Associated Lymphoid Tissue (MALT) Lymphoma

9

Mucosa-Associated Lymphoid Tissue (MALT) Lymphoma

Daisuke Niino and Koichi Ohshima
Department of Pathology, School of Medicine, Kurume University
Japan

1. Introduction

1.1 Definition

Extranodal marginal zone lymphoma of mucosa-associated lymphoid tissue (MALT lymphoma) is an extranodal lymphoma composed of morphologically heterogeneous small B-cells including marginal zone (centrocyte-like) cells, cells resembling monocytoid cells, small lymphocytes, and scattered immunoblasts and centroblast-like cells. There is plasma cell differentiation in a proportion of the cases. The infiltrate is in the marginal zone of reactive B-cell follicles and extends into the interfollicular region. In epithelial tissues, the neoplastic cells typically infiltrate the epithelium forming lymphoepithelial lesions. (Swerdlow et al., 2008) (Isaacson et al., 2004)

1.2 Epidemiology

MALT lymphoma accounts for 7% of all newly diagnosed lymphomas and is therefore one of the more common types of lymphoma (Swerdlow et al., 2008). Most cases occur in adults with a median age of 61 and a slight female preponderance (male:female ratio 1:1.2). (Anon, 1997) There appears to be a higher incidence of gastric MALT lymphomas in north-east Italy (Doglioni et al., 1992) and a special subtype previously known as alpha heavy chain disease and now called immunoproliferative small intestinal disease (IPSID) occurs in the Middle East (Pinkel, 1998), the Cape region of South Africa (Price, 1990) and a variety of other tropical and subtropical locations.

1.3 Etiology

MALT lymphoma is a unique tumor in that it originates from acquired MALT associated with chronic inflammation or autoimmune responses, e.g. *Helicobacter pylori* (*H. pylori*)-associated chronic gastritis, Hashimoto's thyroiditis, and Sjögren's syndrome (Swerdlow et al., 2008, Isaacson, 1999a). MALT lymphoma affects various organs, with the stomach being the most frequently involved (Swerdlow et al., 2008, Isaacson, 1999a, 1999b). Interestingly, the majority of gastric low-grade MALT lymphoma cases, those proven to be neoplastic by detection of monoclonal rearrangement in immunoglobulin heavy chain (IgH) genes, regress after eradication of *H. pylori* (Wotherspoon et al., 1993, Thiede et al., 2000).

1.4 Management

MALT lymphomas have an indolent natural course and are slow to disseminate. Recurrences, that can occur after many years, may involve other extranodal sites and occur more often in patients with extragastric MALT lymphomas than in patients with primary gastric disease (Raderer et al., 2005). The tumors are sensitive to radiation therapy, and local treatment may be followed by prolonged disease-free intervals. Involvement of multiple extranodal sites and even BM involvement do not appear to confer a worse prognosis (Thieblemont et al., 2000). Protracted remissions may be included in H. pylori-associated gastric MALT lymphoma by antibiotic therapy for H. pylori (Neubauer et al., 1997, Wotherspoon et al., 1993). Cases with the t(14;18)(q21;q21) appear to be resistant to H. pylori eradication therapy (Liu et al., 2001). In IPSID, remissions have followed therapy with broad-spectrum antibiotics (Ben Ayed et al., 1989, Lecuit et al., 2004). Antibiotics have also been used to successfully treat selected other MALT lymphomas. Transformation to diffuse large B-cell lymphoma may occur.

2. Regression of rectal MALT lymphoma after antibiotic treatments

2.1 Introduction

MALT lymphoma is less frequently seen in the rectum(Isaacson, 1999b, Morton et al., 1993, Koch et al., 2001), while the presence of *MALT1* gene translocation in rectal MALT lymphoma has occasionally been reported (Motegi et al., 2000, Remstein et al., 2000, Yonezumi et al., 2001). In addition, a few reports have described the regression of rectal MALT lymphomas after antibiotic treatments that are generally found to be successful for gastric MALT lymphomas(Raderer et al., 2000, Matsumoto et al., 1997).

In addition to *H. pylori*, various other infectious agents have been reported to be related to the development of MALT lymphoma, such as *Borrelia burgdorferi* in cutaneous(Roggero et al., 2000), *Chlamydia psittaci* in orbital(Ferreri et al., 2004), and *Campylobacter jejuni* in small intestinal lymphoma(Al-Saleem & Al-Mondhiry, 2005). However, few data are available on the pathogenesis of MALT lymphoma of organs other than the stomach.

In this study, we examined 8 rectal MALT lymphomas to determine whether they regressed after antibiotic treatments. We report here our findings and also discuss the relationship between rectal MALT lymphomas and *MALT1* gene genetic abnormalities (Niino et al., 2010).

2.2 Materials and methods

2.2.1 Rectal MALT lymphoma cases

Formalin-fixed, paraffin-embedded tissues obtained between 2004 and 2007 from 8 cases of rectal MALT lymphoma treated with antibiotic treatments were retrieved from the pathology files at Kurume University School. The patients consisted of 2 men and 6 women, ranging in age from 41 to 80 years (median, 66 years). Lymphomas constituting secondary involvement of the rectum were not included in the study. Clinical data for all cases were obtained from pathological reports and medical reports, and all cases were reviewed to confirm that the histological diagnosis conformed to the criteria of the World Health Organization Classification for Tumors of Hematopoietic and Lymphoid Tissues

(Swerdlow et al., 2008). Diagnosis of rectal MALT lymphomas was based on the following findings: centrocyte-like cells and/or monocytoid cell proliferation, especially at the outside of the mantle zone (marginal zone distribution); presence of plasmacytic differentiation and/or follicular colonization in some cases; and absence of CD5, CD10, and cyclin D1 overexpression. Lymphoepithelial lesions in rectal MALT lymphomas were not as obvious as those in gastric tumors (representative histologies are shown in Fig. 1.). All patients were Japanese. *H. pylori* infection was assessed by rapid- urease test or histological examination.

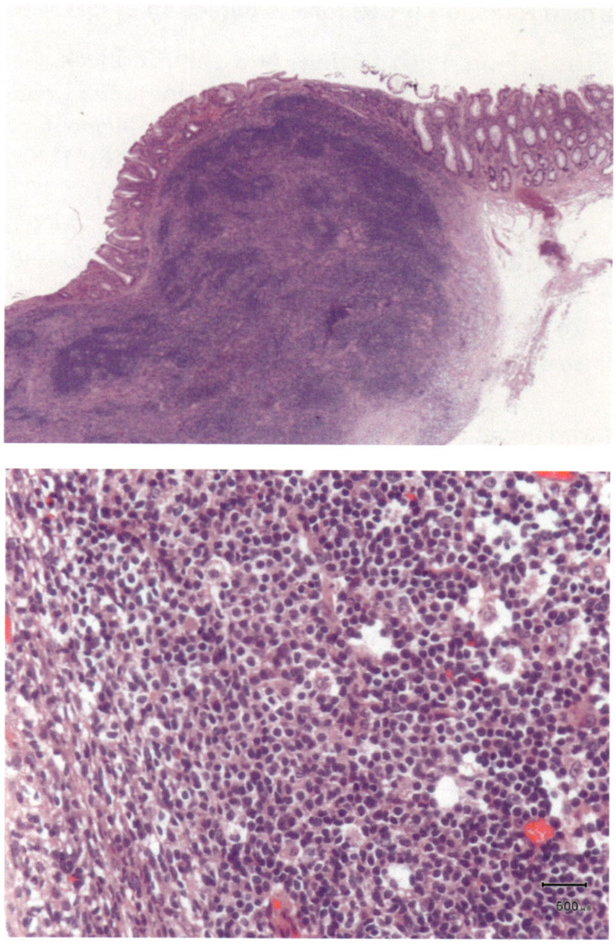

Fig. 1. Hematoxylin and eosin staining show the histopathologic features of rectal mucosa-associated lymphoid tissue (MALT) lymphoma. (A) Dense, diffuse atypical lymphocyte infiltration, mainly in submucosal layer. (B) MALT lymphoma cells showing small nuclei and abundant pale staining cytoplasm, resulting in a monocytoid appearance. (Niino et al., 2010)

Because Inoue and Chiba reported a case without infection of *H. pylori* whose rectal MALT lymphoma regressed after administration of antibiotics(Inoue & Chiba, 1999), the patients were treated with antibiotic treatments. After informed consent had been obtained, 8 patients underwent antibiotic treatments with a combination of antibiotics (clarithromycin and amoxicillin), and follow-up endoscopic examinations including biopsies were performed. Tumor regression after antibiotic treatments was histologically evaluated. Complete regression (CR) was defined as the total disappearance of lymphoma and absence of histopathological evidence of lymphoma on endoscopic biopsy. No regression (NR) was diagnosed when no macroscopic or histologic changes were present. This study was carried out in accordance with the Helsinki Declaration as revised in 1989 and with the ethical guidelines of the participating centers and countries.

2.2.2 Polymerase Chain Reaction (PCR) for the detection of IgH rearrangements

DNA was extracted from 5-µm-thich sections of a paraffin block. Gene amplification of the IgH gene from the framework 2 part of the V segment to the J region by a seminested PCR was performed by using the consensus primers complementary to the framework 2 portion of the VH region (FR2B) and the JH region (CFW1) from genomic DNA. The following primer sequences were used: FR2B, 5′-GTCCTGCAGGC(C/T)(C/T) CC-GG(A/G)AA(A/G)(A/G)GTCTGGAGTGG-3′; CFW1, 5′-ACCTGAGGAGACGGT-GACCAGGGT-3′. The PCR conditions were as follows: after initial denaturation at 95°C for 10 min, 5 cycles (95°C for 30 s, 63°C for 30 s and 72°C for 30 s) followed by 45 cycles (95°C for 30 s, 60°C for 30 s and 72°C for 30 s) with a final extension at 72°C for 10 min. The size of the IgH rearrangement fragments was usually between 250 and 300 bp.

2.2.3 *MALT 1* gene translocation analysis

All cases were analyzed using a *MALT1* break-apart probe (Vysis, Downer's Grove, IL, USA). Interphase fluorescence in situ hybridization (FISH) studies were performed on intact 5-µm sections of formalin-fixed, paraffin-embedded material as previously described in detail(Wongchaowart et al., 2006). Briefly, slides were baked overnight at 60°C, deparaffinized, and subjected to proteinase K treatment. After washing, 10 mL of the probe solution was applied, and probe and target DNA were allowed to codenature at 73°C for 5 minutes and to hybridize overnight at 3°C. Slides were counterstained with DAPI, and signals were visualized on an Axioskop photomicroscope (Zeiss, Oberkochen, Germany). For each probe 100-200 nuclei were scored. Nuclei were considered to be positive for a break-apart probe when a nucleus contained separate red and green signals at least three signal widths apart. Nuclei were scored as positive for +*MALT1* when three or more signals were identified within one nucleus. Cutoffs for interpretation as a positive result were determined for each abnormality based on the analysis of six formalin-fixed, paraffin-embedded sections of benign lymph nodes and tonsils used as control. Cutoff thresholds for each abnormality were established as the mean plus three standard deviations of the mean, so that positivity for *MALT1* translocation, or +*MALT1*, was defined as >4% nuclei with a positive signal pattern.

2.3 Results

2.3.1 Clinical features of rectal MALT lymphoma

Clinical characteristics of this study are shown in Table 1. The clinical records of all cases showed rectal origin. Four of eight patients (50%) were positive and one patient (13%) was negative for *H. pylori*. The remaining patients were not evaluated for *H. pylori*. Five cases occurred as a single tumor, whereas the remaining three cases occurred as multiple tumors. Elevated lesions (polypoid or flat elevation) were formed in 7 cases, whereas circumferential lesion was formed in one case (Case 4). Representative endoscopic image before antibiotic treatment demonstrated multiple small polyps (Case 2) (Fig. 2.). The size of MALT lymphoma ranged from 5 to 100 mm. Seven cases were localized in the submucosa, whereas one case (Case 4) involved the subserosa.

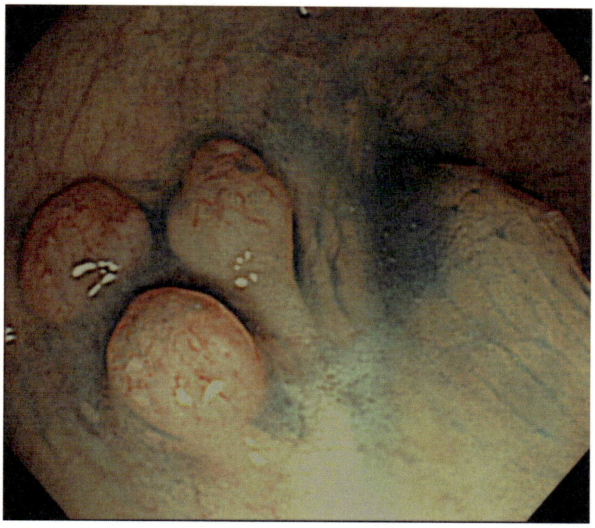

Fig. 2. Representative endoscopic image before antibiotic treatment (Case 2): Colonoscopy demonstrated multiple small polyps. (Niino et al., 2010)

Case no.	Age (y)	Sex	Number	Shape	Size (mm)	Depth	LDH (IU/l)	IL2R (U/ml)	*H.pylori* status
1	67	F	multiple	polypoid	5-10	SM	178	888	positive
2	68	F	single	flat elevation	25	SM	192	NA	positive
3	76	F	single	polypoid	10	SM	NA	NA	NA
4	65	M	single	circumferential	100	SS	NA	NA	NA
5	41	M	multiple	flat elevation	10	SM	215	530	negative
6	80	F	single	polypoid	20	SM	160	369	positive
7	54	F	single	polypoid	15	SM	156	NA	positive
8	46	F	multiple	polypoid	5-7	SM	NA	NA	NA

Abbreviations: LDH, lactate dehydrogenase; IL2R, interleukin 2 receptor; SM, submucosa; *H.pylori, Helicobacter pyroli*; SS, subserosa; NA, not available

Table 1. Clinical characteristics of rectal MALT lymphoma. (Niino et al., 2010)

2.3.2 Detection of IgH rearrangements and *MALT1* gene translocation

PCR for the detection of IgH rearrangement resulted in the identification of a monoclonal band in 7 cases (87.5%) (Table 2).

Results of interphase FISH studies are shown in Table 2 and Fig.3. All cases were successfully analyzed for *MALT1* translocation by FISH. One case demonstrated *MALT 1* gene translocation (one fusion, one orange, and one green signal pattern), while another case demonstrated partial deletion of the *MALT1* gene (one fusion and one green signal pattern). The others showed the normal pattern (two fusion signal patterns). That is, two cases (25%) showed genetic abnormality.

Case no.	PCR-IgH	MALT1 FISH	Response
1	Monoclonal	Negative	CR
2	Monoclonal	Negative	CR
3	Monoclonal	Negative	CR
4	Monoclonal	Partial deletion	NR
5	Monoclonal	Negative	NR
6	Polyclonal	Negative	CR
7	Monoclonal	Rearrangement	NR
8	Monoclonal	Negative	CR

Abbreviations: PCR, polymerase chain reaction;
IgH, immunoglobulin heavy chain;
MALT, mucosa associated lymphoid tissue;
FISH, fluorescence in situ hybridization;
CR, complete regression; NR, no regression.

Table 2. Results and clinical outcomes. (Niino et al., 2010)

2.3.3 Therapeutic outcomes

Therapeutic outcomes are shown in Table 2, 3. Eight patients who had undergone antibiotic treatments were subjected to follow-up colonoscopy after the treatment. Five patients (62.5%) achieved CR after a median follow-up from antibiotic treatments of 5 months (range, 3 to 58 months). Three patients (37.5%) showed NR, among which received further treatment, including chemotherapy. These findings strongly indicate that these cases of rectal MALT lymphoma were responsive to antibiotic treatments. None of the patients who responded to antibiotic treatments harbored *MALT1* gene genetic abnormality, but it was detected in two of the three patients who did not respond. The cases with *MALT1* gene genetic abnormality thus tended to be resistant to antibiotic treatments.

	Antibiotic treatments sensitive cases	Antibiotic treatments resistant cases	Total
Genetic abnormality (+)	0	2	2
Genetic abnormality (-)	5	1	6
Total	5	3	8

Table 3. Relationship between antibiotic treatments sensitivity and *MALT1* gene genetic abnormality. (Niino et al., 2010)

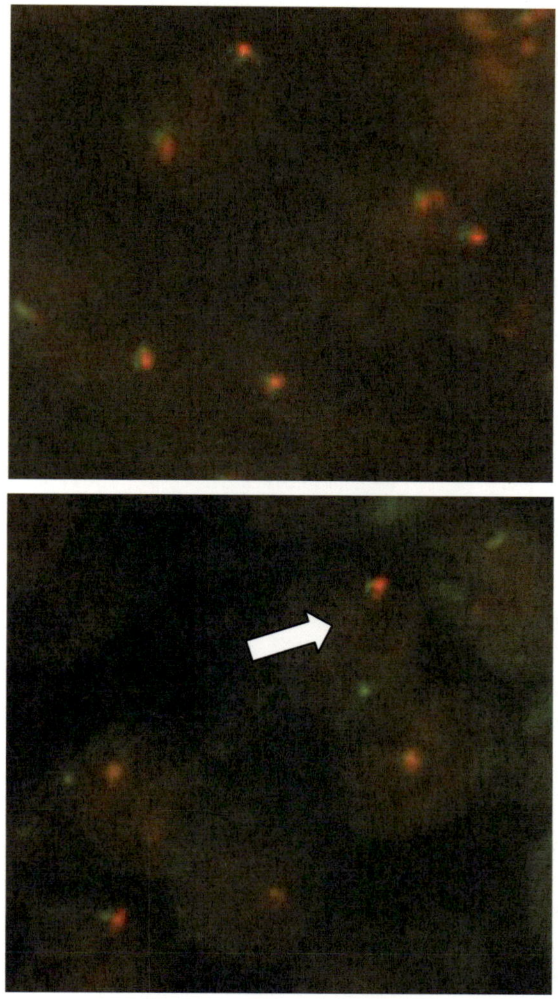

Fig. 3. Interphase fluorescence in situ hybridization (FISH) patterns in representative cases. (A) Normal pattern (two fusion signal patterns). (B) Partial deletion of *MALT1* gene (one fusion and one green signal pattern; arrows). (Niino et al., 2010)

2.4 Discussion

Gastric MALT lymphoma is often associated with infection by *H. pylori*. Eradication of *H. pylori* has therefore been investigated as the first line of treatment for patients with MALT lymphoma of the stomach, and has been found to be highly effective for patients with localized low-grade disease. On the other hand, regression of rectal MALT lymphoma after antibiotic treatments has also been reported. Matsumoto *et al.* reported the first case with rectal MALT lymphoma that regressed after antibiotic treatment in 1997 (Matsumoto et al., 1997). They also stated that the association of MALT lymphoma with *H. pylori* is not limited to the stomach, but involves other organs in which MALT is the predominant tissue for host defense. Inoue and Chiba reported a case without infection of *H. pylori* whose rectal MALT lymphoma regressed after administration of antibiotics(Inoue & Chiba, 1999). Nakase *et al.*

reported three *H. pylori*-negative cases of rectal MALT lymphoma which regressed after antibiotic treatments(Nakase et al., 2002). Regression of rectal MALT lymphoma after administration of quinolones has also been reported (Ferreri et al., 2005). These results suggest that some antigenic stimuli other than *H. pylori* may play a role in the pathogenesis of MALT lymphoma of the rectum, which is constantly exposed to intestinal bacteria and contents. However, for the time being this must remain an unproven hypothesis.

Recently, the *t*(11;18) chromosomal translocation was identified as a specific chromosomal abnormality in some MALT lymphomas, and the *API2-MALT1* fusion gene was found to be associated with this abnormality(Yonezumi et al., 2001). The *MALT1* gene is cloned by 18q21, while *API2*, an apoptosis inhibitor, is present in 11q21. Yonezumi et al. used RT-PCR to test a large series of MALT lymphomas for the presence of the *AP12-MALT1* fusion gene and found that pulmonary MALT lymphomas showed the highest incidence of the *AP12-MALT1* gene (62.5%) while the occurrence rates of MALT lymphomas of the stomach, orbit and large intestine ranged from 10 to 20%(Yonezumi et al., 2001). Sakugawa et al. used RT-PCR to examine 47 colorectal MALT lymphomas, including 27 primary rectal MALT lymphomas, for the *API2-MALT1* fusion gene. *API2-MALT1* fusion gene positivity was observed in 3 (11%) of 27 cases of rectal MALT lymphoma, and in 7 (15%) of 47 cases of colorectal MALT lymphoma(Sakugawa et al., 2003). In our study, the positive ratio for *MALT1* gene genetic abnormality was 2 (25%) of 8 cases of rectal MALT lymphoma. In addition, we found that rectal MALT lymphomas with *MALT1* gene genetic abnormality tend to be resistant for antibiotic treatments.

3. Conclusion

Ours is the first investigation of the regression of rectal MALT lymphoma after antibiotic treatments (Niino et al., 2010). Further follow-up will be needed to determine whether MALT lymphoma of the rectum regresses completely or is actually cured by antibiotic treatments. In addition, a large number of such cases needs to be analyzed to establish suitable standards for antibiotic treatments.

4. References

Al-Saleem, T. & Al-Mondhiry, H. (2005). Immunoproliferative small intestinal disease (IPSID): A model for mature B-cell neoplasms. *Blood,*Vol.105, pp. 2274-2280.

Anon. (1997). A clinical evaluation of the International Lymphoma Study Group classification of non-Hodgkin's lymphoma. The Non-Hodgkin's Lymphoma Classification Project. *Blood,* Vol.89, pp. 3909-3918.

Ben Ayed, F.; Halphen, M.; Najjar, T.; *et al.* (1989). Treatment of alpha chain disease. Results of a prospective study in 21 Tunisian patients by the Tunisian-French intestinal Lymphoma Study Group. *Cancer,* Vol.63, pp. 1251-1256.

Doglioni, C.; Wotherspoon, AC.; Moschini, A.; *et al.* (1992). High incidence of primary gastric lymphoma in north-eastern Italy. *Lancet,* Vol. 339, pp.834-835.

Ferreri, AJ.; Guidoboni, M.; Ponzoni, M.; *et al.* (2004). Evidence for an association between *Chlamydia psittaci* and ocular adnexal lymphomas. *J. Natl. Cancer Inst.,* Vol. 96, pp. 571-573.

Ferreri, AJ.; Ponzoni, M.; Guidoboni, M.; *et al.* (2005). Regression of Ocular Adnexal Lymphoma After *Chlamydia Psittaci*-Eradicating Antibiotic Therapy. *J. Clin. Oncol.,* Vol. 23, pp. 5067-5073.

Inoue, F. & Chiba, T. (1999). Regression of MALT lymphoma of the rectum after anti-H. pylori therapy in a patient negative for H. pylori. *Gastroenterology,* Vol.117, pp. 514–515.

Isaacson, PG. (1999). Mucosa-associated lymphoid tissue lymphoma. *Semin. Hematol.,* Vol.36, pp. 139–147.

Isaacson, PG. (1999). Gastrointestinal lymphomas of T- and B-cell types. *Mod. Pathol.,* Vol.12, pp. 151–158.

Isaacson, PG. & Du, MQ. (2004). MALT lymphoma: from morphology to molecules. *Nat Rev Cancer,* Vol.4, pp. 644-653.

Koch, P.; del Valle, F.; Berdel, WE.; *et al.* (2001). Primary gastrointestinal non-Hodgkin's lymphoma: I. Anatomic and histologic distribution, clinical features, and survival data of 371 patients registered in the German Multicenter Study GIT NHL 01/92. *J. Clin. Oncol.,* Vol.19, pp. 3861–3873.

Lecuit, M.; Abachin, E.; Martin, A.; *et al.*(2004). Immunoproliferative small intestinal disease associated with Campylobacter jejuni. *N Engl J Med,* Vol.350, pp.239-248.

Liu, H.; Ruskon-Fourmestraux, A.; Lavergne-Slove, A.; *et al.*(2001). Resistance of t(11;18) positive gastric mucosa-associated lymphoid tissue lymphoma to Helicobacter pylori eradication therapy. *Lancet,* Vol.357, pp. 39-40.

Matsumoto, T.; Iida, M.; & Shimizu, M. (1997). Regression of mucosa associated lymphoid-tissue lymphoma of rectum after eradication of *Helicobacter pylori. Lancet,* Vol.350, pp. 115–116.

Morton, JE.; Leyland, MJ.; Vaughan Hudson, G.; *et al.*(1993). Primary gastrointestinal non-Hodgkin's lymphoma: a review of 175 British National Lymphoma Investigation cases. *Br. J. Cancer,* Vol.67, pp.776–782.

Motegi, M.; Yonezumi, M.; Suzuki, H.; *et al.* (2000). *API2-MALT1* chimeric transcripts involved in mucosa-associated lymphoid tissue type lymphoma predict heterogeneous products. *Am. J. Pathol.,* Vol.156, pp. 807–812.

Nakase, H.; Ohana, M.; Ikeda, K.; *et al.*(2002). The possible involvement of microorganisms other than *Helicobacter pylori* in the development of rectal MALT lymphoma in *H. pylori*-negative patients. *Endoscopy,* Vol.34, pp. 343-346.

Neubauer, A.; Thiede, C.; Morgner, A.; *et al.*(1997). Cure of Helicobacter pylori infection and duration of remission of low-grade gastric mucosa-associated lymphoid tissue lymphoma. *J Natl Cancer Inst,* Vol.89, pp.1350-1355.

Niino, D.; Yamamoto, K.; Tsuruta, O.; *et al.* (2010). Regression of rectal mucosa-associated lymphoid tissue (MALT) lymphoma after antibiotic treatments. *Pathol Int,* Vol.60, pp. 438-342

Pinkel, D. (1998). Defferentiating juvenile myelomonocytic leukemia from infectious disease. *Blood,* Vol.91, pp.365-367.

Price, SK. (1990). Immunoproliferative small intestinal disease: a study of 13 cases with alpha heavy-chain disease. *Histopathology,* Vol.17, pp.7-17.

Raderer, M.; Pfeffel, F.; Pohl, G.; *et al.* (2000). Regression of colonic low grade B cell lymphoma of the mucosa associated lymphoid tissue type after eradication of *Helicobacter pylori. Gut,*Vol.46, pp. 133–135.

Raderer, M.; Streubel, B.; Woehrer, S.; *et al.* (2005). High relapse rate in patients with MALT lymphoma warrants lifelong follow-up. Clin Cancer Res 11: 3349-3352.
Remstein, ED.; James, CD. & Kurtin, PJ. (2000) Incidence and subtype specificity of *API2-MALT1* fusion translocations in extranodal, nodal, and splenic marginal zone lymphomas. *Am. J. Pathol.*, Vol.156, pp. 1183–1188.
Roggero, E.; Zucca, E.; Mainetti, C.; *et al.* (2000). Eradication of *Borrelia burgdorferi* infection in primary marginal zone B-cell lymphoma of the skin. *Hum. Pathol.*, Vol.31, pp. 263-268.
Sakugawa, ST.; Yoshino, T.; Nakamura, S.; *et al.*(2003). *API2-MALT1* fusion gene in colorectal lymphoma. *Mod. Pathol.*, Vol.16, pp. 1232–1241.
Swerdlow, SH.; Campo, E.; Harris, NL.; *et al.*(2008). WHO Classification of Tumours of Haematopoietic and Lymphoid Tissues. IARC: Lyon.
Thiede, C.; Wündisch, T.; Neubauer, B.; *et al.* (2000). Eradication of *Helicobacter pylori* and stability of remissions in low-grade gastric B-cell lymphomas of the mucosa-associated lymphoid tissue: results of an ongoing multicenter trial. *Recent Results Cancer Res.*, Vol.156, pp. 125–133.
Wongchaowart, NT.; Kim, B.; Hsi, ED., *et al.* (2006). t(14;18)(q32;q21) involving IGH and *MALT1* is uncommon in cutaneous MALT lymphomas and primary cutaneous diffuse large B-cell lymphomas. *J. Cutan. Pathol.*, Vol.33, pp. 286–292.
Wotherspoon, AC.; Doglioni, C.; Diss, TC.; *et al.* (1993). Regression of primary low-grade B-cell gastric lymphoma of mucosa-associated lymphoid tissue type after eradication of *Helicobacter pylori. Lancet,*Vol.342, pp. 575–577.
Yonezumi, M.; Suzuki, R.; Suzuki, H.; *et al.* (2001). Detection of *AP12-MALT1* chimaeric gene in extranodal and nodal marginal zone B-cell lymphoma by reverse transcription polymerase chain reaction (PCR) and genomic long and accurate PCR analyses. *Br. J. Haematol.*, Vol.115, pp. 588–594.

Part 10

Toxic Effects of Hodgkin's Lymphoma Treatment

10

Toxic Effects of Hodgkin Lymphoma Treatment

Alma Sofo Hafizović
Clinical Center University of Sarajevo,
Bosnia and Herzegovina

1. Introduction

In Hodgkin Lymphoma therapy chemotherapy and radiotherapy are applied, and both of them can cause early or late toxicity. Optimal treatment of Hodgkin Lymphoma understands applying "enough therapy, not too few or too much". Early and late toxicities, caused by applying chemotherapy and radiotherapy, will be analyzed with respect to system toxicity (haematological, gastrointestinal, cardiopulmonary toxicity, neurological, etc).

All anti tumour drugs that are used in treatment of this disease will be individually analyzed. These drugs are recommended by protocols suggested in the up to date guidelines. Also early and late toxicity of earlier applied types of radio therapy and Involved field (IF) irradiation will be observed. Late toxicity and development of secondary malignancy and sterility will be discussed separately. This will stress importance of applying special steps that will provide possibility of having offspring even in population of diseased and treated HL patients.

World-wide studies that confirmed toxicity of earlier applied protocols and irradiation treatments (total nodal, subtotal nodal and extended field) will also be discussed. These findings influenced new views of treating HL that understand applying chemotherapy in all clinical stages with or without IF irradiation.

Personal experiences will also be listed based on a studies of patients diagnosed with HL and treated at Haematology Clinic at Clinical Centre University Sarajevo. One such study had primary goal in determining secondary malignancies as a consequence of late toxicity in HL treatment. The study was conducted from 1992 - 2001. In the first group of patients in that study 10 patients (7.9%) were with secondary malignancy out of which one was with myelodysplasia, three with Non Hodgkin Lymphoma, six with solid carcinoma (Ca planocellulare papillae - one patient, Ca planocellulare laringys - one patient, Neo palatum molae - one patient and Ca mammae - three patients). In the same group, epidemiologically observed, the most patients ware aged from 14 to 24 years.

In our country, which is listed as undeveloped, first peak in age bimodal graph was shifted towards younger aged group (15-24 years). This indicates that even maximal success in HL treatment of these patients can, in 15-20 years after the treatment, question this success. This time span is cumulative period needed to develop malignant mutation. Second analyzed period is targeted towards analyzing patients with HL treated from 2002 - 2011 with applying chemotherapy using ABVD and BEACOPP protocol with or without IF irradiation.

To fully understand toxicity of the Hodgkin lymphoma therapy it is necessary to shortly review therapy applications. First therapy approaches in Hodgkin Lymphoma treatment appeared in period from 1932-1950 when treatment was conducted using herbs, X-rays and surgery. Vera Peters and her colleagues from Sanford University pioneered in the field of radiotherapy. They created high dose radiation therapy that was dominant from 1950 to 1970. (Peters M, 1950) Toxicities of such therapy approach were analyzed in the studies conducted in the upcoming years. Those studies changed further chemotherapy approaches from 1970 till 2008. (Kaplan HS, 1996)

Prior to the mid-1960s advanced-stage Hodgkin lymphoma was treated with single-agent chemotherapy. In 1964 Vincent DeVita and George Canellos at the National Cancer Institute (United States) developed the MOPP regimen. National Cancer Institute developed the first combination chemotherapy that cured a number of patients who relapsed after standard radiation therapy. (DeVita V. et al, 1970; De Vita V. et al, 1992.) ABVD was developed as a potentially less toxic end more effective alternative to MOPP. Initial results of ABVD regimen were published at Universita degli Studi di Milano in academic year 1974/1975 (thesis of a student led by Bonadonna Gianni) and these initial results were also published in 1975 by an Italian group led by Bonadonna. (Bonadonna G et al, 1975)

In 1994 German Hodgkin's Lymphoma study Group (GHSG), lead by Volker Dihel, developed a regimen BEACOPP in an attempt to improve the prospect for patients with advanced disease stages. Results were published subsequently for a large prospectively randomised trial HD9 in patients with previously untreated advanced Hodgkin lymphoma. (Diehl V. et al, 1998).

Further improvement of Hodgkin lymphoma treatment is introduction of high dose therapy followed by autologous stem cell transplantation (HDT-ASCT). New findings in the field of immunology and molecular biology, as well as many studies that analyzed response and toxicity of previous therapy options, influenced adoption of contemporary individual treatment approach with application of targeted immunotherapy. This does not conclude HL as there are large numbers of Hodgkin Lymphoma patients that do not achieve required response. Also different treatment complications require constant improvement of therapy approach. Contemporary approach is ever more directed towards researching targeted therapy using antibodies, immunomodulators, HDAC inhibitors and m-TOR inhibitors.

In Hodgkin Lymphoma therapy currently Chemotherapy and Radiotherapy are most often used.

1.1 Chemotherapy

Most often protocol is ABVD which gives 82% CR and 72% OS with follow up of 8 years. On the other side, BEACOPP gives 88% CR1 baseline (B) vs. 96% escalated (E), FFS 76%(B) and 87%(E) and OS of 88% (B) and 91% (E) and follow up of 5 years (Michael C. et al, 2008a; Griffin R. et al., 2010). Up to date treatment options (from 2011) are conducted using EORTC, NCCN and GHSG guidelines. These guidelines state that following protocols (along with ABVD and BEACOPP) are to be used: Stanford V, DHAP, ICE, ASHAP, MINE, Mini-BEAM, HDT+SCT; and rarely: VIM-D, MIME, GVD, GDP, GCD, GEM-P, IGEV, EPOCH, CVP, ABVD/MOPP, COPP/ABVD, COPP, CHLVPP, EVA.

1.2 Radiotherapy

Radiation volume in HL was used in three ways: mantle field, paraaortic region and pelvis. The *mantle field* region encompassed the cervical, supraclavicular, infraclavicular, axillary, mediastinal and hilar nodes. (Sandra J. Horning 2001) *Paraaortic* understands irradiation of spleen and pelvis area individually or in continuity when marked as inverse Y. If all stated areas are used, irradiation is marked as total nodal (TN). If mantle field and paraaortic area are used irradiation is named subtotal nodal (STNI), while only mantle field is marked as extended field (EFRT). There is also involved field (IF) that encompasses lymph node in question and complete lymph drain.(Griffin R. et al., 2010)

Optimal treatment of Hodgkin Lymphoma understands applying "enough therapy, not too few or too much". In creating HL treatment plan, it is very important to define illness and its risks, and fully review patient's condition. Meaning, early favourable and early unfavourable, as well as advanced stage with risk factors (IPS: age, gender, Hgb, albumin < 40g/l, advanced stage IV, white cell count > 15000/mm^2 absolute lymphocyte count) with respect to comorbidity. Pet CT gives significant data regarding disease stage and evaluation of disease location as well as its absence, and hence it gives possibility of optimal therapy dosage. Special attention is required when dealing with younger patients and females younger than 30 years as infertility and secondary malignancies can occur.

1.3 Toxic effects

In Hodgkin Lymphoma therapy, application of chemotherapy and radiotherapy has healing effect but also has different toxic side effects. These side effects can cause early and late toxicity (acute and chronic side effects) which can occur in different systems: haematological, cardiovascular, respiratory, gastrointestinal, renal, urogenital, neurological, reproduction system and skin. These toxicities affect pregnancy and can have carcinogenic effect. Early toxicities are relatively easy to overcome, while late toxicity occurs in the form of: sterility, cardiovascular disease, pulmotoxicity, neurotoxicity and secondary malignancy what poses significant complications. Quality of life and reduction of early and late toxicity represent significant goals in the Hodgkin Lymphoma treatment.

2. Toxicities according to affected system during HL treatment

By applying chemotherapy and radiotherapy different toxicities can occur. Most significant toxicities are named in the remaining of this section and for each of them most important characteristics are listed.

2.1 Hematotoxicity

This toxicity causes *secondary leukaemia, hemolytic anemia* and *myelosuppression* which is most often followed by *neutropenia* which is further most often followed by sepsis. Most difficult cases are when sepsis is caused by gram-negative bacteria or respiratory infection with possibility of ARDS. *Thrombocytopenia* with grade 4 (according to WHO) can cause significant bleedings. A*nemia* can reduce working ability, tissue ischemia or worsened cardiovascular diseases.

2.2 Cardiotoxicity

Pericardium: acute pericarditis, Constrictive pericarditis from 1-6 months of radiotherapy
Myocardium: myocardial fibrosis, Progressive and restrictive cardiomyopathy
Blood vessels: *coronary arterial disease* (CAD) and structural changes in coronary arteries which are similar to atherosclerosis
Valvular disease: Predominantly affects mitral valve and aortic valve (both regurgitation and stenosis possible)
Conduction system: *arrhythmia* (persistent tachycardia) and complete or incomplete atrioventricular block. (Christopher F. 2010)

2.3 Pulmonary toxicity

Most often toxicities are lung fibrosis and pneumonitis.

2.4 Gastrointestinal complications of chemotherapy

Following gastrointestinal complications can occur: nausea, vomiting, emesis, diarrhea, ileus, mucositis, ventricular and colon neoplasm .
Hepatotoxicity: laesio hepatis.

2.5 Urogenital/Renal toxicity

Most often toxicities are cystitis and renal insufficiency.

2.6 Endocrine

Following can occur in the endocrine system: hypothyroidism, Grave's disease, thyroiditis, thyrotoxicosis, thyroid nodule, thyroid malignancies.

2.7 Gonadal complications teratogenicity of cancer therapy

Infertility occurs in both genders. Azoospermia and hormonal elevation occur in male patients while amenorrhoea and FSH elevation occur in females.

2.8 Dermatologic toxicity

Alopecia, erythema and exanthema, striae, hyperpigmentation, oedema, hyperkeratosis, pruritus and nail changes are often dermatologic toxicities.
Local toxicity: Extravasation (necrotizing is possible)

2.9 Secondary malignancies after chemotherapy

Most difficult complications occur on lungs, breast, stomach, colon and thyroid gland. Also malignant melanoma, aggressive and indolent lymphoma and acute secondary leukaemia can occur as secondary malignancies.

2.10 Other

Hypersensitivity reactions are possible to occur.

3. Early and late toxicity of drugs used in HL treatment

When applying drugs it is extremely important to know the cumulative dosage that causes toxicity.

Drug	Cumulative dosage	Substance
Adriamycin / Doxorubicin	450-550 mg/m^2	Anthracyclines
Bleomicin	Pulmotoxicity >300mg (age <15 and >65 years)	Antibiotic
Lomustin/CCNU	Cumulative dosage of nephrotoxicity >1200-1500mg/m^2	Alkylating agent
Dacarbazin/DTIC	standard doze 200-375/m^2 /d i.v, during 3-4 weeks 750-850mg/m^2//d i.v during 4 weeks	non classic Alkylating agent
Carmustin/BCNU	Pulmotoxicity >1000mg/m^2	Alkylating agent
Prokarbazin	>/=4g/m^2	non classic Alkylating agent
Vinkristin	neurotoxicity >20 mg cumulative dosage	Vinca alkaloids
Cisplatin	>100-200 mg/m^2	Alkylating agent
Cyclophosphamide	>7,5g/m^2, Mega dose 16 -19 g/m^2/ (application of these dosages only in specialized haematological and oncology centres)	Alkylating agent
Chlorambucil	Lung fibrosis >2000mg	Alkylating agent
Melphalan	>/=140 mg/m^2	Alkylating agent
Carboplatin	</2g/m^2	Alkylating agent
Rituximab/Mabthera*	standard dosage 375/ m^2	monoclonal antibody

Table 1. Drugs used in HL treatment and their cumulative dosages (Berger D.P. et al, 2002).

3.1 Adriamycin/Doxorubicin

Application of this drug can cause following toxicities:
Hematotoxicity: myelosuppression; *Cardiotoxicity*: acute (arrhythmia, ischemia, infarct) and chronic (dilatative cardiomyopathy) side effects. Risk groups: earlier cardiac illness, younger than 15 and older than 65 years, bolus injection, mediastinum irradiation, cumulative dosage larger than 450-550/mg/m^2; *Gastrointestinal complications of Chemotherapy*: nausea, vomiting, mucositis, stomatitis, diarrhea; *Dermatologic Toxicity:* exanthem, urticaria, alopecia, rarely hyperpigmentation.*Local toxicity*: extravasation; *Gonadal Complications*: infertility; *Second Malignancies after Chemotherapy:* potentially mutagenic, teratogenic and carcinogenic. (Berger D.P. et al, 2002)

3.2 Bleomycin

Application of this drug can cause following toxicities:
Hematotoxicity: myelosuppression; *Pulmonary Toxicity*: interstitial pneumonitis and lung fibrosis; *Gastrointestinal complications of Chemotherapy*: nausea, emesis, loss of appetite,

mucositis, diarrhea; *Dermatologic Toxicity*: alopecia, erythema, exanthem, striae, hyperpigmentation, oedema, hyperkeratosis, pruritus, nail changes; *Other*: fever, myalgia, shivering. (Berger D.P. et al, 2002)

3.3 Carboplatin

Application of this drug can cause following toxicities:
Hematotoxicity: myelosuppression; *Gastrointestinal complications of Chemotherapy*: nausea, emesis, loss of appetite, mucositis. Liver: transitory increase of transaminase; *Renal Toxicity*: rarely nephrotoxicity which appears upon inadequate rehydration; *Dermatologic Toxicity*: alopecia, erythema, dermatitis, allergies, pruritus; *Neurotoxicity*: rarely peripheral neurotoxicity, rarely hearing problems and optic neuritis; *Gonadal Complications*: infertility; *Other*: fever, shivering. (Berger D.P. et al, 2002)

3.4 Carmustin (BCNU)

Application of this drug can cause following toxicities:
Hematotoxicity: myelosuppression; *Pulmonary Toxicity*: interstitial pneumonitis, lung infiltrate and lung fibrosis upon administering cumulative dosage; *Gastrointestinal complications of Chemotherapy*: nausea, emesis, mucositis, diarrhoea, rarely esophagitis, ulcer, gastrointestinal bleeding. Liver: transitory increase of transaminase, veno-occlusive-disease (VOD); *Renal toxicity*: renal insufficiency; *Dermatologic Toxicity*: alopecia, dermatitis, erythema, hyperpigmentation; *Neurotoxicity*: peripheral and central neurotoxicity, psychoorganic syndrome, neuroretinitis, optic neuritis, ataxia; *Gonadal Complications*: infertility, azoospermia, amenorrhoea. (Berger D.P. et al, 2002)

3.5 Chlorambucil

Application of this drug can cause following toxicities:
Hematotoxicity: myelosuppression; *Pulmotoxicity*: lung fibrosis, cumulative dosage larger than 2000mg; *Gastrointestinal complications of Chemotherapy*: nausea, emesis, mucositis. Liver: transitory transaminase increase, rarely heavier liver toxicity; *Dermatologic Toxicity*: alopecia, erythema; *Neurotoxicity*: rarely peripheral and central neurotoxicity; *Gonadal Complications*: infertility (cumulative dose > 400mg) amenorrhoea and azoospermia; *Other*: fever, rarely cystitis; *Second Malignancies after Chemotherapy*: potentially mutagen, carcinogen and teratogenic. (Berger D.P. et al, 2002)

3.6 Cisplatin

Application of this drug can cause following toxicities:
Hematotoxicity: myelosuppression; *Cardiotoxicity*: rarely rhythm disorders, cardiac insufficiency; *Gastrointestinal Complications of Chemotherapy*: nausea, emesis, loss of appetite, mucositis, diarrhoea, enteritis. Liver: transitory transaminase increase; *Renal toxicity*: electrolyte disbalance: decrease of level of Na, K, Ca and Mg. Cumulative dosage – nephrotoxicity followed with tubular insufficiency; *Dermatologic Toxicity*: alopecia, dermatitis, allergy reactions; *Neurotoxicity*: peripheral neurotoxicity, ototoxicity, when applying cumulative dosage > 100-200mg/m^2, dizziness, rarely focal encephalopathy, optic neuritis; *Gonadal Complications*: infertility; *Other*: Local toxicity: local phlebitis, possible necrotizing extravasation. (Berger D.P. et al, 2002)

3.7 Cyclophosphamide

Application of this drug can cause following toxicities:
Hematotoxicity: myelosuppression; *Cardiotoxicity*: high dosage - in 5-10% cases acute myopericarditis, cardio insufficiency, and hemorrhagic myocardium necrosis; *Pulmotoxicity*: high dosage - lung fibrosis, pneumonitis; *Gastrointestinal complications of Chemotherapy*: nausea, emesis, mucositis, stomatitis, loss of appetite Liver: transitory transaminase increase, rarely cholestasis; *Urogenital Toxicity*: hemorrhagic cystitis when applying high therapy doses; *Renal toxicity:* renal insufficiency; *Dermatologic Toxicity*: alopecia, rarely hyperpigmentation, dermatitis, erythema; *Neurotoxicity*: when applying high dosages - acute encephalopathy; *Gonadal Complications*: infertility, azoospermia, amenorrhea; *Other*: fever, allergy reactions. (Berger D.P. et al, 2002)

3.8 Cytarabin

Application of this drug can cause following toxicities:
Hematotoxicity: myelosuppression; *Pulmonary Toxicity*: when applying high dosages - pulmotoxicity, lung oedema, ARDS (acute respiratory distress syndrome); *Gastrointestinal Complications of Chemotherapy*: nausea, emesis, mucositis, diarrhoea, loss of appetite, when applying high dosages rarely pancreatitis, ulcer, esophagitis, colon necrosis Liver: transitory transaminase increase, cholestasis; *Dermatologic Toxicity*: dermatitis, erythema, exanthema, conjunctivitis, keratitis, alopecia; *Neurotoxicity*: peripheral and central neurotoxicity, cerebral and cerebellum disorders at patients > 60 years and high dose therapy (48 g/m2). After intrathecal application - acute arachnoiditis and leukoencephalopathy; *Other*: fever, myalgia, arthralgia, bone pain. (Berger D.P. et al, 2002)

3.9 Dacarbazine (DTIC)

Application of this drug can cause following toxicities:
Hematotoxicity: myelosuppression; *Gastrointestinal complications of Chemotherapy*: nausea, emesis, rarely mucositis, diarrhoea, Liver: transitory transaminase increase, veno-occlusive-disease (VOD); *Renal toxicity*: Kidneys: rarely renal insufficiency; *Dermatologic Toxicity*: alopecia, erythema, exanthem, photosensitivity, allergy reactions; *Neurotoxicity*: rarely CNS disorders (headache, sight disorders, confusion, lethargy, spasms, paresthesia); *Other*: fever, myalgia, shivering. Local toxicity: extravasation, local thromboflebitis. (Berger D.P. et al, 2002)

3.10 Etopozid/VP-16

Application of this drug can cause following toxicities:
Hematotoxicity: myelosuppression; *Cardiotoxicity*: rarely arrhythmia, hypotonia at intravenous application, ischemia; *Gastrointestinal complications of Chemotherapy*: nausea, emesis, rarely mucositis, dysphagia, diarrhea, constipation, Liver: transitory transaminase increase; *Dermatologic Toxicity*: alopecia, rarely erythema, hyperpigmentation, allergy reactions; *Neurotoxicity*: rarely peripheral neuropathy and CNS disorders (somnolence); *Gonadal Complications*: infertility. (Berger D.P. et al, 2002)

3.11 Gemcitabin

Application of this drug can cause following toxicities:

Hematotoxicity: myelosuppression; *Pulmonary Toxicity*: Lung oedema (rarely); *Gastrointestinal complications of Chemotherapy*: nausea, emesis, rarely mucositis, diarrhoea; *Renal toxicity*: proteinuria, hematuria, Liver: transitory transaminase increase; *Dermatologic Toxicity*: rarely erythema, pruritus, rarely alopecia, oedema; *Other*: peripheral oedema. (Berger D.P. et al, 2002)

3.12 Ifosfamid

Application of this drug can cause following toxicities:
Hematotoxicity: myelosuppression; *Gastrointestinal complications of Chemotherapy*: loss of appetite, nausea, emesis, mucositis, diarrhoea. Liver: transitory transaminase increase, rarely cholestasis; *Urogenital*: hemorrhaging cystitis when applying cumulative dosage; *Renal toxicity*: renal insufficiency; *Dermatologic Toxicity*: alopecia, rarely urticaria, hyperpigmentation; *Neurotoxicity*: acute encephalopathy, cerebellum neurotoxicity, confusion, psychosis, ataxia, spasms, somnolence, coma. Prophylaxis natriumbicarbonat, therapy: methylene blue; *Gonadal Complications*: infertility; *Other*: fever, allergy reactions. (Berger D.P. et al, 2002)

3.13 Lomustin (CCNU)

Application of this drug can cause following toxicities:
Hematotoxicity: myelosuppression; *Pulmonary Toxicity*: rarely lung infiltration, lung fibrosis; *Gastrointestinal complications of Chemotherapy*: nausea, emesis, mucositis, diarrhea; *Renal toxicity*: renal insufficiency when applying cumulative dosage; *Dermatologic Toxicity*: alopecia, dermatitis, hyperpigmentation; *Neurotoxicity*: peripheral and central neurotoxicity; *Gonadal Complications*: infertility, amenorrhea, azoospermia. (Berger D.P. et al, 2002)

3.14 Mechlorethamine/Nitrogen mustard

Application of this drug can cause following toxicities:
Hematotoxicity: myelosuppression, hemolytic anemia; *Gastrointestinal complications of Chemotherapy*: nausea, vomiting (almost 100%) onest may be within minutes of drug administration, diarrhea, and anorexia. Liver: hepatotoxicity; *Dermatologic Toxicity*: alopecia, hyperpigmentation of veins, contact and allergic dermatitis (50% with topical use); *Gonadal Complications*: azoospermia, chromosomal abnormalities, delayed menstrual cycle, oligomenorrhea, amenorrhea, impaired spermatogenesis; *Neurotoxicity*: peripheral neuropathy; *Second Malignancies after Chemotherapy*: carcinogenicity, mutagenicity, teratogenicity.

3.15 Melfalan

Application of this drug can cause following toxicities:
Hematotoxicity: myelosuppression; *Pulmonary Toxicity*: rarely lung fibrosis; *Gastrointestinal complications of Chemotherapy*: loss of appetite, nausea, emesis, mucositis, diarrhoea; *Dermatologic Toxicity*: rarely alopecia, exanthem, erythema, urticaria, pruritus, oedema; *Gonadal Complications*: infertility; *Other*: rarely allergy reactions. (Berger D.P. et al, 2002)

3.16 Methotrexat

Application of this drug can cause following toxicities:

Hematotoxicity: myelosuppression; *Gastrointestinal complications of Chemotherapy*: mucositis, nausea, vomiting, emesis, diarrhea, gastrointestinal bleeding; Liver: acute and chronic liver insufficiency; *Renal toxicity*: Renal insufficiency; *Dermatologic Toxicity*: exanthem, dermatitis, pruritus, conjunctivitis, allergy reactions; *Neurotoxicity*: reversible acute encephalopathy after intravenous and intrathecal application, leukoencephalopathy; *Other*: rarely allergies. (Berger D.P. et al, 2002)

3.17 Mitoxantron

Application of this drug can cause following toxicities:
Hematotoxicity: myelosuppression; *Cardiotoxicity*: chronic cardiotoxicity, cardiomyopathy, heart insufficiency; *Gastrointestinal complications of Chemotherapy*: nausea, emesis, mucositis, rarely gastrointestinal bleeding. Liver: transitory transaminase increase, rarely cholestasis *Renal toxicity*: rarely renal insufficiency; *Dermatologic Toxicity:* alopecia, allergy reactions, dermatitis, pruritus; *Gonadal Complications*: infertility; *Second Malignancies after Chemotherapy*: secondary acute leukaemia. (Berger D.P. et al, 2002)

3.18 Prednisone

Application of this drug can cause following toxicities:
Immunosuppression, affects apoptosis in internal signal path, thrombosis with consequential infarct of the affected tissue, suppression adrenal gland, retention Na, decrease of K, iatrogenic diabetes mellitus, psychoses especially severe in older patients.

3.19 Prokarbazin

Application of this drug can cause following toxicities:
Hematotoxicity: myelosuppression; *Cardiotoxicity*: tachycardia, hypotonia; *Gastrointestinal complications of Chemotherapy*: nausea, emesis, rarely mucositis, dysphagia, diarrhoea, Liver: transitory transaminase increase; *Dermatologic Toxicity*: alopecia, erythema, exanthem, photosensitivity, hyperpigmentation, allergy reactions; *Neurotoxicity*: reversible peripheral neurotoxicity, rarely CNS disorders (Somnolence), agitation, depression, hallucinations; *Gonadal Complications*: infertility; *Second Malignancies after Chemotherapy*: secondary malignancies; *Other*: fever, shivering, myalgia, arthralgia, gynecomasty. (Berger D.P. et al, 2002)

3.20 Vinblastin

Application of this drug can cause following toxicities:
Hematotoxicity: myelosuppression; *Cardiotoxicity*: cardiovascular complications, hypertonia, hypotonia; *Pulmonary Toxicity*: acute interstitial pneumonitis, bronchospasm; *Gastrointestinal complications of Chemotherapy*: rarely constipation, ileus, nausea, emesis, diarrhoea, mucositis, rarely gastrointestinal bleeding; *Dermatologic Toxicity*: alopecia, erythema, exanthem, photo sensation; *Neurotoxicity*: peripheral neurotoxicity when applying cumulative dosage, paresthesia, rarely motoric disorders; *Other*: muscle spasms, Local toxicity: necrotizing extravasation. (Berger D.P. et al, 2002)

3.21 Vinkristin

Application of this drug can cause following toxicities:

Hematotoxicity: myelosuppression; *Cardiotoxicity*: cardiovascular complications, hypertonia, hypotonia; *Pulmonary Toxicity*: acute interstitial pneumonitis, bronchospasm; *Gastrointestinal complications of Chemotherapy:* constipation, Ileus, nausea, emesis, mucositis, rarely pancreatitis.*Renal toxicity*: polyuria (decrease of pad secretion ADH), dysuria; *Dermatologic Toxicity*: alopecia, erythema; *Neurotoxicity*: peripheral neurotoxicity (cumulative dosage), CNS disorders: hypesthesia, paresthesia, motoric disorders, areflexia, rarely severe complications like paralysis, ataxia, paralytic ileus, optic atrophia, blindness, spasms; *Gonadal Complications*: infertility. Local toxicity: necrotizing extravasation; *Other*: rarely fever, shivering. (Berger D.P. et al, 2002)

3.22 Vinorelbina

Application of this drug can cause following toxicities:
Hematotoxicity: myelosuppression; *Gastrointestinal complications of Chemotherapy*: rarely constipation, nausea, emesis, diarrhoea, Mucositis; *Dermatologic Toxicity*: alopecia; *Neurotoxicity*: peripheral neurotoxicity when applying cumulative dosage, paresthesia, rarely motoric disorders; *Other*: muscle spasms, Local toxicity: necrotizing extravasation. (Berger D.P. et al, 2002)

4. Toxicities that occur when applying most often used protocols

4.1 Chemotherapy toxicities

Early complications: nausea, vomiting, emesis, alopecia, myelosuppression.
Late complications: Sterility (primarily with MOPP-based regimens, BEACOPP, least with ABVD), Neuropathy (primarily with Vincristine), Cardiomyopathy (primarily with doxorubicin ABVD, COPP/ABVD), Pulmonary fibrosis (primarily with Bleomycin COPP/ABVD, BEACOPP) and Secondary leukaemia (primarily with MOPP, Radiotherapy (RT), BEACOPP escalating more than baseline). (Griffin R. et al., 2010)

4.1.1 ABVD vs. BEACOPP

The most used protocol is ABVD and most studies suggest that it is protocol with least toxicity. One of the largest randomized studies, conducted in multiple centres, is "The GHSG- Successor-trials De-escalation of BEACOPP Advanced stages of Hodgkin lymphoma". It summarized data from three studies (**HD9, HD12 and HD15**) and is still conducted on **HD18**. In analysis of the treatment of advanced HL stages it used data from more than 500 centres including 220 oncologists and over 4500 patients treated with BEACOPP and ABVD. The study confirmed that ABVD had less toxicity (40-90%), lower infertility rate (90% male/52% female in BEACOPP E vs. 34% in ABVD), AML/MDS (1.2% in BEACOPP E vs. <0.5% in ABVD). On the other hand BEACOPP E had higher CR rates (>90%), Higher tumour cell kill PFS (90% vs. 79% in ABVD), Cure rate of 11% (higher at 10 years) and 20% less need for salvage therapy. (Diehl V, 2009)

Study **GHSG HD14** compared BEACOPP with ABVD in early unfavourable HL. Two cycles of BEACOPP escalated followed by 2xABVD and IFRT results in a significant improvement in tumor control compared to 4x ABVD + IFT. Toxicities for ABVD x4+IFT were following: acute grade III/IV toxicity 50.7 %, leucopoenia 24%, thrombocytopenia 0.1%, anemia 1%,

Gr.III/IV infection 3.4% and total of 19 secondary malignancies. On the other hand, toxicity in group 2x BEACOPP E + 2xABVD+IFT were: acute grade III/IV toxicity 87.1%, leucopoenia 79%, thrombocytopenia 22%, anaemia 9%, Gr.III/IV infection 7.3% and total of 16 secondary malignancies. It is important to state that OS was same in the two groups. (Engert A. et al, 2010).

Results from the **HD 2000** - Gruppo Italiano study conducted on patients with advanced stage HL indicate that BEACOPP improved FFS/PFS but has no difference in RFS or OS with increased toxicity, especially hematotoxicity. Hematotoxicity in the BEACOPP group (98 patients) was Gr.3/4 WHO, WBC/Plts 57/22, and in the ABVD group (99 patients) it was 3/34. BEACOPP was associated with higher severe infection rates than ABVD. (Federico M. et al, 2009) In the study "ABVD vs. BEACOPP for Hodgkin's lymphoma when High Dose Salvage Is Planned" Simonetta Viviani also concludes that "Treatment with BEACOPP, as compared with ABVD, resulted in better initial tumour control, but the long-term clinical outcome did not differ significantly between the two regimens". (Simoneta V. et al, 2011).

A randomized trial conducted from 2000 to 2007 by the Michelangelo, GITIL and IIL cooperative group in the analysis of the 3 year outcome ABVD vs. BEACOPP in advanced HL analyzed 321 patients diseased with HL stage IIB/IV and/or ≥3IPS, compared efficiency of 6-8 ABVD cycles vs. BEACOPP 4 escalating cycles + BEACOPP 4 baseline cycles in the first line. It confirmed significant difference of FFP (71±4% vs. 87±3%) but non-significant 3-yr OS (91±3% vs. 90±3%). Results of later relapses and secondary malignancies were not represented due to a longer follow up. (Gianni A.M. et al, 2008).

Other **HD12** study of GHSG at IIB and advanced stage III and IV with IPI ≥ 3 in application of 8 cycles BE vs. 4 BE+ 4BB confirmed that treatment-related toxicity of WHO grade III/IV was observed in 97% of patients. Most prominent differences between pooled chemotherapy (8x BEACOPP escalating + 0 Gy), was anaemia (65% 8BE vs. 51% 4BE+4BB) and thrombopenia (65% vs. 51%). There was 9.9% deaths (22 vs. 32 acute or salvage treatment toxicity; 15 vs. 24 HL; 22 vs. 13 secondary neoplasia). Secondary neoplasias were observed in 77 patients (4.9%). (Diehl V. et al, 2009)

Analysis of BEACOPP baseline vs. BEACOPP escalating confirmed acute haematological toxicity: Leucopoenia gr.4 WHO 37% vs. 93%, thrombocytopenia gr.4 WHA 5% vs. 49%, anemia gr. 3 WHO 17% vs. 50%, anemia gr. 4 WHO 4% vs. 19%. (Diehl V. et al, 1998)

4.1.2 Secondary malignancies

Increased risk of solid tumours was noted by numerous authors (Tucker MA et al, 1988; Boivin JF. Et al, 1984). When applying ABVD protocol, risk of NHL is increased where DLBCL can occur both early and later after treatment. (Van LF. et al, 1989)

After 10 years of follow up of the GHSG **HD9** study final results in the treatment of advanced stage and application of 6 COPP/ABVD vs. 6 BEACOPP baseline vs. 6 BEACOPP escalating, confirmed following toxicity: total of 74 secondary malignancies (6.2%) were documented including acute myeloid leukaemia (0.4%, 1.5% and 3.0%), non Hodgkin Lymphoma (2.7%, 1.7% and 1.0%) and solid tumours (2.7%, 3.4% and 1.9%). Corresponding overall secondary malignancy rates were 5.7%, 6.6% and 6.0% respectively. (Andreas E. et al, 2009). The same study with results published in 2007 confirmed that cardiac toxicity is mostly expressed in COPP/ABVD, pulmotoxicity in COPP/ABVD and baseline BEACOPP. Cardiotoxicity was 1.2%, 0.9% and 0.9%, while pulmotoxicity 0.4%, 0.4% and 0.2%. (Diehl V. et al, 1998)

Preliminary results of the HD9 Causes of Death at 10 years indicate higher death events at COPP/ABVD 24% vs. 19% vs. 12%. (Diehl V. et al, 1998)

When applying MOPP regimen in more than 6 cycles +/- irradiation confirm risk of acute leukaemia. (Kaldor JM, et al, 1990) Early splenectomy increased this risk by two times. (Van LF, et al, 1989; Kaldor JM, et al, 1990) Application of alkylating agents proportional to cumulative dose confirmed 1-10% of cases caused toxicity after 7-10 years. (Boivin JF et al, 1984; Blayney DW, et al, 1987; Arseneau JC, et al, 1972; Coleman CN, et al, 1977)

4.2 Radiotherapy toxicities

Early Complications: Mantle field radiation can cause mouth dryness, pharyngitis, cough, dermatitis. Sub-diaphragmatic radiation can cause anorexia and nausea.

Late Complications: Hyperthyroidism, Graves' ophthalmopathy or thyroid neoplasm was seen after neck radiotherapy. Elevation of TSH level with or without lowered T3 or T4 was seen at 30% of patients which had mantle irradiation with often followed with Hypothyroidism.

4.2.1 Toxicity after lungs irradiation

Pericarditis and pneumonitis can occur. Incidence of radial pneumonitis (characterized by shivering, dyspnoea and cough) depends on volume of lung irradiation and total dose, with recovery seen from 12 to 24 months. (Smith LM, et al, 1989; Horning SJ, et al, 1994; Griffin R, et al, 2010)

4.2.2 Toxicity after heart irradiation

Toxic effect is possible on pericardium, myocardium, blood vessels, cardiac valve and conduction system. Cardiac mortality is significantly improved at patients who were administered with > 30 Gy on mediastinum. Mediastinum radiotherapy is joined with increased risk of heart disease. Increased risk and mortality rate due to coronary arterial disease and acute infarct of myocardium was seen both at adult and child patients. (Hancock SL, et al, 1993; Boivin JF, et al, 1992)

Patients whose heart was irradiated have increased risk of coronary arterial disease. Hence continual monitoring and evaluation is needed together with other risk factors. Follow up of these patients, according to NCCN (National Comprehensive Cancer Network, 2010) predicts basic ECHO of the heart 10 years after treatment with control of the lipid profile once per year. On the other side, according to ESMO base ECHO of the heart should be done 4-10 years after treatment, stress ECHO in patients with earlier RT and follow up of lipid profile at patients which had RT in their therapy. (Bovelli et al. 2010)

4.2.3 Secondary malignancies (solid tumour and secondary acute leukaemia as consequence of irradiation)

According to Stanford study, risk of secondary solid tumours 15 years after treatment was about 18%. (Boivin JF, et al, 1984). Patients that were primarily treated with radiotherapy had increased risk of tumour formation on lungs, breast, bone marrow, soft tissues and thyroid gland.

Possibility of lung cancer, 5 years after irradiation treatment and further during next 20 years, was two to eight times higher what was especially true with patients that smoke. (Griffin R, et al, 2010).

Increased risk of breast cancer was noted at female patients that were treated before age of 30 and was increased in children and adolescent population as well. (Donaldson SS, et al, 1982). Radiotherapy toxicity was especially noted at patients aged from 15-30 years what restricts irradiation of females before age of 30. Average interval of irradiation and diagnostics Ca Thyroid and breast cancer is 10 - 15 years. Hence it is needed to do routine mammography 8 years after completion of irradiation treatment in this group of patients. (Griffin R, et al, 2010) These findings influenced new recommendations in irradiation application by reducing mantle radiotherapy volume. By modifying mantle field and aborting axilla and heart from the radiation area treatments converged towards involved field radiotherapy (IFTT).

Reduction of the radiation area involved exclusion of irradiation of thyroid gland, heart and axilla and decrease risk of Brest Cancer and lung cancer. Low-dose (20Gy) IFRT was associated with decrease risk of Brest Cancer by 77% and lung cancer by 57%. (Hodgson DC, et al, 2007)

Contemporary therapy approach is using IFRT and is preferred for the patients that respond to the first line therapy with PR/SD and/or have bulky. High dose therapy followed by ASCT therapy in large measure suppressed irradiation or it was postponed for after ASCT for unfavourable disease, advanced disease, bulky, borderline zone and transformation.

15 % of patients that were administered with mantle field radiation can develop electric shock sensation radiating down the back of the legs when the head is flexed. This happens 6 to 12 weeks after the treatment due to transitory demyelination of spine cord and what resolves spontaneously. (Griffin R, et al, 2010)

4.2.4 Toxicity after thyroid gland irradiation

The data provided by the Christofer F. suggests that the actual risk of hypothyroidism after radiation therapy for HL at 26 years was 47%. Other less common thyroid abnormalities observed include: Graves's disease, thyroiditis, thyrotoxicosis, thyroid nodules and thyroid malignancies. (Christopher F, 2010).

My personal experience involves a study on patients diagnosed with HL from 1992 to 2001 and treated at Haematology Clinic at Clinical Centre University Sarajevo. The study was aimed to determining secondary malignancies as a consequence of late toxicity in HL treatment. Total of 126 patients were assessed aged from 14 to 75 years (median of 44.5 yr).

Our treatments at that time involved RT for I and IIA stage and for IE, IIB, III and IV stage MOPP or ABVD or ChLVPP with PR+MOPP or RT. In that study 10 patients (7.9%) were with secondary malignancy out of which one was with myelodysplasia, three with Non Hodgkin Lymphoma, six with solid carcinoma (Ca planocellulare papilarae - one patient, Ca planocellulare laringys - one patient, Neo palatum molae - one patient and Brest cancer-three patients). In the same group, epidemiologically observed, the most patients ware aged from 14 to 24 years. In the further follow up of 10 years (2002 to 2011) of the patients diagnosed by 2001, we noted 3 more diseased with secondary malignancy (1 with breast cancer, 1 Myeloma Multiplex and one with MDS). (Sofo Hafizovic A. 2002).

Second analyzed period is targeted towards analyzing patients with HL treated from 2002 - 2011 with applying chemotherapy using ABVD and BEACOPP protocol with or without IFRT. This study is currently being conducted and its results will be published in the upcoming period.

Chemotherapy ± RT 1992 - 2001	Chemotherapy ± RT 2002 - 2011
Hematology complications - total 4 (3.2%) sAML: 0 MDS: 1 (0.8%) NHL: 3 (2.4%)	**Hematology complications - total 2 (1.6%)** MDS: 1 (0.8%) Myeloma Multiplex: 1 (0.8%)
Solid neoplasm - total 6 (4.8%) Ca planocellulare papilarae: 1 Ca planocellulare laringys: 1 Neo palatum molae: 1 Brest cancer 3 (2.4 %)	**Solid neoplasm - total 1 (0.8%)** Brest cancer 1 (0.8%)

Table 2. Therapy toxicity in HL treatment (secondary malignancies) in KCUS.

In follow up of 10 years, secondary malignancies occurred in 10 cases (7.9%) and in follow up of 20 years secondary malignancies occurred in 13 cases (10%).

Case report: One 63 years old patient which had HL (NLP) CS IIA bulky diagnosed in August 2001. In the first line therapy the patient was treated using chemotherapy using ABVD protocol with irradiation of mediastinum and CR1 achieved. After 6 years Myeloma Multiplex was diagnosed and further VAD protocol therapy was applied. Next autologous transplantation of peripheral stem cells was conducted without significant complications. However, in 2010 she develops POEMS (Polyneuropathy Organomegaly Endocrinopathy M-protein Skin-abnormalities) followed with thrombocytopenia immunogene which were successfully treated with Prednisolon and Imuran. On her last control in April 2011 she is still in HL and MM complete remission with good life quality.

5. Gonadal complications in Hodgkin lymphoma treatment

Teratogenic influence of chemotherapy is formed in application of individual, or as a synergy effect of more drugs or in combination with radiotherapy. It is especially stressed in the first trimester of pregnancy. Incidence of difficult congenital malformations in chemotherapy application is 3% from the total number of born and 90% is incidence of minor malformations. (Michael CP. 2008b)

Factors during pregnancy (FDP) determine risk factors from teratogenic effect. According to that Prednisone is in B group, Methotrexte is in X group, Rituximab and Dacarbazine are in C group, and finally Cytosin arabinosid, Gemcitabine, Chlorambucil, Ifosfamid, Mepphalan, busulfan, Cisplatin, carboplatin, Procarbazine, Doxorubicin, Bleomxcin, Mitoxantron, vincristin, Vinblastin, Etoposide, Cytarabine are in D group. (Michael CP. 2008b) [1]

Reproduction effect: about 90% males become permanently sterile if they were administered with 6 cycles of MOPP chemotherapy. (Chapman RM, 1979a) Risk is correlated with cumulative dose of alkylating agents and 2-3 cycles result in azoospermia in about 50% patients. (Da CM, et al, 1984) Fertility in females, after applying MOPP chemotherapy, is in relation to age and treatment and as well as cumulative dosage of alkylating agent dose. (Da CM, et al, 1984; Horning SJ, et al, 1979; Chopman RM, et al,1979b). Also females in the age around 25, which are treated with 6 cycles of MOPP have 80% chance of sterility. ABVD is joined with temporary amenorrhea or azoospermia with total recovery which was noted in 50-90% of patients. (Anselmo AP, et al, 1990; Viviani S, et al, 1985)

Study conducted by Karolin Behringer confirmed teratogenic influence in males and females as follows COPP/MOPP/COPP+ABVD: Azoospermia 86-100%, Recovery of spermatogenesis between 12-20% after 2 years, Dysspermia prior to therapy 70-77%. In treatment of advanced stage HL with use of BEACOPP regimen had 89% azoospermia. In all early stage and use of alkylating agent elevation of FSH is 60%, recovery of fertility 52% and with use of RT recovery was 3%. Using Non-alkylating agent elevation of FSH is 8%, recovery is 82%. Fertility in female HL patients' therapy associated amenorrhea 0-4% ABVD, 51% BEACOPP escalating. (Karolin B. 2008)

Same author states that Ovarion toxicity is 2 years after chemotherapy treatment and in usage of 4xABVD regular cycle 95.9% Amenorrhea 4.1%, 2xABVD regular cycle 98.8% Amenorrhea 1.2%. 4xBEACOPP base regular cycle 87.1% Amenorrhea 12.9%. 8xBEACOPP escalating regular cycle 55% Amenorrhea 45%, 4xBEACOPP baseline +4xBEACOPP escalating regular cycle 81% Amenorrhea 19%. (Karolin B. 2008)

Christopher Flowers discovered that irradiation influenced fertility as follows: 1x dose 0.35 Gy or higher can cause transitory azoospermia (recovery time is longer when higher dose was administered). Dose 2 Gy and higher in germinal epithelium can result in permanent azoospermia. Dose of 15 Gy and higher Leydig cell function can be affected with potential need for testosterone replacement therapy. Ovarion dose of 4 Gy may cause a 30% incidence of sterility in young women but 100% sterility in women ≥ 40 years. (Christopher F. 2010).

Sterility formation stresses importance of applying procedures that will create good conditions for healthy offspring in the population of diseased and treated HL patients. Females should use contraception to protect the unwanted pregnancy on one side, and on

---

[1]FDA category B drugs are those for which studies in pregnant women did not demonstrate a risk to the fetus in any trimester; For C drugs animal reproduction studies have shown an adverse effect on the fetus and even though there are no adequate studies in humans potential benefits justify use in pregnant women; D drugs are those for which studies demonstrated human fetal risk, but the benefit from use in pregnant women patients justify the risk; for X drugs studies demonstrated fetal abnormalities and clearly risk of using this drug in pregnant women outweighs potential benefits. (Michael CP. 2008b)

the other to keep the hormonal level in boundaries that do not cause amenorrhea. Also cryopreservation enables offspring planning even before HL treatment application.

Among adults and adolescents after puberty, semen cryopreservation is proposed before first line treatment with BEACOPP or salvage treatment for relapse, and it is optional in cases of localized Hodgkin lymphoma treated with ABVD and radiotherapy. For women with a stable partner, in vitro fertilization for embryo cryopreservation is a standard procedure but it can be offered to only a small number of patients and requires delayed treatment initiation. Oocyte cryopreservation remains experimental, although its usage is being increased. Ovarian tissue cryopreservation is still experimental. (Harel S. 2011)

6. Conclusion

Optimal treatment of Hodgkin Lymphoma understands therapy application that will achieve complete remission with as few toxic effects as possible. This is especially true for the late toxic effects. Taking care of secondary malignancies and sterility is of uttermost significance and this is the force that drives constant treatment modification and creation of new therapy options of Hodgkin Lymphoma treatment. In current treatment options there is still large percentage of early and late toxicities which reduce life quality of the affected patients. Keeping in mind that high life quality is one of the main goals of any treatment, it should be assessed with appropriate attention and toxicities should be reduced to as low level as possible.

7. References

Andreas Engert, Peter Brichmenn, Annette Pluetschow, Basti Hitz, Zdenek Kral, Richard Greil et al. (2010). Dose-Escalation with BECOPP escalated: combined-Modality Treatment of early unfavourable Final Analysis of the German Hodgkin Study Group. Abstract 765. MondeAy, December 6.

Andreas Engert, Volker Diehl, Jeremy Franclin, Andreas Lohri, Bernard Dorken, Wolf-Dieter Ludwig et al. (2009). Eskalated-dose BEACOPP in the Treatment of Patients with Advanced Stage Hodgkin' s Lymphoma: 10 Years of Follow-Up of the GHSG HD9 Study. Journal of Clinical Oncology 27: (27) 4548-4554.

Anselmo AP, Cartoni C, Bellantuono P, Maurizi ER, Aboulkair N, Ermini M. (1990). Risk of infertility in patients with Hodgkin's disease treated with ABVD vs. MOPP vs. ABVD/MOPP. Hematologica 75:155.

Arseneau JC, Sponzo RW, Levin DL, et al. (1972). Nonlymphomatous malingnant tumors complicating Hodgkin's disease. Possible association with intensive therapy. N Engl J Med 287:1119.

Berger D.P.R, Engeltardt et all. (2002). Das Rote Buch Hamatologie und Internistische Oncologie, Ecomed-Verl-ges. 50-112.

Beutler E, Lichtman MA, Coller BS, Kipps ThJ, Seligsonh U.(2001) Williams Hematology.Hodgkin lymphoma.Chapter 102,Sixth edition.1215-1228.

Blayney DW, Longo DL, Joung RC, et al. (1987). Decreasing risk of leukemia with prolonged follow-up after chemotherapy and radiotherapy for Hodgkin's disease. N Engl J Med 316:710.

Boivin JF, Hutchinson GB, Lubin JH, Mauch P. (1992). Coronary artery disease mortality in patients treated for Hodgkin's disease. Cancer 69:124.

Boivin JF, Hutchinson GB, Lyden M, Godbold J, Chorosh J, Schottenfeld D. (1984). Second primary cancers following treatment of Hodgkin's disease. J Natl Cancer Inst 72:233.

Bonadonna G, Zucali R, Monfardini S,de Lena M, Usllenghi C. (1975). „ Combination chemotherapy of Hodgkin׳ s disease with adriamycin, bleomycin, vinblastin and imidazolecarboxamide versus MOPP". Cancer 36(1):252-9.

Chapman RM, Sutclife SB, Malpas JS. (1979b) Cytotoxic-induced ovarian failure in women with Hodgkin׳ s disease.I.Hormone function. JAMA 242:1877.

Chapman RM, Sutclife SB, Rees LH, Edwards CR, Malpas JS. (1979a). Cyclical combination chemotherapy and gonadal function. Retrospective study in males. Lancet 1:285.

Christopher Flowers. (2010). „ABVD is the Current standard for All patients with Hodgkin Lymphoma" Winship Cancer Institute, Emory University.

Coleman CN, Williams CJ, Flint A, Glatstein EJ, Rosenberg SA, Kaplan HS. (1977). Hematologic neoplasia in patients treated for Hodgkin's disease. N Engl J Med 297:1249.

Da CM, Meistrich ML, Fuller LM, et al.(1984) Recovery of spermatogenesis after treatment for Hodgkin's disease: limiting dose of MOPP chemotherapy. J Clin Oncol 2:571.

De Vita V, Simon R, Hubbard S, Young R, Berard C, Moxley J,Frei E et al. (1992). "Curability of advanced hodgkin׳ s disease with chemotherapy. Longterm follow-up of MOPP-treatment patients athe national Cancer Institute" Ann intern Med 92 (5):587-95.

DeVita V, Serpick A, Carbone P. (1970). Combination chemotherapy in the treatment of advanced Hodgkin's disease. Ann Intern Med 73:881.

Diehl V, Franklin J, Hasenclever D, Tesch H, Pfreundschuh M, Lathan B et al. (1998). „BEACOPP: A now regiment for advanced Hodgkin׳ s disease":Annals of Oncology 9 (Suppl.5):S67-S71.

Diehl V, Haverkamp H, Mueller R, Mueller-Hermelink H,Cerny T,Markova J et al. (2009). "Eight cycles of BEACOPP escalated compared with 4 cycles of BEACOPP escalated followed by 4 cycles of BEACOPP baseline with or without radiotherapy in patients in advanced stage hodgkin lymphoma (HL):Final analysis of the HD12 trial of the German Hodgkin Study Group (GHSG). Journal of Clinical Oncology: ASCO Anual Meeting;27:15s, suppl;abstract 8544.

Donaldson SS, Kaplan HS. (1982). Complications of treatment of Hodgkin's disease in children. Cancer Treat Rep 66:977.

Federico M, Luminari S, Iannitto E, Polimeno G, Marcheselli L, Montanini A et al. (2009). „ABVD compared with BEACOPP compared with CEC fooor the initial treatment of patients with advanced Hodgkins's Lymphoma: results from the HD2000 Gruppo Italiano per lo Studio dei Linfomi Trial. Journal of Clinical Oncology: 10; 27(5):805-811.

Gianni A.M, A.Rampaldi, P.Zinzani,A.Levis, E.Brusamolino, A.Pulsoni et al. (2008). "Comparable 3-year outcome following ABVD or BEACOPP first-line chemotherapy, plus pre-planned high-dose salvage, in advanced Hodgkin lymphoma(HL):A randomised trial of the Michelangelo GITIL and IIL comparative groups". Journal of Clinical Oncology 26: (May suppl; abstract 8506).

Griffin Rodgers, Neal Young. (2010). The Bethesda handbook of Clinical Hematology. Hodgkins Lymphoma: Lipincot Williams & Wilkins second edition; 184-195.

Hancock SL, Donaldson SS, Hoppe RT. (1993). Cardiac disease following treatment of Hodgkin's disease in children and adolescents. J Clin Oncol 11:1208.

Hancock SL, Hoppe RT, Horning SJ, Rosenberg SA. (1988). Intercurrent death after Hodgkin's disease therapy in radiotherapy and adjuvant MOPP trials. Ann Intern Med 109:183.

Hodgson Dc, Koh ES, Tran TH, Heydarion M, Tsabg R, Pintilie M et al. (2007). Individualized estimates of second cancer risks contemporary radiation therapy. Cancer,110(11):2576-86.

Horning SJ, Adhikari A, Rizk N, Hoppe RT, Olshen RA. (1994). Effect of treatmant for Hodgkin's disease on pulmonary function: result of a prospective study. J clin Oncol 12:297.

Horning SJ, Hoppe RT, Kaplan HS, Rosenberg SA: Female reproductive potential after treatment for Hodgkin's disease. N Engl J Med 304:1377.1981.

Kaldor JM, Day NE, Clarke EA, et al. (1990). Leukemia following Hodgkin's disease. N Engl J Med 322:7.

Kaplan HS. (1996). Evidence for a tumoricidal dose level in the radiotherapy of Hodgkin's disease. Cancer Res 26:1221.

Karolin Behringer. (2008). „ Fertility in youn HL patients An overview". German Hodgkin Study group (GHSG), University of Cologne, Germany. ESHRE Campus Symposium, Haidelberg.

Meistrich ML, Fuller LM, et al. (1984). Recovery of spermatogenesis after treatment for Hodgkin's disease: limiting dose of MOPP chemotherapy. J Clin Oncol 2:571.

Michael C. P. (2008). „Chemotherapy of Hodgkin lyphoma". The Chemotherapy Source Book. Fourth Edition. Lippincott Wiliams & Wilkins, Bruce A.Peterson, Chapter 42, S500-514.

Michael C.Perry. (2008). „Chemotherapy in pregnancy". The Chemotherapy Source Book . Fourth Edition. Lippincott Wiliams & Wilkins, Nasir Shahab, Chapter 27,S 274-280.

Peters M. (1950). A study of survivals in Hodgkin's disease treated radiologically. Am. J Roentgenol 63:299.

Simoneta Vivian, Pier Luigi et al. (2011). „ABVD versus BEACOPP for Hodgkin' s Lymphoma When High-Dose Salvage Is Planned". N Engl J Med: 365 203-212.

Smith LM, Mendenhall NP, Cicale MJ, Block ER, Carter RL, Million RR. (1989). Results of a prospective study evaluating the effects of mantle irradiation on pulmonary function. Int J Radiat Oncol Biol Phys 16:79.

Sofo Hafizović A. (2002). Comparative Clinical Study of the Malignant Lymphoma in war and post war period, Master's Dissertation pp. 20-43, Clinical Center University of Sarajevo, Sarajevo

Stephani Harel, Christophe Ferme, Catherine Poirot. (2011). Management of fertility in patients treated for Hodgkin lymphoma. Haematologica 10 3324.

Tucker MA, Coleman CN, Cox RS, Varghese A, Rosenberg SA. (1988). Risk of cecond cancers after gtreatment for Hodgkin's disease. N Engl J Med 318:76.

Van LF, Somers R, Taal BG, et al. (1989). Increased risk of lung cancer, non-Hodgkin's lymphoma, and leukemia following Hodgkin's disease. J Clin Oncol 7:1046.

Viviani S, Santoro A, Ragni G, Bonfante V, Bestestti O, Bonadonna G. (1985). Gonadal toxicity after combination chemotherapy for Hodgkin's disease. Comparative results of MOPP vs ABVD. Eur J Cancer Clin Oncol 21:601.

Part 11

Survivorship in Hodgkin's Lymphoma

11

Survivorship in Hodgkin Lymphoma

Matthew A. Lunning[1] and Matthew J. Matasar[1,2,3]
[1]*Department of Medicine, Memorial Sloan-Kettering Cancer Center, New York, NY*
[2]*Lymphoma and Adult BMT Services,*
[3]*Department of Medicine, New York-Presbyterian Hospital, NY, USA*

1. Introduction

Hodgkin lymphoma (HL), formerly called Hodgkin's disease, is a malignancy of mature B-cell lineage (germinal or post-germinal center), with over 8,000 new cases diagnosed annually in the United States.[1] HL has historically been characterized by many histologic subtypes with the finding of Reed-Sternberg cells unify the diagnosis. HL is well known to have a bimodal distribution of incidence, occurring most frequently in two distinct age groups: young adults (age 15-35) and those ages greater than 55 years old. For the purpose of this chapter, we will focus on the young adults treated for and cured of HL with radiation therapy (RT), chemotherapy, or combined modality therapy (CMT).

HL remains in many ways the archetype within oncology with regards to incremental improvements, established through well-performed clinical trials, turning an incurable and universally fatal illness into one that is, more often than not, cured with first-line therapy. The need for an understanding of how best to care for survivors of HL is predicated upon patients being cured of their HL. This was first achieved in the 1960's when HL was shown to be a curable disease, first with high-dose extended field RT,[2] and subsequently with multi-agent chemotherapeutic regimens such as MOPP (nitrogen mustard, vincristine, procarbazine, and prednisone).[3] Increasingly intensive treatments, however, were handcuffed to increasing toxicity.[4] As the likelihood of cure started to plateau in the 1990's at approximately 80%, the toxic consequences of these intensified treatment regimens - acute as well as late effects - increasingly came into focus.[5] As HL is largely a disease of young, functional, and fertile, with survivors often living long lives (with whatever impairment resulting from disease and treatment), the need to better understand the medical needs of survivors of HL began to receive significant attention from the medical community. Additionally, investigators began to pursue improvement in HL therapy from a very different perspective - seeking not to identify further intensifications of therapy, but rather to attempt to delineate how treatment toxicities could be limited without sacrificing the excellent outcomes gained over the past decades. Accordingly, improvements in radiation delivery have led to preferential use of smaller fields (involved field radiation therapy, and now even involved nodal field radiation in select circumstances.[6, 7] Efforts in the development of systemic chemotherapy for HL have been focused upon not only intensification of therapy, but in the selective application of such treatment. Currently, the management of HL is driven by patient- and disease-specific characteristic including age and gender, stage, bulk, location, and risk models specific for early or advanced stage disease.[8-12] Early-stage patients, particularly those with bulky disease (most often defined as a mass greater than 10 cm in long-axis diameter or encompassing more than a third of the intrathoracic diameter) are commonly treated with combined modality approaches of varying intensity.[13] Advanced disease is frequently treated with chemotherapy alone with consolidation radiation therapy to sites of bulk [14], although here, intensity of treatment is often dictated by risk prediction. The next generation of clinical trials seeks more individualized and specific ways to tailor treatment intensity, particularly using response-adapted strategies with early restaging functional imaging with 18-fluorodeoxyglucose (FDG) positron emission tomography (PET). As treatments continue to emerge, and evolve, the needs of survivors will of course develop in kind. Nonetheless, there exist over 160,000 patients living after being cured of HL; having received treatments with long-term effects, and it is the optimal care of these patients that is the focus of survivorship efforts.[15]

2. Importance of post-treatment care

During the first 10 years following diagnosis of HL, relapse remains the leading cause of death. [16] However, by 15-20 years following diagnosis, risk of death due to causes other than HL will have surpassed those due to the lymphoma itself.[17, 18] By risk stratification, those with early stage disease are more likely to have secondary malignancy and cardiovascular disease when compared to those with advance disease, an observation attributable to improved prognosis as well as effects from RT, more often a component of therapy for early stage disease. As the risk of relapse diminishes after treatment the subsequent quality of life altering comorbidities become apparent and accelerated.[19] Although second primary malignancy and cardiovascular disease are the most frequent causes of non-lymphoma mortality among patients with HL, they are far from the only medical conditions for which they are at risk. Pulmonary, musculoskeletal, endocrine, neurologic, and psychiatric illness all occur at increased frequency among HL survivors, typically as direct sequelae of the disease or its treatment. Tellingly, a single-institution series investigating the global effects of late morbidity found that, among survivors an average of 21 years post-treatment, 94% reported at least one morbidity of any grade severity, 50% at least one morbidity of grade 3 or greater (according to a modification of the Common Terminology Criteria for Adverse Events, version 3), and 23% two or more morbidities of grade 3 or greater.[18] In order for a physician to offer optimal care for survivors of HL, such care should be built upon an understanding of these risks, both individually and collectively.[20]

3. Second primary malignancy

Unfortunately, among those cured of HL, second primary malignancy remains the leading cause of mortality 15 years after disease-free survival.[21] For instance, a risk model approximated that those diagnosed at the age of 30 with HL will have a 30 year cumulative risk of second primary malignancy for men and women at 18% and 26%, respectively, compared to age-matched risks of 7% and 9%.[22, 23] The latency of the various second malignancies seen following therapy for HL varies by histology. Risk for myelodysplastic syndrome (MDS) and acute myelogenous leukemia (AML) peak at three to five years after therapy and return to population baseline, or at most remain minimally elevated, by 10 years after.[24-26] The inverse is true for solid tumor malignancies, where increased risk only first becoming appreciable by 10 years after the completion of therapy.[27]

4. Hematologic malignancies

Already survivors of one hematologic malignancy, the fact that they are at heightened risk for the development of additional hematologic malignancies - particularly MDS, AML, and non-Hodgkin lymphoma (NHL) - are a source of frustration to doctors and patients alike. Treatment-induced MDS or AML is a well-established risk of HL therapy; the relative risk of acute leukemia among patients cured of HL is 80 times greater than the general population, although the absolute excess risk is low.[28] The risk of MDS/AML is largely predicated upon the treatment delivered, as the cumulative dose of potent alkylating chemotherapy (e.g., mechlorethamine) or topoisomerase inhibitors (e.g., doxorubicin or etoposide) and the delivery of radiotherapy account for much of this increased risk.[24, 29] Despite ongoing advancements in the treatment of the acute leukemias, treatment-related AML remains profoundly dangerous, with median survival measured in months.[28] Indeed, it was in part the leukemogenicity of the older MOPP regimen that helped fuel the ascendance of ABVD (doxorubicin, bleomycin, vinblastine, and dacarbazine) as the chemotherapeutic standard of care for average-risk HL. The absolute excess risk of AML following treatment with ABVD is between 0 and 0.4%, whereas with MOPP was 2.8% (and with MOPP and radiotherapy as CMT, 5.5%).[25, 30, 31] The modern intensified regimen, escalated BEACOPP (bleomycin, etoposide, doxorubicin, cyclophosphamide, vincristine, procarbazine, and prednisone), and is associated with a risk of AML of 3.2%. This observation has largely led to the selective use of this highly effective regimen only in high-risk patients - patients in whom the risk of poor outcomes with ABVD merit exposure to more leukemogenic therapy.[32] The risk of secondary acute leukemia in patients receiving consolidative RT for HL appears to be more closely related to the field of therapy than to the delivered dose.[27] This contribution to leukemia risk has been somewhat mitigated, as modern RT strives to limit therapeutic exposure, preferring involved fields to extended fields, although these efforts are not expected to entirely obviate the contribution to risk of leukemia from radiotherapy.

In addition to acute myelogenous leukemia, HL survivors are also at increased risk for the subsequent development of non-Hodgkin lymphoma (NHL).[21, 33, 34] The risk appears to be influenced by the selection of treatment, with alkylator therapy and radiotherapy emerging as the likely causes of oncogenesis. Estimates of the relative risk of NHL among survivors of HL are varied across reports, ranging from 2 to 22, but the absolute risks are low: The 25-year cumulative risk of NHL is less than 4%, and the absolute excess risk (AER) of NHL is less than 10 cases per 10,000 person-years.[21]

5. Solid tumor malignancies

Although the development of a second primary hematologic neoplasms following curative treatment for HL is a potentially life-threatening event, and one for which survivors are at far greater risk than age-matched controls, solid tumors collectively comprise a much greater risk for survivors - 75% of second primary malignancies will not be AML or NHL, but rather will be of solid organ origin, and unlike the risk of AML, the risk (and excess risk) of solid organ malignancy has no apparent plateau among HL survivors. Unlike AML, however, much of the risk of solid tumors arising from treatment of HL is attributable to local genotoxic damage due to radiation therapy; each routine involved field of radiotherapy is associated with potential solid-tumor risks within the given field (Figure 1).

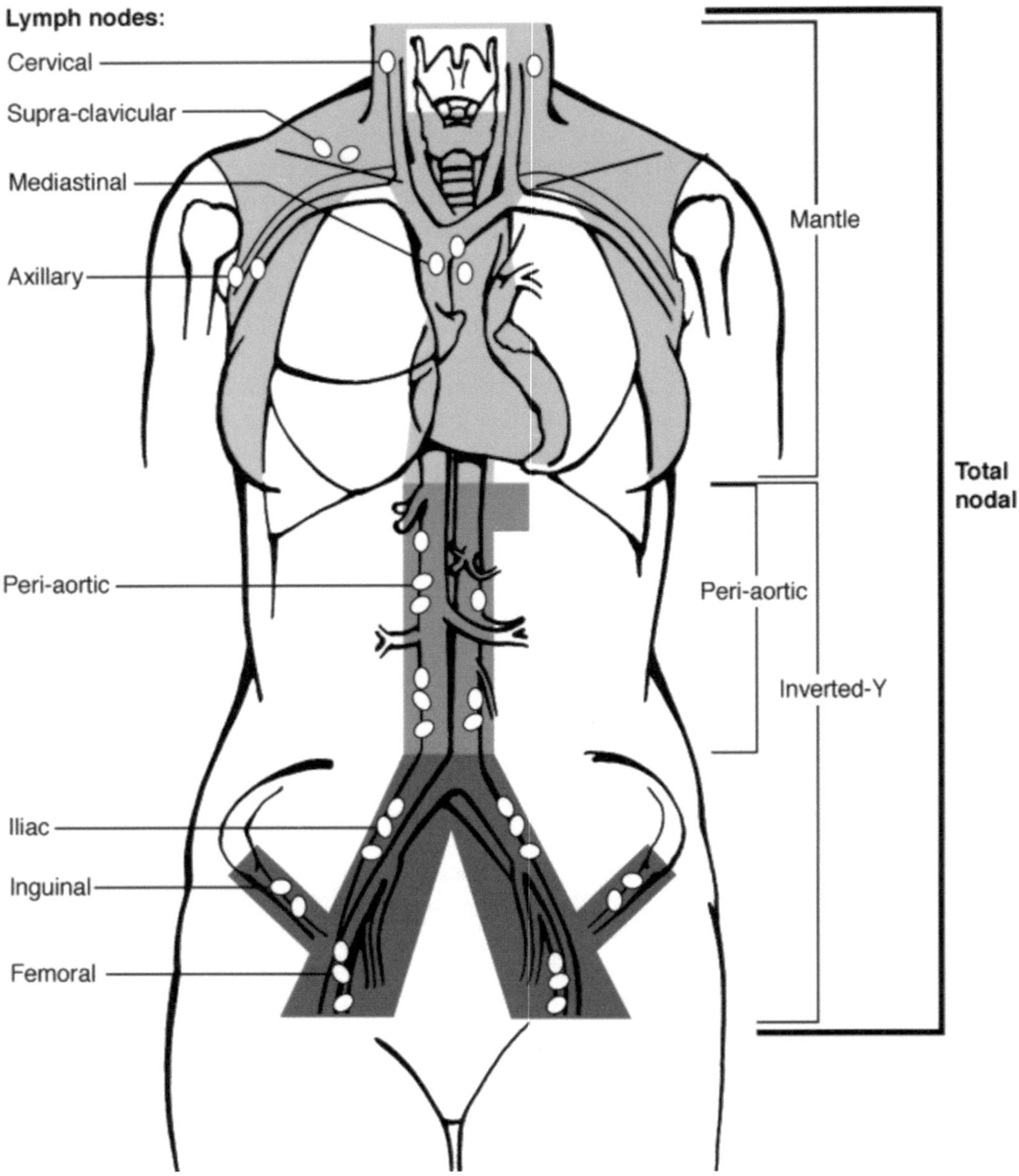

Reprinted with permission from: Stubblefield MD. Radiation fibrosis syndrome: neuromuscular and musculoskeletal complications in cancer survivors. PM&R 2011;3:1041-54.

Fig. 1. Radiation therapy fields in the treatment of classical Hodgkin lymphoma.

6. Lung cancer

HL survivors are at increased risk for developing lung cancer; with a relative risk of 7 and an AER of 7 per 10,000 person-years, lung cancer represents a serious cause of morbidity and mortality.[22, 35-39] This risk is mediated by the volume and dose of lung tissue exposure to ionizing radiation, cumulative dose of alkylating chemotherapy, and environmental factors.[22] HL patients who had a positive smoking history and received radiation therapy as a part of their management have a markedly higher incidence of lung cancer when compared to HL who non-smokers and received radiation therapy, with relative risks as high as 50 times that of the general population.[40] Interestingly, regardless of smoking history, incident lung cancers develop within the radiation-exposed lung parenchyma. HL survivors who develop lung cancer have a median survival of less than a year [41, 42], and recently have been shown to have a 60% less chance of survival than cases of stage-matched *de novo* lung cancer.[43] We continue to adamantly recommend smoking cessation (with the support of a smoking cessation clinic) to patients at the time of diagnosis given the interaction between cigarette smoking and therapy in augmenting the subsequent risk of lung cancer. Whether to screen at-risk patients with a history of HL, and if so, how best to do so, remain unanswered questions. National Comprehensive Cancer Network (NCCN) guidelines recommend annual chest imaging (either X-ray or CT scan) for all patients except those who were treated without alkylator therapy, mediastinal RT, and who have no other risk factors.[44] The recommendation of screening CT has been supported by cost modeling, showing it to be cost effective, particularly in smokers.[45] However, perhaps the greatest impetus, albeit indirect, for lung cancer screening in HL survivors comes from the National Lung Screening Trial.[46] This large randomized trial of non-cancer patients with strong smoking histories demonstrated that, with annual low-dose CT scans of the chest for three consecutive years, lung cancer-specific and overall survival could be improved. How best to extrapolate these findings to the HL survivor population is unclear, and the duration and intensity of screening will require further clarification, but an annual low-dose chest CT scan in at-risk survivors may well emerge as the de facto standard of care, and given the current body of data should be discussed with patients at risk.

7. Breast cancer

After 15 years of follow-up, women treated with mantle field radiation before the age of 20 had a 40-fold increased risk of developing breast cancer compared to age-matched controls.[47] In a retrospective study of HL survivors treated with more modern radiation dose and delivery, doses as low as 4.0Gy to the breast were associated with a 3.2 fold cancer risk compared to women who were treated with lower doses of radiation. This risk increased to 8-fold for women treated with >40 Gy to the breast. Age at radiation dominates the risk assessment for second primary breast neoplasia; in one study, for instance, the actuarial risks of breast cancer for patients receiving mantle radiation by 25 years after treatment were 34%, 22%, and 3.5% for patients under age 20, age 20-30, and over age 30, respectively; radiation therapy to patients over the age of 30 appears to confer at most a minimal risk of subsequent breast cancer.[48] Concomitant use of alkylating agents or pelvic radiation can have protective effects against development of breast cancer, presumably due to the low-estrogen state induced by premature ovarian failure.[47, 49] The question of how best to monitor patients who have received treatment likely to increase breast cancer risk remains unanswered, and an area of active research.

Guidelines for the screening of women for breast cancer continue to evolve, as do recommendations for screening high-risk patients, such as those with hereditary risk for breast cancer due to the inheritance of BRCA1 or BRCA2.[52] Unfortunately, many female HL survivors will also be at an increased risk for subsequent breast cancer, risk that is associated with exposure of breast tissue to ionizing radiation when contained in RT fields. For instance, women treated with mantle radiation under age 20 have a 40-fold increased risk of developing breast cancer compared to age matched controls at a median of 15 years follow-up.[21] Developmental age of breast tissue also strongly influences the risk of radiation induced carcinogenesis, as in patients who received mantle RT under the age of 20, age 20-30, and over 30 the risk of breast cancer was 34%, 22.3%, and 3.5% respectfully at 25 years post treatment.[48] Given the many changes that have taken place in the delivery of RT in the treatment of HL (extended fields giving way to more limited involved fields; efforts at limiting dose; and improved simulation techniques, to name but three), it is hoped that risks of breast cancer following RT may be lower for patients treated in the current era. Nonetheless, recent data suggest that modern radiotherapy techniques may not in fact lead to reductions in second malignancy;[53] estimating risks of breast cancer will require ongoing reassessment so as to permit the most appropriate screening approach for individual patients given their individual risk profiles. Interestingly, concomitant use of alkylating agents or pelvic radiation can have protective effects against development of breast cancer, thought to be related to decreased estrogen production induced by treatment-related ovarian suppression or premature ovarian failure.[54] If efforts at fertility preservation with administration of gonadotropin releasing hormone agonists prove successful, as may be the case in breast cancer therapy[55], it is possible this benefit may be either abrogated or nullified.[56]

The optimal surveillance strategy for patients placed at increased risk for breast cancer by their HL therapy remains a subject of investigation, but standards of care are beginning to emerge. The National Comprehensive Cancer Network (NCCN) and the American Cancer Society (ACS) have recommended that, for those who received mediastinal radiotherapy before the age of 30, breast cancer surveillance should begin between eight and ten years following treatment.[50, 51] Mammography remains an important modality for breast cancer screening in this patient population, although the addition of an annual breast magnetic resonance imaging is reasonable for high-risk patients (particularly those with dense breasts on mammography, a finding that limits the sensitivity of mammography for early detection); the use of MRI in screening is extrapolated from a comparable risk group, women with BRCA1 mutation, in whom breast MRI has been validated as a useful element in screening programs.

Many other types of solid tumor malignancies remain overrepresented in HL survivors. Papillary thyroid carcinoma is the most notable among them and is clearly associated with radiation therapy, although the risk of thyroid cancer decreases with doses above 30 Gy, consistent with increased cell kill of normal thyroid tissue.[58] Other radiation-associated cancers can be seen as well, including gastrointestinal carcinomata and soft tissue sarcomata, as well as a strong association with non-melanoma skin cancer, both basal and squamous cell histologies.[22] Given these risks, surveillance for second primary malignancy should take such risks into account, including modification of colorectal screening for patients receiving infradiaphragmatic radiation, and special attention to skin examination in radiation fields.

8. Cardiovascular toxicities

While secondary malignancies remain the leading cause of mortality in long-term HL survivors, death due to cardiac causes places second and cardiovascular morbidity and mortality is far more common among HL survivors than among comparable untreated individuals. The specific cardiovascular toxicities for which HL survivors are at increased risk can include coronary artery disease (CAD), valvular heart disease, congestive heart failure (CHF), pericardial disease, electrical conduction abnormalities, and cerebrovascular disease.[59]

9. Coronary artery disease

HL survivors who receive radiotherapy to the mediastinum are at increased risk of early onset CAD. A British cohort of HL survivors was found to be 3.2 times more likely to suffer a myocardial infarction (MI) than population controls. [60] In Dutch HL survivors treated with mediastinal radiation, the 20-year cumulative risk of myocardial infraction was 21.2%.[61] In a similar cohort Aleman et al. reported the risk of development of a myocardial infarction at 30 years post-radiation was 12.4%.[62] The selection of chemotherapy, including the use of anthracyclines, does not appear to definitively impact risks of CAD among survivors. Classical CAD risk factors (hypertension, diabetes, cigarette smoking, and hyperlipidemia) continue to play a role in promoting atherosclerosis in HL survivors, necessitating optimal medical management.[63] At present, there have only been two prospective studies of cardiac screening in HL survivors. Heidenreich et al. [64] reported an abnormal stress test (echocardiogram and/or radionucleotide myocardial perfusion scan) in 21% of asymptomatic HL survivors fifty percent of those with an abnormal functional study demonstrated an obstructive lesion at the time of definitive coronary angiography. Furthermore, Kupeli et al. [65] use CT angiogram to detect subclinical CAD in survivors of childhood HL, and found a 6.8 times greater post-radiation HL survivors. CT angiography is felt to represent the non-invasive gold standard for detection of CAD, with sensitivity and specificity of 94% and 97%, respectfully, compared to fluoroscopic angiography.[66] Whether screening CT angiography is appropriate for adult HL survivors remains an open question, and indeed no standard of care yet exists for the surveillance for subclinical CAD in HL survivors.

10. Valvular heart disease

The risk of subsequent valvular heart disease is significantly increased among HL survivors treated with mediastinal RT, again believed due to direct toxic effects on the valve apparatus. Investigators have observed a seven- or eight-fold increase in the likelihood of experiencing significant valvular heart disease among irradiated survivors, risks that appear not to be mediated by chemotherapy agents or dosages.[62, 67] The aortic valve is the most commonly affected, and female gender appears to predispose to disease.[68] Echocardiographic surveillance to assess valvular competence is often included as an element of routine follow-up of HL survivors treated with mediastinal radiation, although as of yet no guidelines for adult survivors have been developed.

11. Congestive heart failure

Although the most common cause of congestive heart failure (CHF) in HL survivors is ischemic cardiomyopathy, significant concerns remain about the risk of late non-ischemic cardiomyopathy. While cumulative dose of anthracycline is associated with risks of CHF, currently the maximum cumulative dose of doxorubicin would not exceed 400 mg/m^2 and typically would not exceed 300 mg/m^2, the dose exposure from 6 cycles of ABVD, dose levels that would be expected to be associated with low risks of cardiomyopathy.[69, 70] Doxorubicin is not the only therapeutic agent for HL associated with CHF; It has long been recognized that mediastinal RT can predispose to CHF as well.[71] The impact of therapy on risk of subsequent CHF has been convincingly elucidated in patients treated as children for HL; data from the Childhood Cancer Survivor Study estimate a hazard ratio of 6.8 in HL survivors, with young age (<10y), female gender, higher doses of doxorubicin, and mediastinal RT all contributing to risk in multivariate modeling.[72] Subclinical LV dysfunction in survivors of childhood HL appears also to be common, although estimates of cumulative incidence are heterogeneous, ranging from 0 to 57% in 25 studies using traditional echocardiographic metrics (studies that were themselves heterogeneous in how subclinical LV dysfunction was defined).[73] Among patients treated for adult HL, long-term survivors are at increased risk for developing CHF, with one set of estimates (among patients who largely did not receive anthracycline-based chemotherapy) of absolute excess risk ranging from 16-35 cases/10,000 person-years.[74] Furthermore, while mediastinal RT appears contributes to the increased cardiac morbidity in HL survivors treated as adults,[59] how this risk interacts with the risk attributable to anthracycline-based chemotherapy has not been well described. How best to monitor the LV function, or even to identify early or subclinical LV dysfunction, in HL survivors needs to be more rigorously investigated if evidence-based screening guidelines are to be developed.

12. Pulmonary toxicity

Beyond the risk of lung cancer (discussed above), therapy for HL has the potential of causing both acute and chronic lung disease. The three most common first-line regimens for HL - ABVD, Stanford V, and BEACOPP - all contain bleomycin, an agent with a well-described association with pneumonitis. Baseline pulmonary function prior to initiation of bleomycin-containing therapy is standard, both to select a group of patients for whom such therapy is inappropriate as well as to establish baselines against which future tests (either routine surveillance in the absence of symptoms or testing to delineate the cause of dyspnea or cough) can be compared. Such complaints are common; as many as 30% of HL survivors will report the symptom of dyspnea during or after treatment.[19] Acute bleomycin pneumonitis is a serious, and potentially life-threatening condition, with mortality rates reported as high as 27%.[75] Patients who experience bleomycin pneumonitis, even when having survived and recovered from the acute episode, are more likely to report chronic fatigue and dyspnea than unaffected patients. Furthermore, when fields include pulmonary parenchyma, radiation therapy can also lead to acute pneumonitis or, later, pulmonary fibrosis, conditions that can compound the damage from bleomycin exposure. Given these risks, many experts will elect to monitor PFT's serially both during treatment as well as periodically among survivors.

13. Endocrinopathies

Endocrine systems are typically characterized by homeostatic balance supported by positive and negative feedback. The organs involved in such systems may be susceptible to damage or disruption from cytotoxic chemotherapy or ionizing radiation, and indeed survivors of HL are at risk for dysfunction of several hormonal systems. Therapy for HL can be toxic to the thyroid and the gonads, resulting in hypothyroidism and compromised fertility, respectively.

14. Thyroid disease

Hypothyroidism is a potential long-term consequence of radiotherapy involving the thyroid bed. Unlike papillary thyroid cancer, an uncommon late sequela of thyroid irradiation, hypothyroidism is seen in at least half of HL survivors who are more then 10 years from treatment cancer having undergone RT involving the thyroid.[76] Risk factors associated with higher rates of hypothyroidism in HL survivors in addition to dose and field of radiation include female gender, treatment with combined-modality therapy, and duration of time since radiation. [77] There is no consensus on the optimal frequency of thyroid stimulating hormone screening or the value at which to initiate thyroid hormone replacement in the absence of symptomatic hypothyroidism, but treatment with thyroid hormone replacement is routine and effective at minimizing the impact of hypothyroidism.

15. Gonadal dysfunction

Given the epidemiology of the disease, survivors of HL are often young, functional, and potentially fertile.[78] Unfortunately, treatments for HL may lead to temporary infertility, primary gonadal failure (azoospermia or primary ovarian failure), or subfertility (dysspermatogenesis or early onset of menopause). Given high cure rates among patients who will often go on to want to have children, investigators have sought to understand the impact of treatment on fertility, as well as how best to safeguard fertility prospectively. While a full discussion of fertility preservation is beyond the scope of this chapter, choice of chemotherapeutic agents, total dose of chemotherapy, radiation field and dose, and age at treatment are influence the outcomes with regards to fertility. The selection of therapy, including alkylating chemotherapy and pelvic radiation, has the potential to impact fertility in both men and women.[79, 80] In male patients, semen cryopreservation when possible should be encouraged before commencing chemotherapy so as to preserve fertility should azoospermia result from treatment, although some patients will be incapable of banking adequate semen, presumed to be due to the cytokine milieu caused by the underlying lymphoma. While ABVD chemotherapy results in temporary azoospermia in approximately one third of patients, permanent azoospermia is rare. This stands in contrast to more intensified regimen using bleomycin, etoposide, doxorubicin, cyclophosphamide, vincristine, procarbazine, and prednisone (baseline or escalated BEACOPP), which typically leads to durable azoospermia.[81]

In female patients, risk of infertility or subfertility is thought to be influenced by delivered therapy, intensity of therapy (number of cycles), and perhaps age at treatment. The leading cause of infertility is related to premature ovarian failure as a result of chemotherapy, radiation or combined modality therapy.[82] While egg preservation is commonly discussed at the time of consultation prior to proceeding to definitive treatment, not infrequently the pace of the disease, financial constraints, or patient choice are barriers to fertility preservation for women. For those who have been treated and subsequently attempt natural pregnancy, the data support optimism regarding likelihood of conception. In females who had received ABVD without pelvic radiation therapy and had no evidence of relapsed at three years were surveyed on their experience on fertility. Hodgson et al. found that of those that attempted to become pregnant 70% were successful with a median time to pregnancy of 2 months.[83] Interestingly, in this report the age at diagnosis or the number of cycles of chemotherapy did not demonstrate an increase risk of subfertility compared to controls. Further data is emerging with patients with aggressive disease by prognostic modeling warranting initial intense treatment with BEACOPP, a regimen felt by most to be significantly more pituitary-gonadal axis. Dann et al. [84] reported that in patients younger than 40 with locally unfavorable or advanced HL whom underwent up to 4 cycles of initial BEACOPP therapy an astounding 94% of had preserved cyclic ovarian function. Furthermore, they reported numerous successful pregnancies in this cohort up to 7 years after commencement of BEACOPP. While this data is encouraging egg preservation or other options to facilitate preservation of fertility in an imperative part of the treatment plan. Recent research into ovarian suppression with gonadotropin releasing hormone agonists prior to initiation of chemotherapy has shown promise, with a recent large randomized clinical trial in women with breast cancer showing a statistically significant decrease in rates of amenorrhea 12 months after completion of adjuvant therapy from 26% to 9%.[55] More definitive efforts at preservation of female fertility include cryopreservation of fertilized embryos or, more recently, unfertilized ova elective oophorectomy with cryopreservation and re-implantation after therapy; and transposition of the ovary outside of pelvic radiotherapy fields.[56] For the survivor of HL, however, pre-treatment fertility preservation is something that was, or was not, done, and there are no established interventions to promote or restore fertility in the post-treatment setting. Recently, however, investigations into the use of anti-Müllerian hormone (AMH) levels to predict both the ability to conceive as well as the likelihood of early menopause in cancer survivors, have offered future promise for a more individualized assessment of fertility prospects and guidance regarding family planning.[85]

16. Health related quality of life

In addition to the medical morbidities that survivors of Hodgkin lymphoma may experience due to their disease and its treatment, there exist significant risks as well of impaired quality of life, with fatigue, anxiety and depression, and impaired vocational success having been well described among HL survivors. An understanding of the global well-being of survivors requires incorporation of psychosocial support into the delivered multi-disciplinary care.

Health related quality of life (HRQOL) encompasses a patient's perception of physical, psychological, and social well-being. In a 10-year follow-up of survivors of early stage HL in

Europe, women tended to have a lower HRQOL and higher symptoms scores than did men. Regardless of gender, younger age was associated with higher functioning and lower symptom severity score, and emotional suffering was generally reported to be more severe than physical symptoms.[86] Of note, results in this study did not demonstrate a relationship between type of treatment and HRQOL outcomes. In a study out of the Southwest Oncology Group in the United States, a comparison of HRQOL in patients treated with either EFRT or CMT found persistent fatigue reported by survivors of each treatment modality, but again without differences according to treatment.[87] Effects seem to wane as length of time post-treatment increases; HL survivor 10 years from treatment continue to report lower general health scores, but many specific QOL domains no longer differ between treated patients and age-matched controls.[88, 89]

17. Chronic fatigue

A common theme among investigations into the quality of life of survivors of HL has been the impact of persistent and pervasive fatigue.[86, 87, 90] Chronic fatigue is three times more likely in HL survivors than in age matched controls, and is less likely to be associated with poor mental health than in untreated patients who experience chronic fatigue.[89, 91] Retrospective studies have attempted to characterize pre-existing risk factors that can predict post-treatment chronic fatigue, and reports have implicated B symptoms at diagnosis, social isolation, and presence of treatment-related pulmonary toxicity.[91, 92] The underlying cause of chronic fatigue in HL survivors remains incompletely understood, although ongoing research suggests a link between chronic fatigue in cancer survivors and inappropriate elevation of proinflammatory cytokines.[93-95] At this time, however, the interventions that have been shown to impact chronic fatigue in HL survivors the most favorably are cognitive behavioral therapy and structured aerobic exercise.[96-98]

18. Psychiatric morbidity

An extensive literature exists describing the frequency and severity of psychological and psychiatric morbidity among cancer survivors in general, and recent investigations have attempted to characterize the impact on mental health resulting from diagnosis and treatment of Single-institution data has found that, at a median follow-up of 21 years, 17% of HL survivors reported having being diagnosed with major depression, and of these 90% had been prescribed one or more anti-depressant medications; an additional 12% denied depression but reported significant anxiety in the post-treatment period.[99] In an analysis of survivors of HL in Norway, both anxiety and depression were overrepresented, and risk of mental illness was associated with lower economic status, having received combined-modality therapy (as opposed to radiation alone), and having had a prior history of a psychiatric diagnosis.[100] It appears the peak risk of depression is at 2 years post diagnosis with a gradual decline thereafter, but the risk of depression, anxiety, and post-traumatic stress disorder can be lifelong and requires collaboration with mental health professionals in the delivery of multi-disciplinary care to HL survivors.[101-103]

19. Occupational outcomes

For many patients diagnosed with HL, symptoms from the illness, time for testing and treatment, and the resultant acute and chronic toxicities from therapy can significantly disrupt careers and limit employment opportunities post-treatment. Several factors including limit the ability to continue working or return to work include disease characteristics at the time of diagnosis (site, stage, treatment, and disease response), patient characteristics (age, gender, comorbidity, socioeconomic status), and work-related factors (physical workload, stress, and social support).[104] Younger patients with good disease control and higher educational attainment are more likely to return to pre-diagnosis socioeconomic stature.[102, 104] Among HL survivors 20 years from treatment, 18% reported that treatment for their HL interfered with their career 11% that it prevented subsequent full-time employment, and 9% that they were incapable even of routinely completing household chores.[99] While employment status in the United States is closely linked to both health and life insurance, HL survivors often suffer a negative impact on their insurance status, even after prolonged remissions.[105] Collectively, these challenges may ultimately disrupt the family support network, but interestingly, despite these challenges HL survivors who were married at the time of diagnosis do not appear to experience higher divorce rates than the general population in either the United States nor the Netherlands, to name but two examples.[102, 106]

20. Future research in the care of survivors

As clinical research in the management of HL continues to develop, with reduction in radiation fields, further limitation of chemotherapy dosages, response-adapted therapy, and possibly eliminating or replacing the most offensive agents in current multi-agent chemotherapeutic programs, opportunities for understanding and discovery in the field of HL survivorship will endure. With the recent FDA approval of brentuximab vedotin in the treatment of relapsed CD30+ HL – the first drug specifically approved for HL – this agent is now be tested earlier in the course of therapy, potentially replacing bleomycin in ABVD.[107] Many additional classes of agents have shown promise in HL, including immunomodulatory agents, histone deacetylase inhibitors, inhibitors of the mammalian target of rapamycin (mTOR), and phosphoinositide-3 kinase (PI3K) inhibitors, to name but four. In this era of rapidly expanding armamentarium of therapeutics, it is imperative that prospective protocols employ thoughtful correlative studies that ask and are powered to answer not only the question regarding acute toxicity, but also late medical morbidity and impact upon quality of life. Also sorely needed are guidelines to aide physicians in monitoring their patients for the myriad late effects associated with therapy – and the data to inform such guidelines. And as HL survival continues to improve (and as oncologists become an increasingly limited resource), models of efficient and effective multi-disciplinary care for survivors of HL need to be developed, tested, and propagated.[108]

21. Conclusion

Survivors of Hodgkin lymphoma represent a unique group of patients who, despite having been cured of an aggressive and life-threatening malignancy, continue to suffer from late medical and psychosocial morbidities associated with their diagnosis, treatment, and the sequelae thereof. Risks of second primary malignancy, cardiovascular disease, pulmonary disease, and endocrine dysfunction are influenced by patient characteristics such as age and gender, and treatment characteristics, such as selected chemotherapy and the inclusion, dose, and field of radiotherapy. Psychosocial challenges appear to be less treatment-dependent, but represent no less of a challenge to well-being among survivors. As treatments continue to evolve, and as our understanding of these risks - who is at risk, how best to identify or screen for them, and even how best to prevent them - evolves as well, the need will only become greater for evidence-based management guidelines. With the appropriate tools, engaged physicians can become all the more capable of promoting and preserving health among patients with, and survivors of, Hodgkin lymphoma.

22. References

[1] Jemal, A., et al., *Cancer statistics, 2010.* CA Cancer J Clin, 2010. 60(5): p. 277-300.
[2] Easson, E.C. and R.N. Grant, *Hodgkin's Disease--a Curable Disease.* CA Cancer J Clin, 1964. 14: p. 150-4.
[3] Devita, V.T., Jr., A.A. Serpick, and P.P. Carbone, *Combination chemotherapy in the treatment of advanced Hodgkin's disease.* Ann Intern Med, 1970. 73(6): p. 881-95.
[4] DeVita, V.T., Jr., et al., *Curability of advanced Hodgkin's disease with chemotherapy. Long-term follow-up of MOPP-treated patients at the National Cancer Institute.* Ann Intern Med, 1980. 92(5): p. 587-95.
[5] Santoro, A., et al., *Long-term results of combined chemotherapy-radiotherapy approach in Hodgkin's disease: superiority of ABVD plus radiotherapy versus MOPP plus radiotherapy.* J Clin Oncol, 1987. 5(1): p. 27-37.
[6] Yahalom, J. and P. Mauch, *The involved field is back: issues in delineating the radiation field in Hodgkin's disease.* Ann Oncol, 2002. 13 Suppl 1: p. 79-83.
[7] Campbell, B.A., et al., *Involved-nodal radiation therapy as a component of combination therapy for limited-stage Hodgkin's lymphoma: a question of field size.* J Clin Oncol, 2008. 26(32): p. 5170-4.
[8] Hasenclever, D. and V. Diehl, *A prognostic score for advanced Hodgkin's disease. International Prognostic Factors Project on Advanced Hodgkin's Disease.* N Engl J Med, 1998. 339(21): p. 1506-14.
[9] Bjorkholm, M., E. Svedmyr, and J. Sjoberg, *How we treat elderly patients with Hodgkin lymphoma.* Curr Opin Oncol, 2011. 23(5): p. 421-8.
[10] Holmberg, L. and D.G. Maloney, *The role of autologous and allogeneic hematopoietic stem cell transplantation for Hodgkin lymphoma.* J Natl Compr Canc Netw, 2011. 9(9): p. 1060-71.
[11] Josting, A., *Prognostic factors in Hodgkin lymphoma.* Expert Rev Hematol, 2010. 3(5): p. 583-92.
[12] Moskowitz, C.H., et al., *Normalization of pre-ASCT, FDG-PET imaging with second-line, non-cross resistant, chemotherapy programs improves event-free survival in patients with Hodgkin lymphoma.* Blood, 2011.
[13] Bonadonna, G., et al., *ABVD plus subtotal nodal versus involved-field radiotherapy in early-stage Hodgkin's disease: long-term results.* J Clin Oncol, 2004. 22(14): p. 2835-41.
[14] Gordon LI, H., *A Randomized Phase III Trial of ABVD Vs. Stanford V +/- Radiation Therapy In Locally Extensive and Advanced Stage Hodgkin's Lymphoma: An Intergroup Study Coordinated by the Eastern Cooperatve Oncology Group (E2496).* ASH Annual Meeting Abstracts 2010 2010. 116: p. 415.
[15] Howlader N, N.A., Krapcho M, et al. *SEER Cancer Statistics Review, 1975-2008.* SEER Cancer Statistics Review, 1975-2008, National Cancer Institute based on November

2010 SEER data submission, posted to the SEER web site, 2011.; http://seer.cancer.gov/csr/1975_2008/].
[16] van Rijswijk, R.E., et al., *Major complications and causes of death in patients treated for Hodgkin's disease.* J Clin Oncol, 1987. 5(10): p. 1624-33.
[17] Ng, A.K., et al., *Long-term survival and competing causes of death in patients with early-stage Hodgkin's disease treated at age 50 or younger.* J Clin Oncol, 2002. 20(8): p. 2101-8.
[18] Matasar MJ, R.E., Ford JS, et al., *Late mortality and morbidity of patients with Hodgkin lymphoma treated in adulthood.* J Clin Oncol, 2009. 27(15s): abstr 8547.
[19] Abrahamsen, A.F., et al., *Late medical sequelae after therapy for supradiaphragmatic Hodgkin's disease.* Acta Oncol, 1999. 38(4): p. 511-5.
[20] Baxi, S.S. and M.J. Matasar, *State-of-the-art issues in Hodgkin's lymphoma survivorship.* Curr Oncol Rep, 2010. 12(6): p. 366-73.
[21] van Leeuwen, F.E., et al., *Second cancer risk following Hodgkin's disease: a 20-year follow-up study.* J Clin Oncol, 1994. 12(2): p. 312-25.
[22] Ng, A.K., et al., *Second malignancy after Hodgkin disease treated with radiation therapy with or without chemotherapy: long-term risks and risk factors.* Blood, 2002. 100(6): p. 1989-96.
[23] Hodgson, D.C., et al., *Long-term solid cancer risk among 5-year survivors of Hodgkin's lymphoma.* J Clin Oncol, 2007. 25(12): p. 1489-97.
[24] Kaldor, J.M., et al., *Leukemia following Hodgkin's disease.* N Engl J Med, 1990. 322(1): p. 7-13.
[25] Schonfeld, S.J., et al., *Acute myeloid leukemia following Hodgkin lymphoma: a population-based study of 35,511 patients.* J Natl Cancer Inst, 2006. 98(3): p. 215-8.
[26] Pedersen-Bjergaard, J., et al., *Risk of therapy-related leukaemia and preleukaemia after Hodgkin's disease. Relation to age, cumulative dose of alkylating agents, and time from chemotherapy.* Lancet, 1987. 2(8550): p. 83-8.
[27] van Leeuwen, F.E., et al., *Leukemia risk following Hodgkin's disease: relation to cumulative dose of alkylating agents, treatment with teniposide combinations, number of episodes of chemotherapy, and bone marrow damage.* J Clin Oncol, 1994. 12(5): p. 1063-73.
[28] Josting A, W.S., Franklin J et al., *Secondary Myeloid Leukemia and Myelodysplastic Syndromes in Patients Treated for Hodgkin's Disease: A Report From the German Hodgkin's Lymphoma Study Group.* J Clin Oncol, 2003 l 21: p. 3440-3446.
[29] Blayney, D.W., et al., *Decreasing risk of leukemia with prolonged follow-up after chemotherapy and radiotherapy for Hodgkin's disease.* N Engl J Med, 1987. 316(12): p. 710-4.
[30] Valagussa, P. and G. Bonadonna, *Hodgkin's disease and the risk of acute leukemia in successfully treated patients.* Haematologica, 1998. 83(9): p. 769-70.
[31] Delwail, V., et al., *Fifteen-year secondary leukaemia risk observed in 761 patients with Hodgkin's disease prospectively treated by MOPP or ABVD chemotherapy plus high-dose irradiation.* Br J Haematol, 2002. 118(1): p. 189-94.
[32] Diehl, V., et al., *Standard and increased-dose BEACOPP chemotherapy compared with COPP-ABVD for advanced Hodgkin's disease.* N Engl J Med, 2003. 348(24): p. 2386-95.
[33] Tucker, M.A., et al., *Risk of second cancers after treatment for Hodgkin's disease.* N Engl J Med, 1988. 318(2): p. 76-81.
[34] Krikorian, J.G., et al., *Occurrence of non-Hodgkin's lymphoma after therapy for Hodgkin's disease.* N Engl J Med, 1979. 300(9): p. 452-8.
[35] van Leeuwen, F.E., et al., *Increased risk of lung cancer, non-Hodgkin's lymphoma, and leukemia following Hodgkin's disease.* J Clin Oncol, 1989. 7(8): p. 1046-58.

[36] Metayer, C., et al., *Second cancers among long-term survivors of Hodgkin's disease diagnosed in childhood and adolescence.* J Clin Oncol, 2000. 18(12): p. 2435-43.
[37] Swerdlow, A.J., et al., *Lung cancer after Hodgkin's disease: a nested case-control study of the relation to treatment.* J Clin Oncol, 2001. 19(6): p. 1610-8.
[38] Dores, G.M., et al., *Second malignant neoplasms among long-term survivors of Hodgkin's disease: a population-based evaluation over 25 years.* J Clin Oncol, 2002. 20(16): p. 3484-94.
[39] Abrahamsen, J.F., et al., *Second malignancies after treatment of Hodgkin's disease: the influence of treatment, follow-up time, and age.* J Clin Oncol, 1993. 11(2): p. 255-61.
[40] Salloum, E., et al., *Second solid tumors in patients with Hodgkin's disease cured after radiation or chemotherapy plus adjuvant low-dose radiation.* J Clin Oncol, 1996. 14(9): p. 2435-43.
[41] Laurie, S.A., et al., *The clinical course of nonsmall cell lung carcinoma in survivors of Hodgkin disease.* Cancer, 2002. 95(1): p. 119-26.
[42] Das, P., et al., *Clinical course of thoracic cancers in Hodgkin's disease survivors.* Ann Oncol, 2005. 16(5): p. 793-7.
[43] Milano, M.T., et al., *Survival after second primary lung cancer: A population-based study of 187 hodgkin lymphoma patients.* Cancer, 2011.
[44] Das, P., et al., *Computed tomography screening for lung cancer in Hodgkin's lymphoma survivors: decision analysis and cost-effectiveness analysis.* Ann Oncol, 2006. 17(5): p. 785-93.
[45] Aberle, D.R., et al., *Reduced lung-cancer mortality with low-dose computed tomographic screening.* N Engl J Med, 2011. 365(5): p. 395-409.
[46] van Leeuwen, F., et al., *Second cancer risk following Hodgkin's disease: a 20-year follow-up study.* J Clin Oncol, 1994. 12(2): p. 312-325.
[47] Aisenberg, A.C., et al., *High risk of breast carcinoma after irradiation of young women with Hodgkin's disease.* Cancer, 1997. 79(6): p. 1203-10.
[48] Travis, L.B., et al., *Cumulative Absolute Breast Cancer Risk for Young Women Treated for Hodgkin Lymphoma.* J. Natl. Cancer Inst., 2005. 97(19): p. 1428-1437.
[49] Saslow, D., et al., *American Cancer Society Guidelines for Breast Screening with MRI as an Adjunct to Mammography.* CA Cancer J Clin, 2007. 57(2): p. 75-89.
[50] Zelenetz, A., et al., *NCCN Clinical Practice Guidelines in Oncology: Non-Hodgkin's Lymphomas.* JNCCN, 2010. 8(3): p. 288.
[51] Balmana, J., et al., *BRCA in breast cancer: ESMO Clinical Practice Guidelines.* Ann Oncol, 2010. 21 Suppl 5: p. v20-2.
[52] O'Brien, M.M., et al., *Second malignant neoplasms in survivors of pediatric Hodgkin's lymphoma treated with low-dose radiation and chemotherapy.* J Clin Oncol, 2010. 28(7): p. 1232-9.
[53] Travis, L.B., et al., *Cumulative absolute breast cancer risk for young women treated for Hodgkin lymphoma.* J Natl Cancer Inst, 2005. 97(19): p. 1428-37.
[54] Del Mastro, L., et al., *Medical approaches to preservation of fertility in female cancer patients.* Expert Opin Pharmacother, 2011. 12(3): p. 387-96.
[55] Beck-Fruchter, R., A. Weiss, and E. Shalev, *GnRH agonist therapy as ovarian protectants in female patients undergoing chemotherapy: a review of the clinical data.* Hum Reprod Update, 2008. 14(6): p. 553-61.
[56] Sigurdson, A.J., et al., *Primary thyroid cancer after a first tumour in childhood (the Childhood Cancer Survivor Study): a nested case-control study.* Lancet, 2005. 365(9476): p. 2014-23.

[57] Adams, M.J., et al., *Cardiovascular status in long-term survivors of Hodgkin's disease treated with chest radiotherapy.* J Clin Oncol, 2004. 22(15): p. 3139-48.

[58] Swerdlow, A.J., et al., *Myocardial infarction mortality risk after treatment for Hodgkin disease: a collaborative British cohort study.* J Natl Cancer Inst, 2007. 99(3): p. 206-14.

[59] Reinders, J.G., et al., *Ischemic heart disease after mantlefield irradiation for Hodgkin's disease in long-term follow-up.* Radiother Oncol, 1999. 51(1): p. 35-42.

[60] Aleman, B.M., et al., *Late cardiotoxicity after treatment for Hodgkin lymphoma.* Blood, 2007. 109(5): p. 1878-86.

[61] Glanzmann, C., et al., *Cardiac lesions after mediastinal irradiation for Hodgkin's disease.* Radiother Oncol, 1994. 30(1): p. 43-54.

[62] Heidenreich, P.A., et al., *Screening for coronary artery disease after mediastinal irradiation for Hodgkin's disease.* J Clin Oncol, 2007. 25(1): p. 43-9.

[63] Kupeli, S., et al., *Evaluation of coronary artery disease by computed tomography angiography in patients treated for childhood Hodgkin's lymphoma.* J Clin Oncol, 2010. 28(6): p. 1025-30.

[64] Schuijf, J.D., et al., *A comparative regional analysis of coronary atherosclerosis and calcium score on multislice CT versus myocardial perfusion on SPECT.* J Nucl Med, 2006. 47(11): p. 1749-55.

[65] Hull, M.C., et al., *Valvular dysfunction and carotid, subclavian, and coronary artery disease in survivors of hodgkin lymphoma treated with radiation therapy.* JAMA, 2003. 290(21): p. 2831-7.

[66] Lund, M.B., et al., *Increased risk of heart valve regurgitation after mediastinal radiation for Hodgkin's disease: an echocardiographic study.* Heart, 1996. 75(6): p. 591-5.

[67] Von Hoff, D.D., et al., *Risk factors for doxorubicin-induced congestive heart failure.* Ann Intern Med, 1979. 91(5): p. 710-7.

[68] Swain, S.M., *Doxorubicin-induced cardiomyopathy.* N Engl J Med, 1999. 340(8): p. 654; author reply 655.

[69] Gottdiener, J.S., et al., *Late cardiac effects of therapeutic mediastinal irradiation. Assessment by echocardiography and radionuclide angiography.* N Engl J Med, 1983. 308(10): p. 569-72.

[70] Mulrooney, D.A., et al., *Cardiac outcomes in a cohort of adult survivors of childhood and adolescent cancer: retrospective analysis of the Childhood Cancer Survivor Study cohort.* BMJ, 2009. 339: p. b4606.

[71] Kremer, L.C., et al., *Frequency and risk factors of subclinical cardiotoxicity after anthracycline therapy in children: a systematic review.* Ann Oncol, 2002. 13(6): p. 819-29.

[72] Aleman, B.M.P., et al., *Late cardiotoxicity after treatment for Hodgkin lymphoma.* Blood, 2007. 109(5): p. 1878-1886.

[73] Martin, W.G., et al., *Bleomycin pulmonary toxicity has a negative impact on the outcome of patients with Hodgkin's lymphoma.* J Clin Oncol, 2005. 23(30): p. 7614-20.

[74] Bethge, W., et al., *Thyroid toxicity of treatment for Hodgkin's disease.* Annals of hematology, 2000. 79(3): p. 114-118.

[75] Abrahamsen, A.F., et al., *Late medical sequelae after therapy for supradiaphragmatic Hodgkin's disease.* Acta oncologica, 1999. 38(4): p. 511-515.

[76] Bloom, J.R., et al., *Psychosocial outcomes of cancer: a comparative analysis of Hodgkin's disease and testicular cancer.* J Clin Oncol, 1993. 11(5): p. 979-88.

[77] Jeruss, J.S. and T.K. Woodruff, *Preservation of fertility in patients with cancer.* N Engl J Med, 2009. 360(9): p. 902-11.
[78] West, E.R., et al., *Preserving female fertility following cancer treatment: current options and future possibilities.* Pediatr Blood Cancer, 2009. 53(2): p. 289-95.
[79] Sieniawski, M., et al., *Fertility in male patients with advanced Hodgkin lymphoma treated with BEACOPP: a report of the German Hodgkin Study Group (GHSG).* Blood, 2008. 111(1): p. 71-6.
[80] Blumenfeld, Z., et al., *Preservation of fertility and ovarian function and minimizing chemotherapy-induced gonadotoxicity in young women.* J Soc Gynecol Investig, 1999. 6(5): p. 229-39.
[81] Hodgson, D.C., et al., *Fertility among female hodgkin lymphoma survivors attempting pregnancy following ABVD chemotherapy.* Hematol Oncol, 2007. 25(1): p. 11-5.
[82] Dann, E.J., et al., *A 10-year experience with treatment of high and standard risk Hodgkin disease: Six cycles of tailored BEACOPP, with interim scintigraphy, are effective and female fertility is preserved.* Am J Hematol, 2011.
[83] Lie Fong, S., et al., *Assessment of ovarian reserve in adult childhood cancer survivors using anti-Mullerian hormone.* Hum Reprod, 2009. 24(4): p. 982-90.
[84] Heutte, N., et al., *Quality of life after successful treatment of early-stage Hodgkin's lymphoma: 10-year follow-up of the EORTC-GELA H8 randomised controlled trial.* Lancet Oncol, 2009. 10(12): p. 1160-70.
[85] Ganz, P.A., et al., *Health status and quality of life in patients with early-stage Hodgkin's disease treated on Southwest Oncology Group Study 9133.* J Clin Oncol, 2003. 21(18): p. 3512-9.
[86] Loge, J.H., et al., *Reduced health-related quality of life among Hodgkin's disease survivors: a comparative study with general population norms.* Ann Oncol, 1999. 10(1): p. 71-7.
[87] Wettergren, L., et al., *Determinants of health-related quality of life in long-term survivors of Hodgkin's lymphoma.* Qual Life Res, 2004. 13(8): p. 1369-79.
[88] Loge, J.H., et al., *Hodgkin's disease survivors more fatigued than the general population.* J Clin Oncol, 1999. 17(1): p. 253-61.
[89] Hjermstad, M.J., et al., *Quality of life in long-term Hodgkin's disease survivors with chronic fatigue.* Eur J Cancer, 2006. 42(3): p. 327-33.
[90] Knobel, H., et al., *Late medical complications and fatigue in Hodgkin's disease survivors.* J Clin Oncol, 2001. 19(13): p. 3226-33.
[91] Bower, J.E., et al., *Inflammatory biomarkers and fatigue during radiation therapy for breast and prostate cancer.* Clin Cancer Res, 2009. 15(17): p. 5534-40.
[92] Bower, J.E., et al., *Inflammation and behavioral symptoms after breast cancer treatment: do fatigue, depression, and sleep disturbance share a common underlying mechanism?* J Clin Oncol, 2011. 29(26): p. 3517-22.
[93] Orre, I.J., et al., *Levels of circulating interleukin-1 receptor antagonist and C-reactive protein in long-term survivors of testicular cancer with chronic cancer-related fatigue.* Brain Behav Immun, 2009. 23(6): p. 868-74.
[94] Gielissen, M.F., C.A. Verhagen, and G. Bleijenberg, *Cognitive behaviour therapy for fatigued cancer survivors: long-term follow-up.* Br J Cancer, 2007. 97(5): p. 612-8.
[95] Gielissen, M.F., et al., *Examining the role of physical activity in reducing postcancer fatigue.* Support Care Cancer, 2011.

[96] Oldervoll, L.M., et al., *Exercise reduces fatigue in chronic fatigued Hodgkins disease survivors--results from a pilot study.* Eur J Cancer, 2003. 39(1): p. 57-63.

[97] Ford J, S., SJ et al., *Psychosocial functining in survivors of Hodgkin lymphom (HL) treated during adulthood.*, in *J Clin Oncol (Meeting Abstracts)*2008. p. 9592.

[98] Loge, J.H., et al., *Psychological distress after cancer cure: a survey of 459 Hodgkin's disease survivors.* Br J Cancer, 1997. 76(6): p. 791-6.

[99] Greil, R., et al., *Retrospective assessment of quality of life and treatment outcome in patients with Hodgkin's disease from 1969 to 1994.* Eur J Cancer, 1999. 35(5): p. 698-706.

[100] Fobair, P., et al., *Psychosocial problems among survivors of Hodgkin's disease.* J Clin Oncol, 1986. 4(5): p. 805-14.

[101] Cameron, C.L., et al., *Persistent symptoms among survivors of Hodgkin's disease: an explanatory model based on classical conditioning.* Health Psychol, 2001. 20(1): p. 71-5.

[102] Mols, F., et al., *Long-term cancer survivors experience work changes after diagnosis: results of a population-based study.* Psychooncology, 2009. 18(12): p. 1252-60.

[103] Kornblith, A.B., et al., *Hodgkin disease survivors at increased risk for problems in psychosocial adaptation. The Cancer and Leukemia Group B.* Cancer, 1992. 70(8): p. 2214-24.

[104] Langeveld, N.E., et al., *Educational achievement, employment and living situation in long-term young adult survivors of childhood cancer in the Netherlands.* Psychooncology, 2003. 12(3): p. 213-25.

[105] Younes, A., et al., *Brentuximab vedotin (SGN-35) for relapsed CD30-positive lymphomas.* N Engl J Med, 2010. 363(19): p. 1812-21.

[106] Bajorin, D.F. and A. Hanley, *The study of collaborative practice arrangements: where do we go from here?* J Clin Oncol, 2011. 29(27): p. 3599-600.